AF597690

Methods in Molecular Biology™

Series Editor
John M. Walker
School of Life Sciences
University of Hertfordshire
Hatfield, Hertfordshire, AL10 9AB, UK

For further volumes:
http://www.springer.com/series/7651

Cardiovascular Development

Methods and Protocols

Edited by

Xu Peng

Department of Systems Biology and Translational Medicine, College of Medicine, Texas A&M Healthy Science Center, Temple, TX, USA

Marc Antonyak

Department of Molecular Medicine, School of Veterinary Medicine, Cornell University, Ithaca, NY, USA

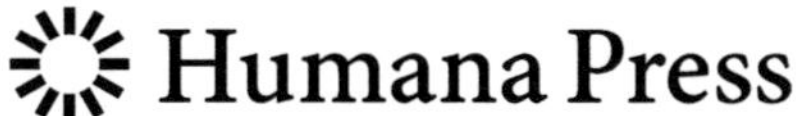

Editors
Xu Peng
Department of Systems Biology
and Translational Medicine
College of Medicine
Texas A&M Healthy Science Center
Temple, TX, USA
xp23@tamu.edu

Marc Antonyak
Department of Molecular Medicine
School of Veterinary Medicine
Cornell University
Ithaca, NY, USA
marcant225@aol.com

ISSN 1064-3745 e-ISSN 1940-6029
ISBN 978-1-61779-522-0 e-ISBN 978-1-61779-523-7
DOI 10.1007/978-1-61779-523-7
Springer New York Dordrecht Heidelberg London

Library of Congress Control Number: 2011944649

Printed on acid-free paper

Humana Press is part of Springer Science+Business Media (www.springer.com)

Preface

Congenital heart disease is the leading cause of infant death and affects approximately one in every 100 babies born in the USA. Aberrant cardiovascular development is the reason for congenital heart diseases and the pathogenesis of majority congenital heart disease remains unclear. Cardiovascular system is the first system to begin functioning and plays critical roles in embryo development. From the lower invertebrate to mammalian animal, the heart morphology is obviously different among Drosophila (one chamber), Zebrafish (two chambers), Xenopus (three chambers), and rodent (four chambers), but the genetic and molecular mechanisms in cardiovascular development are surprisingly conserved. Indeed, the knowledge we get from the invertebrate and vertebrate model organisms can help us understand and explore new strategy for the treatment of human cardiovascular disease.

The study of cardiovascular development has acquired new momentum in last 20 years due to the advancement of modern molecular biology and new available equipments and techniques, and we begin to understand the molecular pathways and cellular interaction in the process of heart induction, rightward looping, chamber formation, and maturation. Heart and vascular developments are sophisticated processes and new information expanded very quickly. It is not difficult to find a text book or review articles to summarize the new advancements in the field of cardiovascular development; however, it is not easy to find a book to describe the comprehensive step-by-step protocols for cardiovascular development research. Owing to the page limitation, the current research articles cannot describe the very detail of the experimental material and methods. The major goal of this book is to provide the step-by-step protocols for both beginner and experience scientist in the field of cardiovascular development research.

Cardiovascular development: methods and protocols cover many new state-of-the-art techniques in the field of cardiovascular development research including in vivo imaging and Bioinformatics. We also described many of the classical methods which are high frequently used in the cardiovascular development research, such as fate mapping and immunohistochemistry staining. This book is divided into three parts. In part I, we summarized using different organisms for cardiovascular developmental research. Part II focused on using cell and molecular biology methods to study cardiovascular development. Part III summarized the new available techniques for cardiovascular development research, such as in vivo imaging and bioinformatics. Our primary audience of this book is for molecular biologists and cell biologists who are working on the cardiovascular development research. It is also a useful reference for clinician, genetic biologist, biochemists, biophysicists, or other field scientists who are interested in cardiovascular development.

Temple, TX, USA *Xu Peng*
Ithaca, NY, USA *Marc Antonyak*

Contents

Contributors

MARC ANTONYAK • *Department of Molecular Medicine, School of Veterinary Medicine, Cornell University, Ithaca, NY, USA*
ERIC A. BRIDENBAUGH • *Department of Systems Biology and Translational Medicine, Texas A&M Health Science Center College of Medicine, Temple, TX, USA*
MORGAN V. CAMERON • *Department of Pathology and McAllister Heart Institute, University of North Carolina, Chapel Hill, NC, USA*
CHING-PIN CHANG • *Department of Medicine, Division of Cardiovascular Medicine, Stanford Cardiovascular Institute, Stanford University School of Medicine, Stanford, CA, USA*
KATHLEEN CHRISTINE • *Department of Genetics, UNC McAllister Heart Institute (MHI), University of North Carolina at Chapel Hill, Chapel Hill, NC, USA*
FRANK L. CONLON • *Department of Genetics, UNC McAllister Heart Institute (MHI), University of North Carolina at Chapel Hill, Chapel Hill, NC, USA*
MICHAEL P. CRAIG • *Department of Molecular and Cellular Physiology, University of Cincinnati College of Medicine, Cincinnati, OH, USA*
MICHAEL CRAVEN • *Biomedical Sciences Department, College of Veterinary Medicine, Cornell University, Ithaca, NY, USA*
RICARDO J. CRISTALES • *Department of Internal Medicine, Division of Molecular Cardiology, College of Medicine, Texas A&M Health Science Center, Temple, TX, USA*
DAVID E. DOSTAL • *Department of Internal Medicine, Division of Molecular Cardiology, College of Medicine, Texas A&M Health Science Center, Temple, TX, USA; Central Texas Veterans Health Care System, Temple, TX, USA*
YONGHE DING • *Department of Biochemistry and Molecular Biology, Mayo Clinic, Rochester, MN, USA; Department of Medicine, Division of Cardiovascular Diseases, Mayo Clinic, Rochester, MN, USA*
MINGUI FU • *Department of Basic Medical Science and Shock/Trauma Research Center, School of Medicine, University of Missouri Kansas City, Kansas City, MO, USA*
ANATOLIY A. GASHEV • *Department of Systems Biology and Translational Medicine, College of Medicine, Cardiovascular Research Institute Division of Lymphatic Biology, Texas A&M Health Science Center, Temple, TX, USA*
FNU GERILECHAOGETU • *Department of Internal Medicine, College of Medicine, Division of Molecular Cardiology, Texas A&M Health Science Center, Temple, TX, USA*
HONEY B. GOLDEN • *Department of Internal Medicine, Division of Molecular Cardiology, College of Medicine, Texas A&M Health Science Center, Temple, TX, USA*

Deepika Gollapudi • *Department of Internal Medicine, Division of Molecular Cardiology, College of Medicine, Texas A&M Health Science Center, Temple, TX, USA*

Zeenat S. Hakim • *Department of Pathology and McAllister Heart Institute, University of North Carolina, Chapel Hill, NC, USA*

Calvin T. Hang • *Department of Medicine, Division of Cardiovascular Medicine, Stanford Cardiovascular Institute, Stanford University School of Medicine, Stanford, CA, USA*

Tiffany Hoage • *Department of Biochemistry and Molecular Biology, Mayo Clinic, Rochester, MN, USA; Department of Medicine, Division of Cardiovascular Diseases, Mayo Clinic, Rochester, MN, USA*

Melinda B. Holland • *Department of Cell and Molecular Physiology, Curriculum in Genetics and Molecular Biology, McAllister Heart Institute, University of North Carolina at Chapel Hill, Chapel Hill, NC, USA*

Jay R. Hove • *Department of Molecular and Cellular Physiology, University of Cincinnati College of Medicine, Cincinnati, OH, USA*

Jennifer James • *Laboratory of Stem Cell and Neuro-Vascular Biology, Genetics and Developmental Biology Center, National Heart, Lung, and Blood Institute, National Institutes of Health, Bethesda, MD, USA*

Suk-Won Jin • *Department of Cell and Molecular Physiology, Curriculum in Genetics and Molecular Biology, McAllister Heart Institute, University of North Carolina at Chapel Hill, Chapel Hill, NC, USA*

Yixin Jin • *Department of Systems Biology and Translational Medicine, College of Medicine, Texas A&M Healthy Science Center, Temple, TX, USA*

Michael I. Kotlikoff • *Biomedical Sciences Department, College of Veterinary Medicine, Cornell University, Ithaca, NY, USA*

Jieli Li • *Department of Systems Biology and Translational Medicine, College of Medicine, Texas A&M Health Science Center, Temple, TX, USA*

Yang Liu • *Department of Systems Biology and Translational Medicine, College of Medicine, Texas A&M Healthy Science Center, Temple, TX, USA*

Gerald A. Meininger • *Department of Medical Pharmacology and Physiology, Dalton Cardiovascular Research Center, University of Missouri-Columbia, Columbia, MO, USA*

Richard P. Metz • *Department of Systems Biology and Translational Medicine, Texas A&M Health Science Center, College of Medicine, College Station, TX, USA*

Yoh-suke Mukouyama • *Laboratory of Stem Cell and Neuro-Vascular Biology, Genetics and Developmental Biology Center, National Heart, Lung, and Blood Institute, National Institutes of Health, Bethesda, MD, USA*

Mariappan Muthuchamy • *Department of Systems Biology and Translational Medicine, Texas A&M Health Science Center College of Medicine, College Station, TX, USA*

Alyson S. Nadworny • *Biomedical Sciences Department, College of Veterinary Medicine, Cornell University, Ithaca, NY, USA*

Joseph Nam • *Laboratory of Stem Cell and Neuro-Vascular Biology, Genetics and Developmental Biology Center, National Heart, Lung, and Blood Institute, National Institutes of Health, Bethesda, MD, USA*

ANUPAMA NATARAJAN • *Department of Biology, Seminole State College of Florida, 100 Weldon Blvd, Sanford, FL, USA*
JAN L. PATTERSON • *Department of Systems Biology and Translational Medicine, Texas A&M Health Science Center, College of Medicine, College Station, TX, USA*
XU PENG • *Department of Systems Biology and Translational Medicine, College of Medicine, Texas A&M Healthy Science Center, Temple, TX, USA*
WILLIAM T. PU • *Department of Cardiology, Children's Hospital Boston, Boston, MA, USA; Harvard Stem Cell Institute, Cambridge, MA, USA*
DONGFEI QI • *Department of Basic Medical Science and Shock/Trauma Research Center, School of Medicine, University of Missouri Kansas City, Kansas City, MO, USA*
MAY J. REED • *Department of Medicine, University of Washington, Harborview Medical Center, Seattle, WA, USA*
DOMENICO RIBATTI • *Department of Basic Medical Sciences, Section of Human Anatomy and Histology, University of Bari Medical School, Policlinico, Bari, Italy*
L. BRUNO RUEST • *Department of Biomedical Sciences, Texas A&M Healthy Science Center-Baylor College of Dentistry, Dallas, TX, USA*
CHRISTOPHER E. SCHMITT • *Department of Cell and Molecular Physiology, Curriculum in Genetics and Molecular Biology, McAllister Heart Institute, University of North Carolina at Chapel Hill, Chapel Hill, NC, USA*
CHRIS SHOWELL • *Department of Genetics, UNC McAllister Heart Institute (MHI), University of North Carolina at Chapel Hill, Chapel Hill, NC, USA*
OLIVER SMITHIES • *Department of Pathology and McAllister Heart Institute, University of North Carolina, Chapel Hill, NC, USA*
ZHE SUN • *Department of Medical Pharmacology and Physiology, Dalton Cardiovascular Research Center, University of Missouri-Columbia, Columbia, MO, USA*
SURAJ SUNDER • *Department of Internal Medicine, Division of Molecular Cardiology, College of Medicine, Texas A&M Health Science Center, Temple, TX, USA*
PANNA TANDON • *Department of Genetics, UNC McAllister Heart Institute (MHI), University of North Carolina at Chapel Hill, Chapel Hill, NC, USA*
DAVID G. TAYLOR • *Department of Biology, Seminole State College of Florida, Sanford, FL, USA*
JOAN M. TAYLOR • *Department of Pathology and McAllister Heart Institute, University of North Carolina, Chapel Hill, NC, USA*
YUTAKA UCHIDA • *Laboratory of Stem Cell and Neuro-Vascular Biology, Genetics and Developmental Biology Center, National Heart, Lung, and Blood Institute, National Institutes of Health, Bethesda, MD, USA*
VINCENT VANBUREN • *Department of Systems Biology and Translational Medicine, College of Medicine, Texas A&M Healthy Science Center, Temple, TX, USA*
ROBERT B. VERNON • *Hope Heart Program, Benaroya Research Institute at Virginia Mason, Seattle, WA, USA*
EMILY WILSON • *Department of Systems Biology and Translational Medicine, Texas A&M Health Science Center, College of Medicine, College Station, TX, USA*
XIN WU • *Department of Systems Biology and Translational Medicine, Texas A&M Health Science Center College of Medicine, College Station, TX, USA*

YIQIN XIONG • *Department of Medicine, Division of Cardiovascular Medicine, Stanford Cardiovascular Institute, Stanford University School of Medicine, Stanford, CA, USA*

XIAOLEI XU • *Department of Biochemistry and Molecular Biology, Mayo Clinic, Rochester, MN, USA; Department of Medicine, Division of Cardiovascular Diseases, Mayo Clinic, Rochester, MN, USA*

BRITNI ZAJAC • *Department of Pathology and McAllister Heart Institute, University of North Carolina, Chapel Hill, NC, USA*

DAVID C. ZAWIEJA • *Department of Systems Biology and Translational Medicine, College of Medicine, Cardiovascular Research Institute Division of Lymphatic Biology, Texas A&M Health Science Center, Temple, TX, USA*

SHENYUAN ZHANG • *Department of Systems Biology and Translational Medicine, College of Medicine, Texas A&M Healthy Science Center, Temple, TX, USA*

YANPING ZHANG • *Department of Biomedical Sciences, Texas A&M Healthy Science Center-Baylor College of Dentistry, Dallas, TX, USA*

HONGYING ZHENG • *Department of Systems Biology and Translational Medicine, College of Medicine, Texas A&M Healthy Science Center, Temple, TX, USA*

BIN ZHOU • *Department of Cardiology, Children's Hospital Boston, Boston, MA, USA; Harvard Stem Cell Institute, Cambridge, MA, USA; Key Laboratory of Nutrition and Metabolism, Institute for Nutritional Sciences, Shanghai Institutes for Biological Sciences, Chinese Academy of Sciences, Shanghai, China; Department of Genetics, Albert Einstein College of Medicine, Bronx, NY, USA*

Part I

Model Organisms

Chapter 1

Use of Whole Embryo Culture for Studying Heart Development

Calvin T. Hang and Ching-Pin Chang

Abstract

Congenital heart defects occur in approximately 1% of newborns and are a major cause of morbidity and mortality in infants and children. Many adult cardiac diseases also have developmental basis, such as heart valve malformations, among others. Therefore, dissecting the developmental and molecular mechanisms underlying such defects in embryos is of great importance in prevention and developing therapeutics for heart diseases that manifest in infants or later in adults. Whole embryo culture is a valuable tool to study cardiac development in midgestation embryos, in which ventricular chambers are specified and expand, and the myocardium and endocardium interact to form various cardiac structures including heart valves and trabecular myocardium (Cell 118: 649–663, 2004; Dev Cell 14: 298–311, 2008). This technique is essentially growing a midgestation embryo *ex utero* in a test tube.

One of the strengths of embryo culture is that it allows an investigator to easily manipulate or add drugs/chemicals directly to the embryos to test specific hypotheses in situations that are otherwise very difficult to perform for embryos *in utero*. For instance, embryo culture permits pharmacological rescue experiments to be performed in place of genetic rescue experiments which may require generation of specific mouse strains and crosses. Furthermore, because embryos are grown externally, drugs are directly acting on the cultured embryos rather than being degraded through maternal circulation or excluded from the embryos by the placenta. Drug dosage and kinetics are therefore easier to control with embryo culture. Conversely, drugs that compromise the placental function and are thus unusable for *in utero* experiments are applicable in cultured embryos since placental function is not required in whole embryo culture. The applications of whole embryo culture in the studies of molecular pathways involved in heart valve formation, myocardial growth, differentiation, and morphogenesis are demonstrated previously (Cell 118: 649–663, 2004; Dev Cell 14: 298–311, 2008; Nature 446: 62–67, 2010). Here we describe a method of embryo culture in a common laboratory setting without using special equipments.

Key words: Whole embryo culture, Myocardium, Trabeculation, Endocardial cushion, Heart valve

Xu Peng and Marc Antonyak (eds.), *Cardiovascular Development: Methods and Protocols*, Methods in Molecular Biology, vol. 843, DOI 10.1007/978-1-61779-523-7_1,

1. Introduction

Whole embryo culture is fundamentally growing a complete mid-gestation embryo *ex utero* under specific atmospheric and culture conditions in a test tube (1–3). The embryo grows best starting at E8.5 and can be cultured up to late E10. During this period, osmosis is sufficient for nutrient uptake and gas exchange for proper embryo growth and development. Past late E10, osmosis is not adequate to meet the metabolic needs of a growing embryo, which then requires circulation supplied through the placenta for proper growth.

Whole embryo culture consists of three parts: dissection, incubation, and analysis. Individual uterine deciduas are carefully dissected so that the resulting embryos are enclosed by intact yolk sac. Then they are placed into whole embryo culture media in vials and incubated under specific gas composition and at 37°C. During incubation, drugs or other reagents can be added and gas is periodically refilled. At the end of culture, embryos are inspected for viability and experimental analysis.

2. Materials

2.1. Instruments/ Equipment

1. Dissecting forceps.
2. Plastic transfer pipettes.
3. Petri dishes.
4. Long forceps (Fisher, 10–316C), or similar extra-long forceps.
5. 2-dram vials (VWR, 66011–085).
6. 1-L Gas roller bottles (Fisher, 02-924-6F), or similar narrow-necked 1-L roller bottles.
7. Gas mixture of O_2, CO_2, and N_2 (See Subheading 3.4. for specific composition).
8. Roller/rocker/incubator.

2.2. Media

1. Hank's Balanced Salt Solution (HBSS): 400 mg/L KCl, KH_2PO_4, 60 mg/L KH_2PO_4, 350 mg/L $NaHCO_3$, 8,000 mg/L NaCl, 48 mg/L Na_2HPO_4 (anhydrous), 1,000 mg/L d-Glucose. Kept at room temperature, but prewarmed to 37°C prior to dissection.
2. Rat whole embryo culture serum. Kept at –20°C, but thaw to 37°C prior to dissection, refreeze afterwards. Aliquot rat serum into 1 mL to prevent freeze–thaw cycles (see Note 1).
3. 100× Penicillin/Streptomycin. Kept at 4°C. Working concentration at 100 U/mL penicillin and 100 μg/mL streptomycin.

4. 100× Glucose in Phosphate Buffer Saline (PBS): 140 mM NaCl, 10 mM phosphate buffer, 3 mM KCl, pH7.4. Make a 200 mg/mL glucose stock, and dilute to 2 mg/mL working concentration. Filtered and kept at 4°C. Make fresh every few months.

3. Methods

3.1. Preparation of Media and Other Materials

1. Prewarm HBSS and thaw embryo culture rat serum to 37°C in a water bath prior to dissection. If necessary, sterilize 2-dram vials by laying them on the side under UV in any cell culture hood during dissection. Wipe all surfaces and equipment with 70% ethanol. Cut the mouth of the transfer pipette to widen it so that the embryos can be easily aspirated in without being compressed or damaged.
2. 5–10 petri dishes are needed. One will act as a reservoir in which all undissected deciduas are stored, and another will be where dissected embryos are kept. All other petri dishes are for the dissection itself. If the dissection dish becomes cloudy with blood and uterine tissue, use a new one with fresh HBSS for the next dissection. Also, keep the embryos reasonably warm, therefore it may be necessary to transfer dissected embryos to fresh warm HBSS periodically. Usually a litter of 10–15 embryos will take about 1 h from start to finish.

3.2. Harvesting Embryos

Appearance of coital plug is counted as E0.5, and gestation age is staged by ultrasonography (4) if available. E8.5 to late E10 embryos are best suitable for whole embryo culture. Uterine horns are removed from the mother and placed into prewarmed HBSS in a petri dish. Individual deciduas are carefully cut away from one another (see Note 2).

3.3. Dissection

1. For the purpose of illustrating dissection, the embryo is surrounded by four layers that are visually distinctive and torn off in order (Fig. 1). The outermost layer is a very fibrous and opaque membrane; the next layer is composed of thick spongy uterine tissue; the third layer is thin and spotted red and is called Reichert's membrane; and finally the innermost is the yolk sac. The three outer layers are carefully removed in sequence to generate an embryo enclosed by an intact yolk sac (see Note 3).
2. To start, grasp the decidua at one end with a pair of forceps and carefully use the other pair to tear off in a lateral motion along the decidua in a piecemeal fashion. The outermost fibrous layer should be torn away at multiple different places, not at a single place. Because the embryos are under higher pressure within the yolk sac, tearing the fibrous membrane at only one place and expanding that hole will cause the underlying

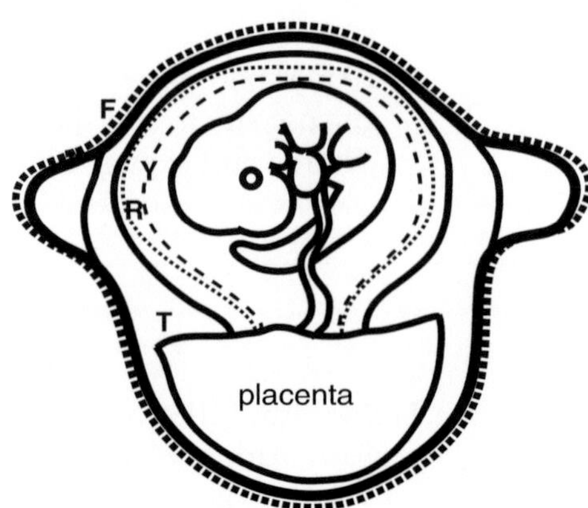

Fig. 1. Schematic diagram of a single decidua and embryonic membranes to be dissected in sequence, from the outermost: Fibrous membrane (F); thick uterine tissue (T) that is spongy in texture; Reichart's membrane (R), which is spotted red and may be attached to the underlying yolk sac (Y). Note that the embryo lies on the side of the two small protrusions where one decidua connects to its neighboring deciduas.

embryo to suddenly extrude or pop from that single hole, resulting in tissue damage. Cutting at multiple places gradually relieves the inner pressure of the tightly enclosed embryo. At the end, the decidua becomes bigger when the fibrous layer is completely removed and pressure is released.

3. Follow the same procedure as before to tear away the uterine spongy layer piece by piece. Because this layer is thicker, always start by grasping the spongy layer at the surface and do not dig deep. Also, beware where the embryo proper lies, and to be safe, start tearing away the spongy layer opposite to that. Each decidua has two minor "horns" or cuts where it connects to two neighboring deciduas. Embryos lie on that side with the horns, and at the opposite is the placenta. Start by tearing spongy tissues at the placental side and work towards the horned side. It is not necessary to tear away the entire spongy layer at the placenta, but it is important to remove the spongy layer enclosing the embryo proper. Take note to leave some spongy tissue at the placental end, since removing it all will puncture the yolk sac.
4. The third layer to be teased away is the Reichert's membrane and is the most difficult to remove without damaging the underlying yolk sac. Depending on embryonic age, this thin membrane may be physically connected to the yolk sac. To create an opening to remove this layer, grasp it lightly with a pair of forceps at the surface and not deep. Then gently pull the membrane up vertically so that a small portion is above the dissecting media. A small "tent" is formed at where the forceps are grasping the membrane. Use the other pair of forceps to make small tears on

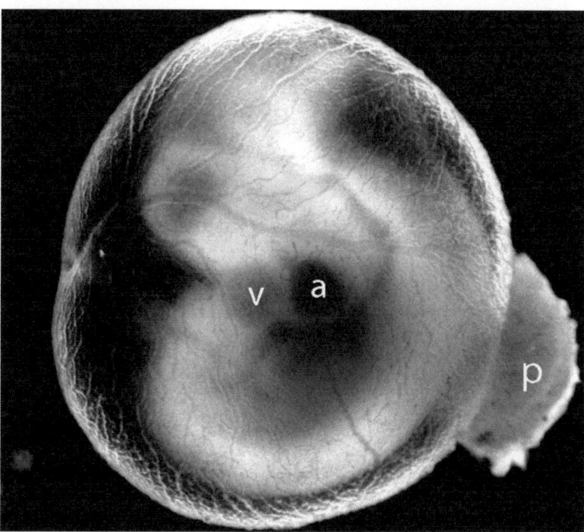

Fig. 2. An embryo cultured from early E9 to E10.5. A small piece of placental tissue (p) still attached to preserve an intact yolk sac. Note that the yolk sac and the embryo are well-vascularized, and the atrium (a) and ventricle (v) are engorged with blood.

that "tent," and at no other places. Then carefully tease away the Reichart's membrane (see Note 4). The resulting embryo is enclosed only by the yolk sac, with some remnant uterine tissue at the placental position connected to the yolk sac.

5. Lastly, trim the placental tissues so only a small piece is still attached to the yolk sac (Fig. 2). Any maternal or uterine tissue left will not grow in culture and may be detrimental to the development of the embryo itself. But be careful not to trim too much of placenta that a hole is formed on the yolk sac. Use a plastic transfer pipette to carefully move the dissected embryo to warm HBSS for storage until ready for incubation.

3.4. Incubation

1. Use a plastic transfer pipette to move the dissected embryos from HBSS into 2-dram vials. It is acceptable if HBSS is also transferred along with the embryos. Each vial holds 3–5 embryos adequately. Then carefully aspirate or pipette out the HBSS in the vial and put in 1 mL of thawed 37°C embryo culture media. A 2-dram vial holds 1 mL of media optimally, as anything higher than that may cause leakage during incubation. Add glucose so the working concentration is 2 mg/mL. Also add Penstrip antibiotics at 100 U/mL penicillin and 100 μg/mL streptomycin working concentration. Drugs or other reagents can be directly added into the media as well. Use filtered pipette tips for all subsequent procedures.
2. Embryos at different gestational stages require different gas composition. E8.5 embryos require 20% O_2, 5% CO_2, 75% N_2

(20/5/75), E9.5 embryos need 70/5/20, and E10.5 embryos, 95/5/0. Fill 1-L plastic bottles with the appropriate gas and cap them to prevent leakage. Each 1-L plastic bottle holds only one 2-dram vial. Use a pair of extra-long forceps, hold the mouth of the open vial, and gently but quickly place it into the bottle. Cap the bottle and put it horizontally onto a roller platform in a 37°C incubator and slowly roll the bottle (see Note 5).

3. The bottles should be gassed every 8–12 h or when the embryos reach the next gestational day. Vials can be taken out and media can be changed or reagents added, and then placed back into incubation.

3.5. Analysis

The embryos should look healthy if the culture is successful. For instance, the embryo should resemble that *in utero*, although they may be a slightly slower in growth in comparison. Furthermore, the heart should beat rapidly when the embryos are first taken out from culture, although the rate slows down overtime at room temperature. Also, if cultured starting at E8.5, a successful embryo taken out later at E10 may have strong vasculature in the yolk sac and in the embryo itself.

4. Notes

1. Please use the rat embryo culture serum supplied by Harlan Laboratories, BT-4520.
2. Because embryos are enclosed by a fibrous outermost membrane, they are under higher pressure than normal. Therefore, when there is a cut on the surface of the decidua, the underlying tissue has a tendency to extrude from that cut and the embryo may suddenly pop out. When separating individual deciduas from an uterine horn, it is necessary to do it carefully under the microscope. Also, tearing away small pieces of fibrous membrane (just some stretches, not all the fibrous membrane) before cutting out individual deciduas can relieve the problem.
3. Do not use new pairs of forceps or those that are too sharp, as embryos can be easily punctured or damaged. It is better to use forceps whose ends slightly curve up, and during dissection, hold them so that the curve points upward to the microscope objective. This also prevents unwanted damages and is useful in dissecting away Reichert's membrane. Furthermore, always use one pair to hold (keep this hand stationary), and use the other to tear away in a lateral motion. Also, to make dissection easier, fill the petri dish with just enough HBSS to cover the whole decidua so that it does not float around. Likewise, it is possible to dissect a whole embryo in a drop of HBSS, although care must be taken not to allow that droplet to cool down too fast.

4. To remove larger tissues away in a controlled manner, hold the unwanted part not only with the tip, but also with the middle of the forceps. Then use another pair of forceps and run or slide its tip down the groove formed by the pair that is holding the tissue. This removes the tissue precisely without damaging unintended parts.
5. If no roller incubator is available, simply secure the roller bottles horizontally onto a suitable platform mixer and place the whole assembly into a 37°C regular cell culture incubator. Set shaking speed to slow.

Acknowledgments

C.P.C. is supported by funds from National Institute of Health (NIH), March of Dimes Foundation, Children's Heart Foundation, Office of the University of California (TRDRP), American Heart Association (AHA), California Institute of Regenerative Medicine, Kaiser Foundation, Baxter Foundation, Oak Foundation, and Stanford Cardiovascular Institute; CTH by predoctoral fellowships from AHA and NIH.

References

1. Chang, C. P., Neilson, J. R., Bayle, J. H., Gestwicki, J. E., Kuo, A., Stankunas, K., Graef, I. A., and Crabtree, G. R. (2004) A field of myocardial-endocardial NFAT signaling underlies heart valve morphogenesis. *Cell 118*, 649–63.
2. Stankunas, K., Hang, C. T., Tsun, Z. Y., Chen, H., Lee, N. V., Wu, J. I., Shang, C., Bayle, J. H., Shou, W., Iruela-Arispe, M. L., and Chang, C. P. (2008) Endocardial Brg1 represses ADAMTS1 to maintain the microenvironment for myocardial morphogenesis. *Dev Cell 14*, 298–311.
3. Hang, C. T., Yang, J., Han, P., Cheng, H. L., Shang, C., Ashley, E., Zhou, B., and Chang, C. P. (2010) Chromatin regulation by Brg1 underlies heart muscle development and disease. *Nature 466*, 62–7.
4. Chang, C. P., Chen, L., and Crabtree, G. R. (2003) Sonographic staging of the developmental status of mouse embryos in utero. *Genesis 36*, 7–11.

Chapter 2

Quantifying Cardiac Functions in Embryonic and Adult Zebrafish

Tiffany Hoage, Yonghe Ding, and Xiaolei Xu

Abstract

Zebrafish embryos have been extensively used to study heart development and cardiac function, mainly due to the unique embryology and genetics of this model organism. Since most human heart disease occurs during adulthood, adult zebrafish models of heart disease are being created to dissect mechanisms of the disease and discover novel therapies. However, due to its small heart size, the use of cardiac functional assays in the adult zebrafish has been limited. To address this bottleneck, the transparent fish line *casper;Tg(cmlc2:nuDsRed)* that has a red fluorescent heart can be used to document beating hearts in vivo and to quantify cardiac functions in adult zebrafish. Here, we describe our methods for quantifying shortening fraction and heart rate in embryonic zebrafish, as well as in the juvenile and adult *casper;Tg(cmlc2:nuDsRed)* fish. In addition, we describe the red blood cell flow rate assay that can be used to reflect cardiac function indirectly in zebrafish at any stage.

Key words: Zebrafish, Physiology, Shortening fraction, Heart rate, Flow rate

1. Introduction

Uniquely suitable for developmental and chemical genetic studies, the zebrafish is quickly becoming a popular model organism for studying cardiogenesis and heart disease (1, 2). The zebrafish embryo develops ex utero in a clear sac (the chorion), has a beating heart (including an outflow tract, a ventricle, and an atrium) by 24 h postfertilization, and hatches on day 3–4 postfertilization (3). Due to the embryo's transparency, heart growth and cardiac function can be studied at single-cell resolution. Morpholino knockdown and mRNA overexpression are two convenient tools to study gene function during embryogenesis (4). Stable knockout fish can also be established via TILLING or zinc finger nuclease

Xu Peng and Marc Antonyak (eds.), *Cardiovascular Development: Methods and Protocols*,
Methods in Molecular Biology, vol. 843, DOI 10.1007/978-1-61779-523-7_2,

(ZFN)-based technology (5–7). Unlike in cardiac gene knockout mouse models, zebrafish knockout phenotypes will not be complicated by secondary defects associated with lack of oxygen, because their small body size allows adequate oxygenation by diffusion without a beating heart for the first 5 days (8). The Tol2 transposon system allows novel genetic lines to be created in 50–70% of embryos injected (9), making zebrafish a very convenient model organism to generate transgenics (2). Like Drosophila, zebrafish is the only vertebrate model that is feasible to perform a mutagenesis screen in a standard lab (10, 11). Hundreds of cardiac mutants have already been identified, and cloning of the corresponding genes has revealed insights in both heart development and cardiac function (3, 12–14). Once established, the zebrafish-based disease models can be utilized for rapid and efficient downstream modifier screens or small molecule discovery efforts, with the goal of identifying new therapies (15–19).

Since most heart disease, such as cardiomyopathy and heart failure, occurs in adulthood (20), it is important to establish adult zebrafish models of heart disease and cardiac functional assays. Cardiomyopathy-like responses do exist in the adult zebrafish, as has been reported in the anemia-induced cardiac hypertrophy model *tr265* (21). Simplified ECG technology has been developed to monitor heart beating in the adult zebrafish heart, and electrophysiological studies have revealed adult zebrafish have similar action potentials as humans (22, 23). Due to the small size of the adult zebrafish heart (about 1 mm in diameter), the resolution of classic ultrasound-based technology is not satisfactory for reliable measurements of shortening fraction. A high-frequency ultrasound system for use in small animals has been developed, but can only reach a resolution of 25 μm (24, 25). Optical coherence tomography, with a higher resolution of 9–23 μm, has been applied to quantify cardiac functions in Xenopus, chicken embryos, and Drosophila (26–28). It remains unclear whether this technology will be useful to quantify cardiac functions in adult zebrafish.

We have taken advantage of the relatively transparent *casper* zebrafish line to develop a tool that allows us to quantify cardiac functions in adult zebrafish. The *casper* line contains two mutated genes (*nacre* and *roy* lines) that inhibit the formation of melanocytes and iridophores, which give the fish a certain degree of transparency into adulthood (29). To improve imaging of the heart, we crossed the *casper* line to *Tg*(*cmlc2:nuDsRed*) (30), which has a red fluorescent heart. A beating heart can be observed during the lifespan of the *casper*;*Tg*(*cmlc2:nuDsRed*) fish, which allows one to quantify shortening fraction as well as heart rate in vivo in both the embryo and adult zebrafish. In this chapter, we describe our imaging-based, cardiac function quantification methods in both embryos and adults. In addition, we have included the red blood cell flow rate assay that can be used in most fish as an indirect measure of cardiac function (21, 31).

2. Materials

1. 1× E3: 60 mL 5 M NaCl, 10 mL 1 M KCl, 20 mL 1 M $CaCl_2$, and 20 mL 1 M $MgSO_4$ are mixed with 890 mL ddH_2O. pH is adjusted to 7 based on (32).
2. 5 mM (10×) PTU: 0.76 g 1-Phenyl-2-thiourea (Sigma, St. Louis, MO) is added to 1 L of E3 in a glass bottle wrapped in tin foil. For 1× PTU, dilute 50 mL stock solution in 450 mL E3 in a glass bottle wrapped in tin foil. Both solutions can be stored at room temperature (see Note 1).
3. 25× Tricaine solution: 400 mg Tricaine powder (Aquatic Eco-Systems, Inc., Apopka, FL) is mixed with 97.9 mL ddH_2O and 2.1 mL 1 M Tris (pH 9). pH is adjusted to 7. The stock solution is stored in the freezer. For 1× Tricaine, 4.2 mL 25× Tricaine solution is diluted in 96 mL E3 based on (32). Working solution can be stored at room temperature for up to 1 week.
4. 3% Methyl Cellulose: 15 mg Methyl Cellulose (Sigma) is added to 500 mL ddH_2O and agitated at 80°C until the particles have dissolved and dispersed. After aliquoting, store at 4°C. Use at room temperature.
5. Equipment: light and fluorescent microscopes connected to a digital camera.

3. Methods

Videos taken of the zebrafish hearts in vivo are used to calculate shortening fraction and heart rate, while the red blood cell flow rate assay consists of direct observation and a picture of the area observed. Shortening fraction and heart rate can be calculated in most fish lines until 4 weeks postfertilization, when pigmentation of the skin begins to obscure direct observation of the heart. The *casper;Tg(cmlc2:nuDsRed)* line allows the documentation of a beating heart in fish beyond 4 weeks through adulthood. In fact, we have been able to image fish at 10 months by selecting those fish that have less opaque skin. Because of the limited fluorescence in the atrium of the *casper;Tg(cmlc2:nuDsRed)* fish, only the shortening fraction for the ventricle is measured. Ventricular shortening fraction is calculated from maximum diastole and maximum systole measurements. Although not discussed in this chapter, a software program is now available to semiautomate the analysis of shortening fraction in larvae, as well as calculate other parameters associated with the heart (33, 34). Heart rate can be directly observed throughout the lifespan of the *casper;Tg(cmlc2:nuDsRed)* fish by counting the beats in 15 s and extrapolating it to beats per minute.

Unlike shortening fraction and heart rate, the red blood cell flow rate can be obtained in most zebrafish during embryogenesis and adulthood. Red blood cell flow rate (mm/s) is found by timing a red blood cell between two specified points and dividing the distance by the time.

Our basic setup consists of a Nikon COOLPIX 8700 digital camera (Melville, NY) connected to either a Zeiss Axioplan two microscope (Carl Zeiss, Thornwood, NY) with differential interference contrast for embryological studies or a Leica MZ FLI III fluorescence stereomicroscope (Bannockburn, IL) for older fish. The video files obtained are in QuickTime (.MOV) at 30 frames per second (see Note 2) and picture files are in JPEG. For quantification, a millimeter ruler should be recorded in a video or picture, depending on which assay is used: video for the shortening fraction assay or a JPEG image for the red blood cell flow rate assay. Directions for quantifying distances and areas using the free graphical analysis software ImageJ (National Institutes of Health, Bethesda, MD) are included in the protocols below. To reduce variation in the assays, at least six different fish should be analyzed. Three separate data per fish should be obtained and averaged. The final average (reflecting all the averages in the group tested) and standard deviation are suggested for reporting in publications.

3.1. Heart Imaging of Zebrafish Up to Four Weeks Old

1. Tricaine fish for a desired amount of time before placing on a microscope slide in a thin layer of Methyl Cellulose or E3 water (see Notes 1 and 3–5).
2. Position the fish horizontally to obtain a lateral view under a microscope connected to a digital camera (see Note 2). The right eye should be facing downward for optimal viewing of the heart (see Fig. 1a).
3. Choose a magnification such that the heart fills at least 50% of the camera screen (e.g., up to 400× for embryological studies and as low as 50× for older fish) (see Fig. 1b).
4. Record the heart beating for at least 15 s.
5. For cross-sectional area and volume measurements, take a video of a millimeter ruler at the same magnification.
6. If Methyl Cellulose was used, add E3 water to remove the zebrafish.

3.2. Heart Imaging of Zebrafish Older than Four Weeks

1. Tricaine fish for a desired amount of time before placing in a moist sponge (see Fig. 1d and Notes 4 and 5).
2. Position the fish vertically to obtain a ventral view under a microscope connected to a digital camera (see Note 2).
3. Choose a magnification such that the heart fills at least 50% of the camera screen (e.g., 30×).

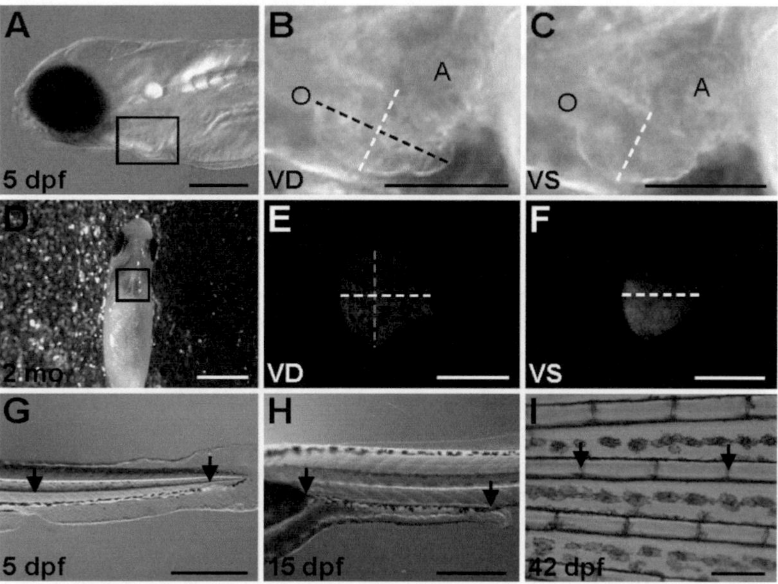

Fig. 1. Orientations and measurement locations for shortening fraction, heart rate, and red blood cell flow rate assays. (**a**) For cardiac imaging, zebrafish up to 4 weeks old are placed on their right side in 3% methyl cellulose or E3, as shown with the 5-dpf zebrafish. (**d**) Fish older than 4 weeks are placed on a moist sponge, ventral-side up. (**b**, **c**, **e** and **f**) Maximum ventricular diastole (VD) and ventricular systole (VS) are shown, with the width depicted as a *white dashed line* and the length as a *black* or *gray dashed line*. Outflow tract (O) and atrium (**A**) are labeled in images (**b**, **c**). For the red blood cell flow rate assay, (**g**) 5-dpf, (**h**) 15- and 21-dpf, and (**i**) 6-week fish are placed horizontally on their right side. *Arrows* refer to specific locations used for starting and stopping the stopwatch. Scale bars for (**a–i**) are 0.25, 0.125, 0.125, 3, 1, 1, 0.5, 0.5, and 0.5 mm, respectively. (Images (**g-i**) are reproduced from (21)).

4. Record the heart beating for at least 15 s.
5. For cross-sectional area and volume measurements, take a video of a millimeter ruler at the same magnification.

3.3. Quantifying Shortening Fraction (and Ventricle Size)

1. In the video file, use the arrow keys to move between frames.
2. Save the maximum ventricular systole (VS) and ventricular diastole (VD) frames (see Fig. 1b, c, e, and f) as JPEGs.
3. In pixels, measure the width of the heart (depicted as a white dashed line in Fig. 1b, c, e, and f) at maximum diastole and systole of the ventricle.
   (a) Open the file with ImageJ.
   (b) Select the Straight tool.
   (c) Hold in a left click for the width of the ventricle.
   (d) Select Analyze → Measure.
   (e) Record ImageJ's "Length" value for the width measurement (in pixels).

Table 1
Example of calculations for ventricular shortening fraction, cross-sectional area, and volume

Parameter	Calculation	Result
Width at VD (pixels)	–	136.74
Width at VS (pixels)	–	111.72
Ventricular SF (%)	=(100)(136.74–111.72)/136.74	18.3
Cross-sectional area of ventricle (pixels^2)	–	25,780
Pixels in 1 mm	–	838
Cross-sectional area of ventricle (mm^2)	=(25780)/(838)^2	0.037
Width at VD (mm)	=(136.74)/(838)	0.163
Length at VD (pixels)	–	224.93
Length at VD (mm)	=(224.93)/(838)	0.268
Volume of the ventricle (mm^3)	=(0.523)(0.163^2)(0.268)	0.004

4. Calculate the shortening fraction (%) for the ventricle (see Table 1 for a sample calculation): (100)(width at diastole–width at systole)/(width at diastole).
5. For calculating cross-sectional area and approximating the volume of the ventricle, proceed with the following steps (see Table 1 for sample calculations).
6. Cross-sectional area can be found by using ImageJ:
   (a) Open the file containing a picture of the ventricle in diastole with ImageJ.
   (b) Select the Polygon selections tool.
   (c) Left click around the perimeter of the ventricle.
   (d) Select Analyze → Measure.
   (e) Record ImageJ's "Area" value for the ventricle cross-sectional area (in pixels^2).
   (f) Save a picture of the ruler (from the video) as a JPEG.
   (g) Open the file with ImageJ.
   (h) Select the Straight tool.
   (i) Hold in a left click for the length of 1 mm.
   (j) Select Analyze → Measure.
   (k) Record ImageJ's "Length" value for the number of pixels in 1 mm.
   (l) For cross-sectional area (mm^2), use the following formula: (cross-sectional area in pixels^2)/(pixels in 1 mm)^2.

7. To approximate the volume of the ventricle, proceed with the following:
   (a) Determine the width (in mm) of the ventricle at maximum diastole by dividing the length in pixels (found above) by the pixels in 1 mm.
   (b) Use ImageJ to find the length (in mm) of the ventricle at maximum diastole (see Fig. 1b, e), and then convert the value to mm.
   (c) Calculate the approximate volume of the ventricle (mm^3) using the following formula (see Note 6): (0.523)(width in mm)^2(length in mm).

3.4. Quantifying Heart Rate

1. From either a video or live, count the number of beats in 15 s.
2. To calculate heart rate (beats/min), multiply the number of beats counted by four. For example, if the beats counted in 15 s is 25, the heart rate is 100 beats/min.

3.5. Red Blood Cell Flow Rate

1. If necessary, anesthetize the zebrafish in Tricaine solution before placing on a microscope slide in a thin layer of Methyl Cellulose or E3 water (see Notes 4 and 7).
2. Position the fish horizontally to obtain a lateral view under a microscope connected to a digital camera, as shown in Fig. 1h. The right eye should be facing down.
3. Using a millisecond stopwatch, determine the time in seconds it takes a red blood cell to travel between two arbitrary points. Examples of arbitrary points are shown in Figs. 1g–i (see Note 8).
4. Take a picture of the area observed.
5. With the same magnification, take a picture of a millimeter ruler.
6. Using ImageJ, determine the number of pixels in 1 mm.
   (a) Open the file with ImageJ.
   (b) Select the Straight tool.
   (c) Hold in a left click for the length of 1 mm.
   (d) Select Analyze → Measure.
   (e) Record ImageJ's "Length" value for the number of pixels in 1 mm.
7. In pixels, measure the distance traveled by the red blood cell.
8. Calculate the distance traveled in mm by dividing the number of pixels traveled by the number of pixels in 1 mm (see Table 2 for a sample calculation).
9. To calculate the red blood cell (RBC) flow rate (mm/s), divide the distance traveled (in mm) by the time (in seconds) (see Table 2 for a sample calculation).

Table 2
Example of calculations for RBC flow rate

Parameter	Calculation	Result
Time (seconds)	–	1.172
1 mm (pixels)	–	1,659
Distance traveled (pixels)	–	932.09
Distance traveled (mm)	=932.09/1659	0.562
RBC flow rate (mm/s)	=0.562/1.172	0.48

4. Notes

1. To prevent pigment formation, PTU treatment should begin at 24 h postfertilization. PTU is not necessary for imaging embryos less than 3 days postfertilization (dpf) or *casper* embryos.
2. Higher frames per second increases the accuracy of the measurements. A minimum of 30 frames per second is recommended.
3. A paintbrush can be used to position the young zebrafish in Methyl Cellulose.
4. Consistency in handling the fish, positioning of the fish, time of anesthesia, and duration between anesthesia and measurement is crucial for consistent results.
5. We anesthetize 4–6-week zebrafish for 2 min and 16-week zebrafish for 2.5 min in 1× Tricaine and image the heart by 3 or 3.5 min, respectively.
6. The volume of the ventricle is based on the assumption that the shape of a ventricle is an approximate ellipsoid: $(4/3)(\pi)$ (width in $mm^2)^2$(length in mm^2), which can be simplified to (0.523)(width in $mm)^2$(length in mm).
7. For the red blood cell flow rate assay, day-5 zebrafish are not anesthetized. Week-6 zebrafish are anesthetized in 1× Tricaine for 2 min and timed between 2.75 and 3 min, while 16-week fish are anesthetized for 2.5 min and timed between 3.25 and 3.5 min.
8. When measuring red blood cell flow rate in the tail fin, we measure within the area of the fourth main ray from the ventral side.

Acknowledgments

We thank Dr. Leonard Zon at Children's Hospital, Boston, for sharing with us the *casper* fish; Dr. Geoff Burns at Massachusetts General Hospital, Boston, for the *Tg*(*cmlc2:nuDsRed*) fish; Jomok Beninio for his help with zebrafish husbandry; and Dr. Jingchun Yang and Dr. Xiaojing Sun for their advice on the shortening fraction methodology for zebrafish larvae.

References

1. Chico, T. J., Ingham, P. W., and Crossman, D. C. (2008) Modeling cardiovascular disease in the zebrafish. *Trends Cardiovasc Med 4*, 150–155.
2. Lieschke, G. J., and Currie, P. D. (2007) Animal models of human disease: zebrafish swim into view. *Nat Rev Genet 8*, 353–367.
3. Glickman, N. S., and Yelon, D. (2002) Cardiac development in zebrafish: coordination of form and function. *Semin Cell Dev Biol 13*, 507–513.
4. Nasevicius, A., and Ekker, S. C. (2000) Effective targeted gene 'knockdown' in zebrafish. *Nat Genet 26*, 216–220.
5. Ekker, S. C. (2008) Zinc finger-based knockout punches for zebrafish genes. *Zebrafish 5*, 121–123.
6. Moens, C. B., Donn, T. M., Wolf-Saxon, E. R., and Ma, T. P. (2008) Reverse genetics in zebrafish by TILLING. *Brief Funct Genomic Proteomic 7*, 454–459.
7. Foley, J. E., Maeder, M. L., Pearlberg, J., Joung, J. K., Peterson, R. T., and Yeh, J. R. (2009) Targeted mutagenesis in zebrafish using customized zinc-finger nucleases. *Nat Protoc 4*, 1855–1867.
8. Pelster, B., and Burggren, W. W. (1996) Disruption of hemoglobin oxygen transport does not impact oxygen-dependent physiological processes in developing embryos of zebra fish (Danio rerio). *Circ Res 79*, 358–362.
9. Kawakami, K., Takeda, H., Kawakami, N., Kobayashi, M., Matsuda, N., and Mishina, M. (2004) A transposon-mediated gene trap approach identifies developmentally regulated genes in zebrafish. *Dev Cell 7*, 133–144.
10. Stainier, D. Y., Fouquet, B., Chen, J. N., Warren, K. S., Weinstein, B. M., Meiler, S. E., Mohideen, M. A., Neuhauss, S. C., Solnica-Krezel, L., Schier, A. F., Zwartkruis, F., Stemple, D. L., Malicki, J., Driever, W., and Fishman, M. C. (1996) Mutations affecting the formation and function of the cardiovascular system in the zebrafish embryo. *Development 123*, 285–292.
11. Stainier, D. Y. (2001) Zebrafish genetics and vertebrate heart formation. *Nat Rev Genet 2*, 39–48.
12. Warren, K. S., Wu, J. C., Pinet, F., and Fishman, M. C. (2000) The genetic basis of cardiac function: dissection by zebrafish (Danio rerio) screens. *Philos Trans R Soc Lond B Biol Sci 355*, 939–944.
13. Chen, J. N., and Fishman, M. C. (2000) Genetics of heart development. *Trends Genet 16*, 383–388.
14. Dahme, T., Katus, H. A., and Rottbauer, W. (2009) Fishing for the genetic basis of cardiovascular disease. *Dis Model Mech 2*, 18–22.
15. MacRae, C. A., and Peterson, R. T. (2003) Zebrafish-based small molecule discovery. *Chem Biol 10*, 901–908.
16. Milan, D. J., Kim, A. M., Winterfield, J. R., Jones, I. L., Pfeufer, A., Sanna, S., Arking, D. E., Amsterdam, A. H., Sabeh, K. M., Mably, J. D., Rosenbaum, D. S., Peterson, R. T., Chakravarti, A., Kääb, S., Roden, D. M., and MacRae, C. A. (2009) Drug-sensitized zebrafish screen identifies multiple genes, including GINS3, as regulators of myocardial repolarization. *Circulation 120*, 553–559.
17. Kaufman, C. K., White, R. M., and Zon, L. (2009) Chemical genetic screening in the zebrafish embryo. *Nat Protoc 4*, 1422–1432.
18. Zon, L. I., and Peterson, R. T. (2005) In vivo drug discovery in the zebrafish. *Nat Rev Drug Discov 4*, 35–44.
19. Peterson, R. T., Shaw, S. Y., Peterson, T. A., Milan, D. J., Zhong, T. P., Schreiber, S. L., MacRae, C. A., and Fishman, M. C. (2004) Chemical suppression of a genetic mutation in a zebrafish model of aortic coarctation. *Nat Biotechnol 22*, 595–599.
20. AHA (2010) Heart Disease and Stroke Statistics – 2010 Update. Dallas, Texas
21. Sun, X., Hoage, T., Bai, P., Ding, Y., Chen, Z., Zhang, R., Huang, W., Jahangir, A., Paw, B.,

Li, Y. G., and Xu, X. (2009) Cardiac hypertrophy involves both myocyte hypertrophy and hyperplasia in anemic zebrafish. *PLoS One 4*, e6596.

22. Nemtsas, P., Wettwer, E., Christ, T., Weidinger, G., and Ravens, U. (2010) Adult zebrafish heart as a model for human heart? An electrophysiological study. *J Mol Cell Cardiol 48*, 161–171.
23. Milan, D. J., Jones, I. L., Ellinor, P. T., and MacRae, C. A. (2006) In vivo recording of adult zebrafish electrocardiogram and assessment of drug-induced QT prolongation. *Am J Physiol Heart Circ Physiol 291*, H269–273.
24. Sun, L., Xu, X., Richard, W. D., Feng, C., Johnson, J. A., and Shung, K. K. (2008) A high-frame rate duplex ultrasound biomicroscopy for small animal imaging in vivo. *IEEE Trans Biomed Eng 55*, 2039–2049.
25. Sun, L., Lien, C. L., Xu, X., and Shung, K. K. (2008) In vivo cardiac imaging of adult zebrafish using high frequency ultrasound (45-75 MHz). *Ultrasound Med Biol 34*, 31–39.
26. Boppart, S. A., Tearney, G. J., Bouma, B. E., Southern, J. F., Brezinski, M. E., and Fujimoto, J. G. (1997) Noninvasive assessment of the developing Xenopus cardiovascular system using optical coherence tomography. *Proc Natl Acad Sci U S A 94*, 4256–4261.
27. Choma, M. A., Izatt, S. D., Wessells, R. J., Bodmer, R., and Izatt, J. A. (2006) Images in cardiovascular medicine: in vivo imaging of the adult Drosophila melanogaster heart with real-time optical coherence tomography. *Circulation 114*, e35–36.
28. Manner, J., Thrane, L., Norozi, K., and Yelbuz, T. M. (2008) High-resolution in vivo imaging of the cross-sectional deformations of contracting embryonic heart loops using optical coherence tomography. *Dev Dyn 237*, 953–961.
29. White, R. M., Sessa, A., Burke, C., Bowman, T., LeBlanc, J., Ceol, C., Bourque, C., Dovey, M., Goessling, W., Burns, C. E., and Zon, L. I. (2008) Transparent adult zebrafish as a tool for in vivo transplantation analysis. *Cell Stem Cell 2*, 183–189.
30. Mably, J. D., Mohideen, M. A., Burns, C. G., Chen, J. N., and Fishman, M. C. (2003) heart of glass regulates the concentric growth of the heart in zebrafish. *Curr Biol 13*, 2138–2147.
31. Brutsaert, D. L. (2006) Cardiac dysfunction in heart failure: the cardiologist's love affair with time. *Prog Cardiovasc Dis 49*, 157–181.
32. Westerfield, M. (2000) The zebrafish book. A guide for the laboratory use of zebrafish (Danio rerio). 4th ed. Univ. of Oregon Press, Eugene, Oregon.
33. Ocorr, K., Fink, M., Cammarato, A., Bernstein, S., and Bodmer, R. (2009) Semi-automated Optical Heartbeat Analysis of small hearts. *J Vis Exp 31*.
34. Fink, M., Callol-Massot, C., Chu, A., Ruiz-Lozano, P., Izpisua Belmonte, J. C., Giles, W., Bodmer, R., and Ocorr, K. (2009) A new method for detection and quantification of heartbeat parameters in Drosophila, zebrafish, and embryonic mouse hearts. *Biotechniques 46*, 101–113.

Chapter 3

Analysis of the Patterning of Cardiac Outflow Tract and Great Arteries with Angiography and Vascular Casting

Ching-Pin Chang

Abstract

Formation of the cardiac outflow tract and great arteries involves complex morphogenetic processes, whose abnormities result in several clinically important diseases. Studies of these developmental processes are therefore important for understanding congenital vascular defects. However, the three-dimensional structure of arteries makes it challenging to analyze the pattern of vasculature using conventional histological approaches. Here we describe a vascular casting method to visualize the branching and connections of great arteries in developing embryos as well as in adult mice. This technique can be used to study the development of cardiac outflow tract, semilunar valves, and great arteries as demonstrated previously (Circ Res, 2008; Development 135: 3577–3586, 2008).

Key words: Great arteries, Cardiac outflow tract, Persistent truncus arteriosus, Tetralogy of Fallot, Overriding aorta, Bicuspid aortic valve, Pulmonic stenosis, Heart valve, Heart development, Vascular patterning

1. Introduction

Development of the cardiac outflow tract requires several developmental steps that include the division of a common arterial trunk (truncus arteriosus) into two arteries (aorta and main pulmonary artery), alignment of these two arteries to their respective cardiac chambers (left and right ventricles), and formation of heart valves at the base of each artery (aortic and pulmonic valves) (1). This septation and alignment of cardiac outflow tract links the left ventricle to aorta, which is further connected to a set of arteries originating from five pairs of primitive branchial arch arteries (2, 3). These branchial arch arteries, after extensive remodeling, develop into a distinct set of arteries that receive blood from the aorta to supply the head, neck, and upper limbs of the body. These arteries

Xu Peng and Marc Antonyak (eds.), *Cardiovascular Development: Methods and Protocols*,
Methods in Molecular Biology, vol. 843, DOI 10.1007/978-1-61779-523-7_3,

include ductus arteriosus, aortic arch, brachiocephalic, common carotid, and subclavian arteries.

Abnormalities in cardiac outflow tract development result in congenital heart diseases, including persistent truncus arteriosus, tetralogy of Fallot, overriding aorta with ventricular septal defect, bicuspid aortic valve, and pulmonic valve stenosis (2, 4, 5). On the other hand, malformations of branchial arch arteries can cause aberrant arteries and abnormal vascular connections that may require surgical corrections (3). For identifying these defects, angiography or vascular casting provides an effective way to visualize the pattern of cardiac outflow tract and arterial connections. This angiographic technique, using dyes and resin to outline the heart and blood vessels, consists of the following steps: resin preparation, embryo harvest, embryo preparation for the procedure, angiography and vascular casting, and tissue maceration.

2. Materials

2.1. Instruments/ Equipment

1. Dissecting microscope.
2. Dissecting forceps.
3. Plastic pipettes.
4. Petri dishes.
5. 33-gauge needle (Hamilton).
6. Styrofoam platform wrapped with aluminum foil (ex. Reynolds Wrap).
7. Pins.
8. Glass vials.
9. A chemical hood.

2.2. Reagents

1. Acrylic resin (methyl methacrylate monomer, Polyscience, Inc.), stored in the cold room or 4°C until use (see Note 1).
2. Blue pigment (Batson's #17 Blue Pigment, Polyscience, Inc.), stored at room temperature.
3. Maceration Solution (Polysciences, Inc.), stored at room temperature.
4. Phosphate-buffered saline (PBS).
5. Potassium hydroxide (Maceration Solution, Polysciences, Inc.).
6. 4% paraformaldehyde (PFA).
7. India ink (undiluted, water-insoluble form).
8. Benzyl alcohol/benzyl benzoate solution: Mix one volume of Benzyl alcohol with two volumes of benzoate.

3. Methods

3.1. Resin Preparation

Prepare the resin in a chemical hood.

1. Add the acrylic resin (clear liquid) by pipetting into a glass vial.
2. Use a tooth pick to transfer a small amount of blue pigment into the vial.
3. Mix the resin with the pigment by inverting the vial a few times.
4. Add more blue pigment if deeper color is desired. Please note that the pigment increases the viscosity of the resin.
5. Cap the vial and keep it on ice. If stored at 4°C, the blue resin remains stable for vascular casting for at least several months.

3.2. Embryo Harvest

Mouse embryos are harvested in cold PBS by the standard method. The resin-based vascular casting technique can be applied to E12.5-E18.5 embryos as well as neonatal and adult mice (see Subheading 3.3–3.5) (4, 5). For younger embryos at E10.5 or E11.5, we perform India ink-based angiography to visualize the vasculature (see Subheading 3.6).

3.3. Embryo Preparation for Angiography and Vascular Casting

1. Pin the harvested embryo to an aluminum foil-wrapped styrofoam platform for dissection under the microscope.
2. Spread the upper limbs of the embryo horizontally and pin each upper limb to the platform to expose the chest wall.
3. Pin the tail or the lower limbs to the platform to position the embryo.
4. Cut open the chest wall at the midline with two pairs of forceps under the dissecting microscope (see Note 2). Pin each half of the chest wall to the platform to expose the heart.

3.4. Angiography and Vascular Casting

1. Load a 1-mL tuberculin syringe with the blue resin prepared in Subheading 3.1. Keep the loaded syringe on ice (see Note 3).
2. Mount a 33-gauge needle (Hamilton) on the syringe.
3. Squirt a small amount of the resin through the needle to eliminate air bubbles.
4. Insert the needle into the right ventricle of the embryonic mouse heart with the bevel facing up (see Note 4).
5. Gently inject the blue resin into the right ventricle. Make sure that the bevel is entirely within the right ventricular chamber before injecting (see Note 5). Carefully observe the dynamic flow of resin into the right ventricle, main pulmonary artery, ductus arteriosus, aortic arch, ascending aorta, and descending aorta (see Note 6). This angiographic flow can be videotaped if necessary.

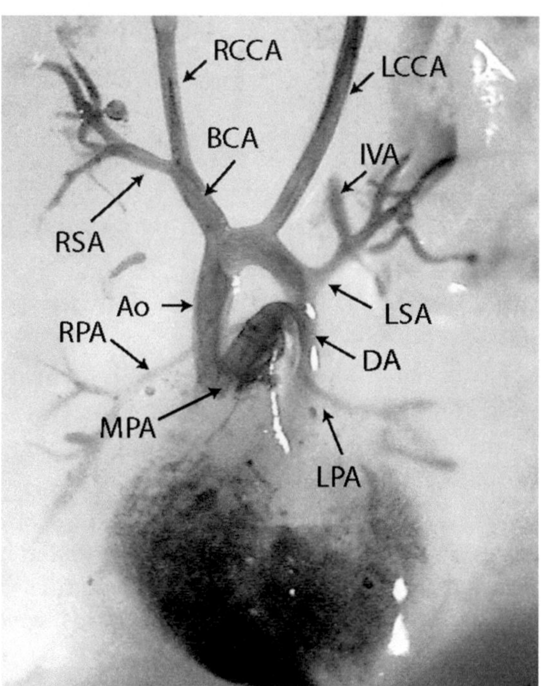

Fig. 1. Vascular casting of great arteries in an E14.5 embryo. *Ao* aorta; *MPA* main pulmonary artery; *DA* ductus arteriosus; *RPA, LPA* right and left pulmonary arteries; *RSA, LSA* right and left subclavian arteries; *RCCA, LCCA* right and left common carotid arteries; *BCA* brachiocephalic artery; *IVA* internal vertebral artery.

6. Remove residual resin spilled onto the surface of the heart or tissues surrounding the arteries (see Note 7). After the cleaning, the resin-filled arteries within the embryo are ready for imaging in situ (Fig. 1) (see Note 8). Alternatively, the embryo can be transferred to a petri dish on ice for imaging later, while another embryo is prepared for angiography and vascular casting.
7. After the procedure, embryos are kept at 4°C for 2–6 h to allow the resin to polymerize and harden within the vessels (see Note 9). The vascular tree can then be photographed in their normal position within the embryo. Alternatively, the soft tissues of embryos can be removed by maceration to expose and isolate the vascular cast for photography.

3.5. Tissue Maceration

1. Dissolve the soft tissues of the embryo in potassium hydroxide at 55°C for 1–3 h to expose the vascular cast (see Note 10).
2. Clean the vascular cast in water with forceps to remove residual soft tissues. After the cleaning, the vascular cast is ready for imaging (4, 5).

3.6. Angiography of Younger Embryos at E10.5 or E11.5

India ink-based angiography is performed for younger embryos at E10.5 or E11.5 (5, 6) (see Note 11).

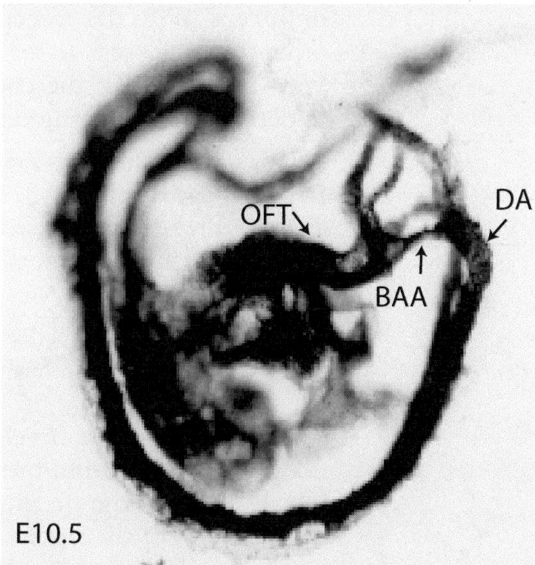

Fig. 2. India ink-based angiography of an E10.5 embryo. *OFT* cardiac outflow tract; *BAA* brachial arch (or pharyngeal arch) artery; *DA* dorsal aorta.

1. Embryos are harvested and fixed overnight in 4% PFA in PBS (see Note 12).
2. Inject india ink into the left ventricle using a fine glass micropipette controlled by a mouth pipette while the embryos rest in PBS.
3. Dissect the embryos to expose the branchial arch arteries for imaging.
4. Alternatively, embryos can be cleared in 1:2 benzyl alcohol/ benzyl benzoate before imaging (Fig. 2).

4. Notes

1. The Batson's #17 Anatomical Corrosion Kit from Polysciences, Inc (Catalog #07349) contains monomer base, catalyst, promotor, pigment red, and pigment blue. Our method of vascular casting does not require the catalyst or promoter. The only two required components are the monomer base (methyl methacrylate monomer, Catalog #02599) and the blue pigment (Catalog #07352), which can be purchased separately. We do not use the red pigment because the color does not contrast well with the blood or tissue color of the embryos.
2. Use one pair of forceps to cut into the subxiphoid space. Then grasp the sternum and lift the chest wall slightly with this pair

of forceps. With this forceps as an anchor and balance, use the other pair of forceps to tear open the chest wall along the midline. The lifting of the chest wall is to prevent injury of the underlying heart during dissection of the chest wall.

3. Keeping the resin cold slows down the polymerization process. It helps to maintain the resin in a fluid state to facilitate the angiographic flow. The viscosity of resin can be adjusted by adding different amounts of blue pigment, which increases resin viscosity.

4. When inserting the needle into the right ventricle, use the left hand to hold and steady the syringe (bevel facing up) and use the right hand to hold the plunger. Then squirt a tiny amount of resin through the bevel to eliminate air bubble. Angle the needle at 30–45° from the anterior wall of the right ventricle. Slowly advance the needle with both hands to penetrate the anterior wall of the right ventricle. Stop advancing the needle when the entire bevel is within the right ventricular chamber. Use the left hand to stabilize the position of the syringe and needle. Use the right hand to gently push the plunger and inject resin into the heart. It is important to steady the syringe and needle while injecting the resin, particularly for smaller embryonic hearts. Additional movement of the bevel within the heart may puncture the posterior or inferior wall of the heart, resulting in resin leakage and failure of angiography.

   Hearts of different sizes may require adjustment of the insertion angle. The key for the adjustment is to have the bevel entirely within the ventricular chamber without perforating the posterior or inferior wall of the heart. A bevel facing up within the right ventricle directs the resin flow to the right ventricular outflow tract, the main pulmonary artery, the ductus arteriosus, and then the aorta. In contrast, a bevel facing down directs the flow to the posterior or inferior wall of the right ventricle, preventing filling of the great arteries.

5. A partially exposed bevel causes leakage of the resin during injection, resulting in ineffective vascular casting. The bevel size relative to the cardiac chamber size, therefore, determines the age of embryos whose great vessels can be casted using this method.

6. Observation of the resin flow may identify abnormal connections of arteries or shunting between cardiac chambers and arteries.

7. Because the injection of resin increases the pressure within the right ventricular chamber, the resin may leak from the puncture or insertion site of the right ventricle. This does not affect the procedure as long as the great arteries are successfully filled with the blue resin. However, it is important to clean up the resin spill to have a high-quality image of the casted arteries.

Wait for 1–5 min or longer before removing the resin spilled onto tissues surrounding the heart or arteries. The spilled resin will harden partially within a few minutes and form a thin film, which is easier to remove than the liquid resin. Hardened resin also prevents further leakage from the insertion site. In case the leakage becomes so severe as to drain the resin from the great vessels, reinsert the needle into the right ventricle through the original insertion site, and then inject more resin to fill the vessels.

8. Imaging the vascular tree in situ allows the investigator to identify the position, course, origin, and destination of each vessel within the embryo based on anatomical landmarks. This information is useful for identifying normal or aberrant blood vessels, which are often named by their course through the tissue or by the tissues they supply.
9. Keeping embryos in a covered petri dish at 4°C slows down the drying and degeneration of soft tissues, which provide anatomical landmarks for identifying the casted vessels. Embryos thus stored remain good for imaging within 2–4 days after casting.
10. The amount of maceration solution should be at least two to three times the volume of tissue mass. Mouse embryonic tissues can be removed within 1–3 h of maceration, while maceration of adult tissues may take 8–24 h. When macerating the adult tissues, remove the specimen from the solution every 2–3 h, rinse it in water, and clean up the tissue debris before further maceration. If the solution becomes very cloudy with debris floating, change the solution to facilitate the maceration process.
11. The hearts of E10-E11 embryos are too small to accommodate a 33-gauge Hamilton needle for the resin-based angiography and casting. Glass micropipettes with fine tips (used for injecting DNA transgenes into mouse eggs) are necessary for cannulating the E10 or E11 hearts. However, because the resin is too viscous to pass smoothly through the fine tip of a micropipette, we use India ink to deliver the contrast for angiography using micropipettes.
12. For the resin-based angiography on older embryos, we prefer fresh to fixed embryos. PFA-fixed tissues become stiff and brittle, resulting in suboptimal vascular casting. In contrast, for the fragile E10-E11 embryos, we fix embryos with PFA before conducting the India ink-based angiography. Fixed tissues are less fragile and more resistant to the pressure of ink injection.

Acknowledgments

C.P.C. is supported by funds from National Institute of Health (NIH), March of Dimes Foundation, Children's Heart Foundation,

Office of the University of California (TRDRP), American Heart Association (AHA), California Institute of Regenerative Medicine, Kaiser Foundation, Baxter Foundation, Oak Foundation, and Stanford Cardiovascular Institute.

References

1. Harvey, R. P., and Rosenthal, N. (1999) *Heart Development*, Academic Press.
2. Kirby, M. L. (2007) *Cardiac Development.* Oxford University Press, New York.
3. Sadler, T. (2004) *Langman's Medical Embryology*, Ninth ed., Williams & Wilkins, Baltimore.
4. Stankunas, K., Shang, C., Twu, K. Y., Kao, S. C., Jenkins, N. A., Copeland, N. G., Sanyal, M., Selleri, L., Cleary, M. L., and Chang, C. P. (2008) Pbx/Meis Deficiencies Demonstrate Multigenetic Origins of Congenital Heart Disease. *Circ Res.*
5. Chang, C. P., Stankunas, K., Shang, C., Kao, S. C., Twu, K. Y., and Cleary, M. L. (2008) Pbx1 functions in distinct regulatory networks to pattern the great arteries and cardiac outflow tract. *Development 135*, 3577–86.
6. Jia, Q., McDill, B. W., Li, S. Z., Deng, C., Chang, C. P., and Chen, F. (2007) Smad signaling in the neural crest regulates cardiac outflow tract remodeling through cell autonomous and non-cell autonomous effects. *Dev Biol 311*, 172–84.

Chapter 4

Morpholino Injection in *Xenopus*

Panna Tandon, Chris Showell, Kathleen Christine, and Frank L. Conlon

Abstract

The study of gene function in developmental biology has been significantly furthered by advances in antisense technology made in the early 2000s. This was achieved, in particular, by the introduction of morpholino (MO) oligonucleotides. The introduction of antisense MO oligonucleotides into cells enables researchers to readily reduce the levels of their protein of interest without investing huge financial or temporal resources, in both *in vivo* and *in vitro* model systems. Historically, the African clawed frog *Xenopus* has been used to study vertebrate embryological development, due to its ability to produce vast numbers of offspring that develop rapidly, in synchrony, and can be cultured in buffers with ease. The developmental progress of *Xenopus* embryos has been extensively characterized and this model organism is very easy to maintain. It is these attributes that enable MO-based knockdown strategies to be so effective in *Xenopus*. In this chapter, we will detail the methods of microinjecting MO oligonucleotides into early embryos of *X. laevis* and *X. tropicalis*. We will discuss how MOs can be used to prevent either pre-mRNA splicing or translation of the specific gene of interest resulting in abrogation of that gene's function and advise on what control experiments should be undertaken to verify their efficacy.

Key words: *Xenopus*, *Laevis*, *Tropicalis*, Morpholino, Microinjection, Knockdown, Inhibition, Translation, Splicing, Splice, Antisense

1. Introduction

Understanding of the molecular and genetic control of cardiogenesis has advanced rapidly in recent years through the use of several complementary model systems, including oviparous vertebrate model organisms such as the zebrafish (*Danio rerio*) and the frog (principally *Xenopus laevis*). *Xenopus* species have numerous advantages in addition to the external nature of their embryonic development and ease of use. They are largely transparent at tadpole stages, allowing anatomical defects in the heart to be easily seen; their

Xu Peng and Marc Antonyak (eds.), *Cardiovascular Development: Methods and Protocols*, Methods in Molecular Biology, vol. 843, DOI 10.1007/978-1-61779-523-7_4,

hearts undergo the process of atrial septation similarly to higher vertebrates; they can survive to advanced developmental stages in the absence of a functioning circulatory system, allowing for more detailed studies of early cardiovascular defects; and they have a well-defined fate map at the 32-cell stage (6 h post-fertilization) that allows the blastomeres that will give rise to the heart to be identified and manipulated. These features have enabled many investigators to examine events in cardiac development in the frog, but it has only been with the advent of effective antisense techniques that significant advances have been made linking these events to the genes that control them. The most extensively used of these techniques is the use of morpholino (MO) oligonucleotides to inhibit the function of specific genes by preventing translation or splicing of their corresponding messenger RNA (mRNA). This has led to the publication of many studies of heart development in *Xenopus* that have advanced our understanding of this process in vertebrates (1–9).

The use of MOs began in the mid-1990s, when morpholine-based oligonucleotides were introduced into cultured cells to achieve inhibition of gene function (Partridge et al., 1996). Since then, MOs have been utilized extensively in vertebrate embryos, particularly those of the frog *Xenopus* and the zebrafish (*Danio rerio*) to achieve successful inhibition of specific genes (10–12). This type of experiment is invaluable in characterizing the function of a gene and also for confirming the results of genetic mapping studies by phenocopying the biological effects of mapped loss-of-function mutations isolated in genetic screens.

MO antisense oligonucleotides are synthetic nucleic acid analogs that consist of a six-membered morpholine ring instead of the normal five-membered sugar ring (13). These neutrally charged oligonucleotides are thereby stable, soluble, and bind to RNA with high-affinity. In addition, they are resistant to nuclease-degradation and have limited interaction with proteins (14–16). Consisting of 25 bases, MOs are designed to reduce gene function in two ways. First, the MO can be designed to target sequences in the 5′ untranslated region (UTR), close to the translation initiation codon of the gene. By binding to this location, the MO can sterically block the attachment of the ribosomal machinery and inhibit protein translation (11). Alternatively, they can be made to target the splice junctions within the pre-mRNA strand. When a MO complimentary to the splice donor site is used, this typically prevents the associated intron from being spliced out of the mRNA. This results in the incorporation of intron-encoded amino acids and, in many cases, early termination of translation due to the presence of stop codons present within the intron itself or created by a shift in the reading frame of subsequent sequences. MOs complimentary to the splice acceptor site tend to cause exon skipping, which occurs when the splice donor of the preceding exon cannot splice with the targeted acceptor site and instead splices with the acceptor of a more 3′ exon. This results in the targeted exon and its flanking introns being spliced out. Other aberrant splicing events have also been detected and the results of mRNA mis-splicing can vary in different instances, so these events should always be characterized for the particular MO used (17).

The decision to use a translation-blocking versus a splice-blocking MO strategy is often based on the availability of effective antibodies against the targeted gene product, as this determines the type of assay that can be used to demonstrate MO efficacy *in vivo*. When an antibody is available, a reduction in endogenous protein levels can be assayed by western blotting of electrophoresed embryo lysates (see Subheading 2.3). This is perhaps the best assay of MO efficacy and is ideal for translation-blocking strategies. When antibodies are not available, specific activity of a translation-blocking MO against its targeted sequence can be demonstrated *in vivo* through co-injection of targeted mRNA encoding a fusion with an epitope tag to which an antibody is available, or *in vitro* through the use of cell-free translation systems (see Subheading 2.4). Alternatively, a suitable splice-blocking MO may be used. In this case, reverse transcription polymerase chain reaction (RT-PCR) is used to monitor mis-splicing of the endogenous targeted mRNA (see Subheading 2.5).

Proper design of MOs is a critical factor in their effectiveness. Translation-blocking MOs should be designed against 25-bp target sequences within the 50-bp region centered on the translation initiation site. Similarly, splice-blocking MOs should be designed against 25-bp target sequences within a 50-bp region centered on either the splice donor or splice acceptor site. It is recommended that self-complementarity be avoided in order to prevent intrastrand pairing and/or dimer formation. In most cases, MO sequences will be suggested by the vendor based on these considerations and the submitted sequence. To demonstrate that a phenotype results from depletion of a particular targeted mRNA, it is advisable to use at least two independent MOs designed to target unique regions of the same mRNA, as these are unlikely to share off-target effects. Control MOs are also useful for validating the observations made in MO experiments. MOs containing five mismatched nucleotides distributed across their sequence are commonly used in negative control experiments, as are MOs targeting sequences from other species with no significant similarity to orthologous sequences in *Xenopus*, such as MOs against the human *β-globin* mRNA. Well-characterized MOs such as those against *β-catenin* may serve as positive controls for the MO microinjection procedure, should these be necessary.

Strategies other than MOs have been employed to inhibit gene function. These include RNA interference (RNAi), whereby the RNA is targeted for degradation by the binding of small-inhibitory

RNA (siRNA) molecules and recruitment of the RNA-induced silencing complex (RISC), phosphorothioate-linked DNA (S-DNA) that employs cellular RNase H to cleave the target RNA strand, and peptide nucleic acid nucleotides (PNAs) that, similarly to MOs, sterically block RNA translation (14, 18). However, due to their few off-target effects, low cost, and binding success, MOs have become the favored tool for studying gene knockdown in vertebrate models (14, 19). In this chapter, we describe methods for conducting MO-mediated knockdown experiments in both *Xenopus laevis* and *Xenopus tropicalis*, together with associated methods for determining their efficacy.

2. Materials

2.1. Obtaining X. laevis and X. tropicalis Embryos

1. 1-mL syringe.
2. Syringe needles (25-gauge, 5/8-in.).
3. Human chorionic gonadotropin (hCG) (Sigma, St. Louis, Missouri). 1,000 U/mL stock in dH_2O. Store at 4°C.
4. Benzocaine (ethyl ρ-amino benzoate). 10% (w/v) stock solution in ethanol. Dilute to 0.05% in distilled water (dH_2O) for use.
5. Dejellying solution: 2% (w/v) cysteine hydrochloride in water, pH adjusted to 8.0 with sodium hydroxide. Make fresh each day.
6. Kitchen shears.
7. Testis buffer: Leibovitz L-15 medium supplemented with 0.3 g/L l-glutamine (Sigma), 10% (v/v) bovine calf serum (defined, iron-supplemented, sterile-filtered; e.g., Hyclone), 50 μg/mL gentamycin sulfate. Store at 4°C.
8. 10× Marc's Modified Ringers (MMR) solution (20): 0.1 M NaCl, 2 mM KCl, 1 mM $MgSO_4$, 2 mM $CaCl_2$, 5 mM HEPES pH 7.4. Store at room temperature. Dilute stock to 1× in dH_2O for use. Store at room temperature.
9. 10× Modified Barth's Saline (MBS) pH 7.8: 880 mM NaCl, 10 mM KCl, 10 mM $MgSO_4$, 50 mM HEPES pH 7.8, 25 mM $NaHCO_3$. 1× MBS solution is made by mixing 100 mL of 10× stock solution with 700 μL 1 M $CaCl_2$ and adjusting the volume to 1 L with dH_2O. Dilute to 0.1× working solution with dH_2O for storing developing embryos. Store at room temperature.

2.2. Microinjection of Morpholinos

1. Microinjection buffer: 1× MBS, 4% (w/v) Ficoll 400 (Sigma). Store at 16°C for up to a week.
2. Sterile nuclease-free H_2O.

3. Mineral oil.
4. Glass capillaries (0.8–1.0 × 102-mm Kwik-Fil Borosilicate glass capillaries, 1B100F-4, World Precision Instruments).
5. Micropipette puller (Sutter Instrument Co., model P-87).
6. Micromanipulator (Narishige M-152 and Kanetec USA Corp. magnetic base, or Singer Instruments Mk1).
7. Microinjector (Narishige IM 300).
8. Stereo dissecting microscope (Leica MZ6).
9. Petri dishes (35-mm, 5-cm, and 10-cm).
10. Microinjection dish: 5-cm dish with nylon mesh glued to inner surface (approximate mesh diameter 0.8 mm, Small Parts, Inc.).
11. Plastic transfer pipettes.
12. Parafilm.
13. Graticule with 100-μm divisions.
14. Fine-tipped forceps.

2.3. Embryo Lysis and Western Blotting

1. Embryo lysis buffer: 50 mM Tris pH 7.6, 150 mM NaCl, 6 mM EDTA, 10% Triton X-100, protease inhibitor cocktail tablets (Roche) in distilled water. Use within 1 day if adding protease inhibitors. Store at 4°C.
2. Sonicator (Bioruptor, Diagenode.)
3. Loading buffer: 4× NuPAGE LDS Sample buffer (Invitrogen). Dilute to 1× with lysis sample and add 1 μL β-mercaptoethanol per sample.
4. Precast SDS-PAGE gel, e.g., NuPAGE 4–12% Bis-Tris Gel, 1.0 mm × 12 well (Invitrogen).
5. Xcell SureLock Mini-Cell electrophoresis system (Invitrogen).
6. Running buffer: 20× MES buffer (Invitrogen).
7. Protein molecular weight standards.
8. Nitrocellulose membrane, PVDF membrane.
9. Transfer apparatus, Mini Trans-blot Cell (BioRad).
10. Transfer buffer: 15 g Glycine, 3 g Tris-base in 1 L dH_2O. Add 200 mL 100% methanol once dissolved. Make fresh on the day and chill before use.
11. 20× TBST: 200 mM Tris–HCl pH 8, 3 M NaCl, 2% v/v Tween-20 in distilled water. Dilute in 1 L distilled water for 1× TBST working solution.
12. Blocking buffer: 5% skimmed milk powder in 1× TBST.
13. Whatman filter paper (Whatman Ltd.).
14. Appropriate primary and secondary antibodies.

15. Chemiluminescent substrate, e.g., ECL chemiluminescent visualization (Thermo Scientific).
16. Autoradiography film.

2.4. In Vitro Translation Blocking Assay

1. m^7G-capped mRNA of gene of interest.
2. Nuclease-free sterile water.
3. Dry-block heater.
4. RNasin RNase inhibitor (Promega).
5. Nuclease-treated rabbit reticulocyte lysate translation system (Promega).

2.5. Total RNA Purification and RT-PCR

1. TRIzol reagent (Invitrogen) or RNeasy mini column(s) (Qiagen).
2. DNase I, e.g., RQ1 DNase (Promega).
3. SuperScript reverse transcription system (Invitrogen).
4. RNasin RNase inhibitor (Promega).
5. Magnesium chloride solution, 25 mM in nuclease-free water, filter-sterilized.
6. Deoxynucleotide triphosphate (dNTP) mix: dATP, dCTP, dTTP, and dGTP, each at 10 μM in nuclease-free water.
7. 10× Taq polymerase buffer: 500 mM potassium chloride, 100 mM Tris hydrochloride, pH 9.0, 1% (v/v) Triton X-100, 25 mM magnesium chloride.
8. Taq polymerase.
9. Thin-walled PCR tubes.
10. DNA molecular weight standards.
11. Thermal cycler, e.g., GeneAmp PCR System 9700 (Applied Biosystems).

3. Methods

3.1. Obtaining X. laevis and X. tropicalis Embryos

The day before you intend to inject embryos, adult females must be induced to lay eggs by administration of hCG, a procedure termed "priming." This procedure is similar for both *X. laevis* and *X. tropicalis.* Once collected, eggs are fertilized *in vitro* to provide synchronously cleaving early embryos. Haste is important when fertilizing *Xenopus* embryos, therefore all materials required should be made ready beforehand.

1. For *X. laevis*, inject 500 U of hCG into a dorsal lymph sac of each adult female (see Note 1) and keep them in aquatic system water overnight (approximately 16 h) at 16°C in the dark.

2. For *X. tropicalis*, inject 20 U of hCG into a dorsal lymph sac of each adult female and male required, then keep in aquatic system water overnight (approximately 20 h) at 23–28°C (see Notes 2 and 3). Inject a second dose of 100 U of hCG the next morning.
3. The next morning, replace the water in the tanks with 1× MMR solution (3 inches depth for *X. laevis*, 2 inches depth for *X. tropicalis*) and leave the frogs at room temperature for ovulation. Remove debris or feces from tank to limit pollution of eggs. The eggs can remain in the tank until there are a sufficient number to fertilize.
4. Kill a male by immersion in 0.05% benzocaine for 30 min, followed by decapitation and pithing. Dissect out the testes into 10 mL of testis buffer. Testes may be stored at 16°C for up to a week in 10 mL testis buffer.
5. Collect eggs from the tank into a 10-cm Petri dish (approximately 300–500 *X. laevis* eggs, approximately 600–800 *X. tropicalis* eggs) and remove as much MMR as possible, allowing the eggs to form a monolayer (see Note 4).
6. Take 1/3rd *X. laevis* testis, or both *X. tropicalis* testes and macerate using forceps.
7. Carefully pass the macerated testis tissue over the eggs, ensuring that all eggs come into contact with it. Once done, allow the eggs to sit undisturbed for 3 min.
8. Flood the fertilized eggs with 0.1× MBS (approximately 30 mL) and allow to sit undisturbed for 10–15 min at room temperature. Contraction of the dark pigment at the animal pole and/or rotation of the egg within its vitelline membrane so that the animal pole is uppermost are both signs of fertilization.
9. Once fertilization has occurred, the outer jelly coat should be removed by treatment with dejellying solution. Add approximately 20–30 mL of solution to the embryos and gently agitate to mix. Do not swirl as this may lead to the formation of a duplicated anteroposterior axis in the embryos (see Note 5). Once the jelly coats have been removed, pour off the solution and wash the embryos thoroughly (approximately five times) in 0.1× MBS. *X. laevis* embryos may be incubated at 16°C, *X. tropicalis* at 23°C, prior to microinjection (see Notes 6 and 7).

3.2. Microinjection of Morpholinos

We utilize microinjection techniques to introduce MOs into the fertilized egg at the one-cell stage; however, it is also possible to use other transfection methods, e.g., Endo-porter (21) and electroporation (22).

1. Prepare several glass capillary needles using a micropipette puller at settings to give a fine gauge (Fig. 1b). We use a Sutter

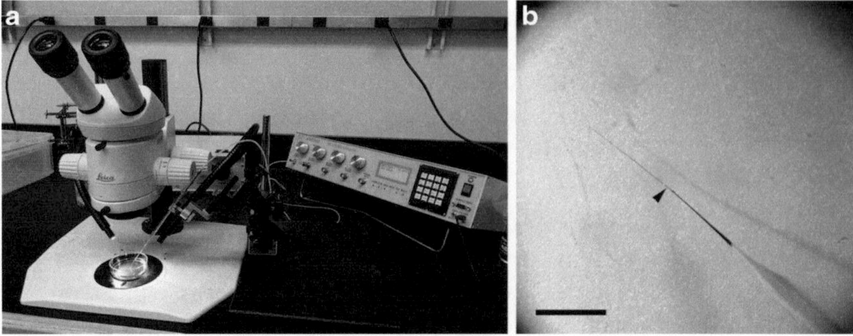

Fig. 1. Microinjection apparatus and glass capillary needle tip gauge. (**a**) Photograph of the assembled microinjection apparatus with a stereo dissecting microscope. (**b**) Image of a pulled glass capillary needle. The optimal breakage position is indicated (*arrowhead*). The needle is stained for visualization. Scale bar is 2 mm.

Instrument Co. model P-87 flaming/brown micropipette puller at the following settings: heat 781, pull 50, velocity 80, time 150, and pressure 200. The settings required may vary between instruments and between individual tungsten filaments and may need adjustment. Store needles in a safe box to limit breakage.

2. Set up instruments for microinjection beside a suitable stereo dissecting microscope. Place the needle in the holder of a three-axis micromanipulator mounted onto a magnetic base (Fig. 1a).
3. Lower the needle onto the floor of the dish gently so that its tip slightly bends. Using fine-tipped forceps, break the tip of the glass pipette at this point. Figure 1b shows a needle suitable for microinjecting *Xenopus* embryos.
4. After breaking the tip, equilibrate (or "balance") the pressure in the needle using the injector apparatus before drawing up any solution (see Note 8).
5. Fill the needle with approximately 1 μL of sterile water dispensed onto Parafilm on the microscope stage.
6. To calibrate the needle by droplet volume: Fill a 35-mm petri dish with a thin layer of mineral oil. Place the dish on top of a graticule. Lower the tip of the needle into the oil and inject a droplet of water. Measuring the diameter (d) of the droplet against the graticule allows its volume to be calculated as $4/3\pi(1/2d)^3$, assuming that the droplet is spherical. A 10-nL volume is suitable for microinjection into *Xenopus*, corresponding to a droplet with a diameter of 268 μm. Adjust the volume by either altering the injection time (typically 200–500 ms) or pressure (typically 9–12 psi). Calibration may be verified by comparing the actual and expected numbers of injections required to expel a known volume of solution from the needle.

7. Once calibrated, fill the needle with an appropriate volume of MO solution from a drop dispensed onto Parafilm.
8. Transfer embryos into the microinjection dish containing microinjection buffer. The embryos will orient themselves with their animal pole uppermost.
9. Inject into the animal hemisphere at an angle of approximately 30° from the equator of the embryo (see Note 9). Withdraw the needle gently from the embryo after each injection to minimize damage.
10. Collect injected eggs and place into a petri dish filled with microinjection solution.
11. Incubate the embryos at 16°C while they undergo early cleavage cycles, then transfer into 10 cm petri dishes containing 0.1× MBS. Culture embryos at 16–18°C until gastrulation is complete, and at 16–23°C thereafter.

3.3. Embryo Lysis and Western Blotting

The efficacy with which a MO inhibits translation of a specific mRNA in embryos can be demonstrated directly using several approaches, all of which utilize the immunoblotting (or western blotting) technique. When a suitable antibody raised against the targeted gene product is available, the levels of the endogenous protein can be assayed in embryo lysates. If an antibody is not available, mRNA encoding an epitope-tagged form of the protein may be coinjected with the MO, followed by western blotting of embryo lysates with an antibody against the epitope tag. In this case, the injected mRNA must contain the target site for MO binding. The following details the methods for preparing whole-embryo lysates of *X. laevis* and *X. tropicalis*, and for western blotting analysis of protein levels.

1. Collect 10–15 embryos per stage, per condition to be analyzed, and remove as much buffer as possible using a micropipette. At this point, embryos may be snap-frozen in a dry ice-ethanol bath and stored at –80°C for later processing.
2. Add 100 μL lysis buffer per sample. Pipette to homogenize the embryos and sonicate at 4°C for 15 min with a 30-s on/30-s off cycle to shear genomic DNA (see Note 10).
3. Centrifuge samples at 18,000 ×*g* for 5 min at 4°C to remove cellular debris. Transfer the supernatant to a clean 1.5-mL microfuge tube and either keep on ice (if it will be used immediately) or store at –80°C.
4. Prepare SDS-PAGE gels in the apparatus. Remove the protective strip and well comb. Pour 800 mL 1× MES buffer into the apparatus. Gently wash any excess storage buffer/residual acrylamide out of the wells with 1× MES buffer using a pipette.

5. 10–15 μg of embryo-equivalent protein lysate should be adequate to visualize protein depletion by western analysis. Mix the sample with 4× NuPAGE sample buffer in a new tube. Add 1 μL β-mercaptoethanol to each tube and mix. Boil sample in a water bath at 95°C for 5 min. Centrifuge briefly to collect the sample.
6. Load the samples into the wells, alongside appropriate protein molecular weight standards.
7. Run the gel at 150 V for approximately 1 h until the standard has separated appropriately.
8. While the gel is running, cut Whatman filter paper and PVDF membrane to an appropriate size, slightly larger than the gel. Prepare transfer buffer and prechill. Before the gel has finished running, pour some of the transfer buffer into a tray large enough to assemble the transfer sandwich cassette.
9. Once the gel is run, crack open the gel casting and discard. Gently place the gel in the tray with chilled transfer buffer. Excise and discard the wells and the thickened gel at the base.
10. Prewet the PVDF membrane for 10 s in 100% methanol, then store in transfer buffer. Use tweezers to handle the membrane.
11. Place the transfer cassette in the tray. The proteins will transfer from the gel onto the nitrocellulose membrane electrophoretically, hence the proteins will move from the cathode (usually marked black) to the anode (red) in the transfer apparatus. You must ensure to correctly prepare the transfer sandwich with the nitrocellulose membrane between the gel and the anode. First, lay down a sponge prewet with transfer buffer, then one piece of prewet filter paper. Roll out any bubbles with a glass rod from the center outwards. Place the gel gently on the filter paper, ensuring no bubbles are trapped. With tweezers, place the membrane onto the gel and add another prewet filter paper on top. Roll out any bubbles, and then add the last prewet sponge. Close the cassette securely and place into the transfer module, ensuring the gel-membrane sandwich is in the correct orientation with the membrane towards the anode.
12. Pour in the remaining transfer buffer and place at 4°C (see Note 11). Run at a current of 400 mA for 1 h.
13. Before the transfer is complete, prepare a washing container with 1× TBST. Prepare a sufficient amount of blocking buffer to cover the membrane.
14. Once the transfer is complete, open up the cassette and discard the filter paper. If using a prestained protein standard, the transfer of these bands to the membrane will indicate a successful transfer (see Note 12).

15. Quickly place the membrane into 1× TBST. Ensure it does not dry out. Rinse gently with 1× TBST, then replace the TBST buffer with sufficient blocking buffer to cover the membrane (approximately 10 mL for a 100 × 80 mm membrane). Incubate for 1 h at room temperature on a rocking platform.
16. Discard the blocking buffer, dilute the primary antibody in an appropriate volume of fresh blocking buffer, and add it to the membrane, ensuring it is sufficiently covered (see Note 13). Incubate for 1 h at room temperature or overnight at 4°C on a rocking platform.
17. Wash the membrane in 30 mL 1× TBST at room temperature on a rocking platform for 20 min. Repeat four times (see Note 14).
18. Prepare a 1:10,000 dilution of secondary horseradish peroxidase-conjugated antibody in an appropriate volume of blocking buffer. Discard the final 1× TBST wash. Add the blocking buffer with secondary antibody to the membrane and incubate for 20–60 min at room temperature on a rocking platform.
19. Discard antibody solution and wash the membrane as in step 17.
20. To visualize the protein, place the membrane on a dry plastic surface. With haste, pipette 500 μL of each ECL substrate component directly onto the membrane. Gently hand-rock the membrane to mix the solutions and ensure complete coverage. Wait 30 s before gently blotting the excess substrate from the membrane. Place the membrane between acetate sheet protectors or Saran-wrap and place into a light-tight developing cassette.
21. In a darkroom with safelight, carefully place a piece of autoradiography film on top of the membrane and close the cassette. An initial exposure time of 1 min will indicate whether subsequent exposures, of shorter or longer duration, are required. An example of a western blot of *X. laevis* embryos coinjected with mRNA encoding a V5-tagged protein and specific translation-blocking MOs is given in Fig. 2.

3.4. *In Vitro* Translation-Blocking Assay

The ability of a MO to bind to its target mRNA and inhibit translation can be tested *in vitro* through the use of cell-free translation systems, such as reticulocyte lysate or wheatgerm extract, providing an alternative to the *in vivo* assays described in Subheading 3.3. The method described here uses purified m7G-capped mRNA in a reticulocyte lysate translation system, but can be easily adapted to use coupled transcription-translation systems (e.g., TnT, Promega). A second MO designed to target an unrelated mRNA, or a 5-bp mismatched MO serves as negative controls to demonstrate the sequence specificity of the inhibitory effect.

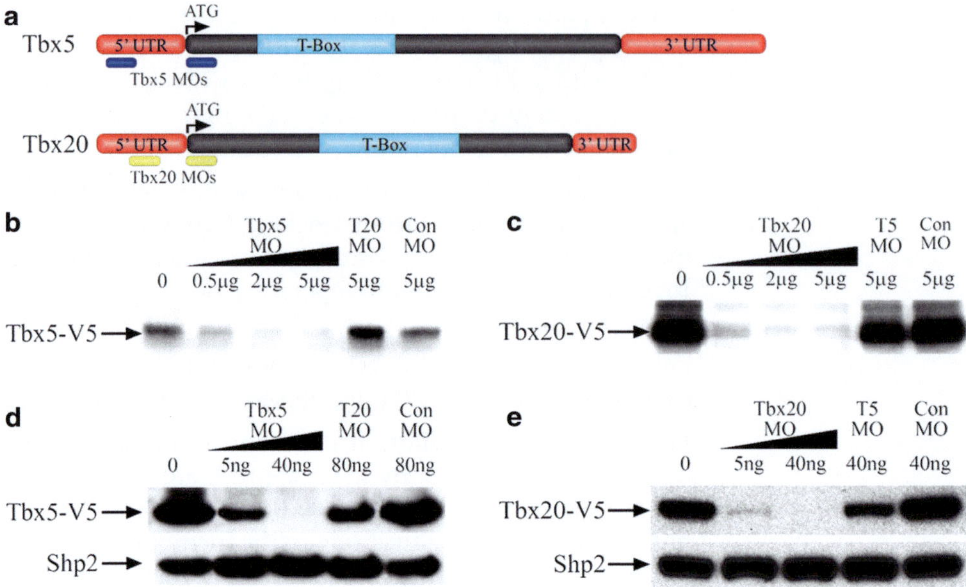

Fig. 2. An example of translation-blocking MOs targeting the 5′UTR region of *X. laevis* genes *Tbx5* and *Tbx20*. (**a**) Schematics showing the MO target locations on *Tbx5* and *Tbx20* mRNA. (**b–e**) Western blot analysis of Tbx5 and Tbx20 translation inhibition by specific MOs using V5 antibody. (**b**) Tbx5 MOs inhibit the in vitro translation of *Tbx5* RNA fused with V5 epitope in a dose-dependent manner. Both Tbx20 (T20) MO and Con MO are unable to inhibit *Tbx5-V5* translation. (**c**) Tbx20 MOs inhibit the in vitro translation of *Tbx20* RNA tagged with V5 epitope in a dose-dependent manner. Both Tbx5 (T5) MO and Con MO cannot inhibit *Tbx20-V5* translation. (**d**) Embryos were injected with 2 ng *Tbx5-V5* RNA and Tbx5 MOs. Translation of *Tbx5* was inhibited in vivo by Tbx5 MO in *X. laevis* animal caps in a dose-dependent manner as assessed by anti-V5 western blot. Tbx20 and Con MO are unable to reduce Tbx5-V5 protein expression. The membrane was reprobed with anti-Shp2 antibody as a loading control. (**e**) Translation of 2 ng *Tbx20-V5* RNA is inhibited by Tbx20 MOs in *X. laevis* animal caps in a dose-dependent manner. Tbx5 and Con MO are unable to reduce Tbx20-V5 protein expression, assayed by western blot with anti-V5 antibody. Reproduced from (24) with permission from The Company of Biologists.

1. Approximately 1.5 μg of m^{7}G-capped mRNA encoding the targeted protein (including the site for MO binding) should be denatured before assembling the translation reaction. Mix the capped mRNA with nuclease-free water to a final volume of 11 μL. Heat at 95°C in a dry-block heater for 2 min, then chill immediately in an ice-water bath. Keep on ice until adding it to the reaction.
2. Add 2 μL of MO (0.5–5 μg) to 35 μL of nuclease-treated rabbit reticulocyte lysate on ice and mix by gentle pipetting (see Note 15).
3. Add 1 μL amino acid mix (see Note 16) and 1 μL RNasin to the reaction. Mix by gentle pipetting.
4. Add the 11 μL of denatured capped mRNA prepared in step 1 and incubate at 30°C for 90 min (see Notes 16 and 17). Samples may be stored at −80°C.

5. Analyze the 5–15 μL samples of translation products by SDS-PAGE and western blotting (see Note 16) (Fig. 2), as described in Subheading 3.3, steps 4–21.

3.5. Total RNA Purification and RT-PCR

If using splice-blocking MOs, the reverse transcription polymerase chain reaction (RT-PCR) can be used to characterize mis-splicing of the transcript in vivo. The design of primers for RT-PCR will depend upon the intron-exon structure of the gene and the predicted mis-splicing products, but in general they should amplify a minimum of 150 bp of the correctly spliced transcript along with either larger fragments resulting from intron inclusion (when the splice donor site is targeted), or differently sized fragments resulting from exon skipping (when the splice acceptor is targeted). This may necessitate the use of more than one pair of primers simultaneously in a multiplex RT-PCR reaction and may also require primers to be designed against introns as well as exons. These primers should be tested against cDNA or genomic DNA templates to ensure that they effectively amplify their predicted targets. It should be noted that standard RT-PCR can only provide a semiquantitative assay of the relative abundance of different splice forms of a transcript. Quantitative RT-PCR (qPCR) techniques may provide a more accurate measure, if required. The products of RT-PCR reactions may be cloned, sequenced, and aligned with a reference sequence from the targeted gene to confirm their origin.

1. Collect ten embryos at an appropriate stage (based on the temporal expression profile of the targeted gene) per condition for RT-PCR analysis.
2. Isolate total RNA using either TRIzol reagent or RNeasy mini columns, following the manufacturer's protocol for RNA purification from animal cells.
3. Following RNA isolation, treat samples with DNase to remove all genomic DNA. Add 2 U of DNase (e.g., RQ1 DNase, Promega) to each sample, mix, centrifuge briefly, and incubate at 37°C for 1 h. To heat-inactivate the enzyme, incubate at 65°C for 10 min. Place samples on ice. Subsequent RNA-clean up may be required using RNeasy spin columns following manufacturer's protocol.
4. Dilute RNA samples to 250 ng/μL final concentration with sterile, nuclease-free water.
5. To synthesize first-strand cDNA with SuperScript reverse transcriptase: Mix 1 μL of 250 ng/μL random primers, 2 μL 250 ng/μL total RNA, 1 μL 10 mM dNTP mix, 8 μL sterile, nuclease-free water. Incubate at 65°C for 5 min. Chill in ice water and centrifuge briefly (<20 s) before adding 4 μL first-strand buffer, 2 μL 0.1 M DTT and 1 μL RNase inhibitor. Incubate at 42°C for 2 min before adding 1 μL of reverse transcriptase (see

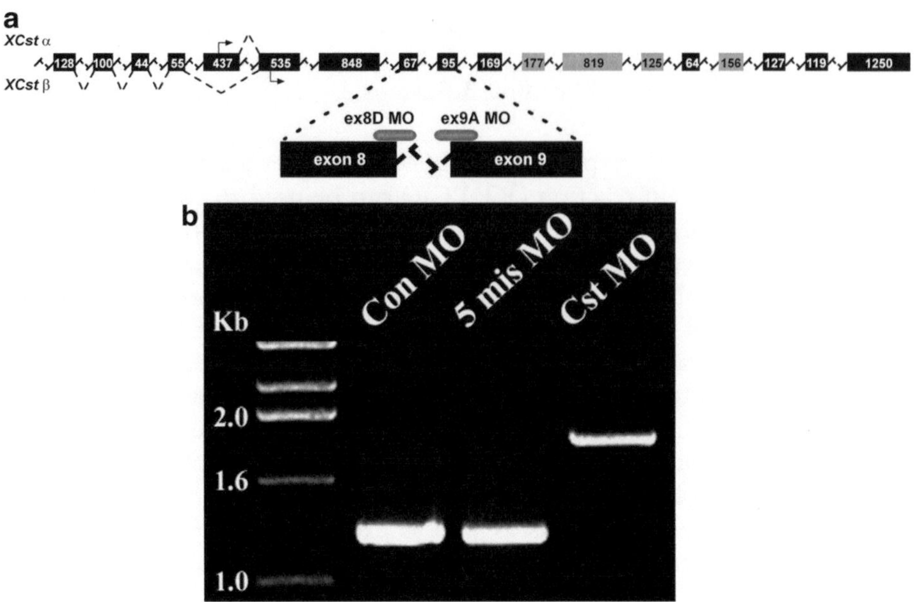

Fig. 3. An example of a splice-blocking MO targeting the *X. laevis* gene *Castor* (*Cst*). (**a**) The position of the *Cst* splice junction morpholinos relative to the pre-mRNA transcript. These MOs target the splice donor site on exon 8 (ex8D MO) and the splice acceptor site on exon 9 (ex9A MO). (**b**) RT-PCR analysis of stage 42 *X. laevis* tadpoles injected at the one-cell stage with both the ex8D and ex9A MOs, demonstrating the inhibition of proper splicing of Cst pre-mRNA and the inclusion of a 679-bp intron, as indicated by the larger amplified product compared to control (Con) MO and 5-mismatch (5-mis) MO. Abrogation of splicing in this context introduced a stop codon after the second amino acid following exon 8. Reprinted from Christine and Conlon (23), Copyright (2008), with permission from Elsevier.

Note 18). Incubate for 50 min at 42°C, then for 15 min at 70°C. Add 1 μL of RNase H and incubate at 37°C for 20 min. Store the reaction at –20°C until ready to carry out PCR.

6. To perform PCR: Select thin-walled PCR tubes of an appropriate size for the thermal cycler to be used and assemble the reactions on ice. Mix 0.5 μL of first-strand cDNA reaction, 5 μL of 10× Taq polymerase buffer, 5 μL 25 mM $MgCl_2$, 1 μL 10 mM dNTP mix, 25 picomoles of each sequence-specific primer, sufficient nuclease-free water to bring the final volume to 49 μL, and 1 μL Taq polymerase. Cycle as appropriate for synthesis.

7. Analyze the reaction products by electrophoresis on a 1% (w/v) agarose gel, alongside suitable molecular weight standards. An example of how RT-PCR can be used to determine the efficacy of splice-blocking MOs is given in Fig. 3.

4. Notes

1. Chorionic gonadotropin is considered biohazardous so caution must be used, gloves must be worn at all times when handling the hormone, and needles must be disposed of in the correct manner.
2. Mild anesthesia can help to subdue very active *X. tropicalis* for injection, reducing the risk of injury. Immerse frogs for 25 min in a 0.025% (w/v) solution of ethyl 3-aminobenzoate methanesulfonate salt in water. Monitor anesthesia carefully and remove frogs from the anesthetic solution once they become sufficiently inactive for safe handling and injection.
3. Exposing *X. tropicalis* to temperatures below 23°C can be lethal to them.
4. Check egg quality under a microscope to assess for dead or dying eggs (larger and white), color density on animal pole (should be solid and not speckly, with a noticeable defined border between the two poles), and shape abnormalities (eggs should be roughly spherical).
5. Watch closely to see the jelly coats dissolve from the embryos. This should take approximately 3–5 min at room temperature. Embryos will appear to cluster more tightly without the jelly coats. Do not leave embryos in dejellying solution for too long as this may damage them and can also affect the firmness of the embryo, making microinjection more difficult.
6. Eggs that did not successfully fertilize will normally stick to the plate and have a slightly flattened appearance. Fertilized eggs will generally be free-floating and spherical.
7. The time window between dejellying and the first embryonic cleavage is typically 30–40 min for *X. laevis*, 25–30 min for *X. tropicalis* (depending upon temperature). Subsequent cleavages occur at approximately 30 and 20 min intervals for *X. laevis* and *X. tropicalis,* respectively. This should be taken into account when planning microinjections.
8. Each time the needle is replaced or rebroken, it must be rebalanced to ensure that there is no net positive or negative pressure on the injection solution in the needle. Positive pressure causes the injection solution to leak from the tip of the needle, while negative pressure causes the needle to take up buffer from the injection dish resulting in a decreased concentration of MO in the injection solution.
9. Generally it is not advised to inject >80 ng of MO per embryo. We test our MOs by initially injecting a range of concentrations, e.g., 20, 40, and 80 ng per *X. laevis* embryo in a 10-nL volume,

and assessing the efficacy of the MO by the methods described. MOs are aliquoted and stored at −20°C. Before injection allow the aliquot to reach room temperature to resolubilize the oligonucleotide. Other sources state storing MOs at room temperature is adequate. Should the MO come out of solution, it is suggested to heat the aliquot to 65°C for 5 min and allow to cool to room temperature. Centrifuge the aliquot for 30 s at 18,000 × *g* prior to injection (http://www.gene-tools.com/node/25).

10. Unsheared genomic DNA in the samples will lead to significant difficulties when loading the polyacrylamide gel.
11. Alternatively, the apparatus may be set in a tray of ice with an ice pack placed in the module for transferring at room temperature.
12. When unstained standards are used, other staining procedures can be performed on the membrane to determine transfer success, such as Coomassie and Ponceau staining.
13. An antibody against a standard protein can serve as an internal loading control. This incubation can be performed simultaneously with the target antibody if the sizes of the corresponding proteins are known to be sufficiently different, otherwise it may be necessary to either run two separate gels to transfer and blot separately, or to strip the blot and reprobe with the second primary antibody after ECL visualization. To strip the blot, there are two methods; low and high stringency incubations. First, wash the membrane in water for 5 min. For low stringency stripping, incubate the membrane in 0.2 M NaOH for 20 min at room temperature; for high stringency prepare a 62.5 mM Tris pH6.8 buffer with 2% w/v SDS. Before use, add β-mercaptoethanol to a final concentration of 100 mM. Incubate the membrane in this buffer for 30 min at 55–65°C. After incubation, wash the membrane in water for 5 min, followed by three washes in 1× TBST, before proceeding with the western procedure (blocking and primary antibody incubation).
14. The primary antibody-blocking solution can be reused at least once. Store at 4°C for subsequent uses.
15. The MO should be added to the translation reaction before adding the capped mRNA to ensure maximal inhibition of translation.
16. If a suitable antibody is not available for western blotting, the translation products can be radiolabeled by incorporation of ^{35}S methionine (in presence of amino acid mix lacking methionine) and analyzed by SDS-PAGE and autoradiography.
17. If radiolabeling will be used, reduce the volume of the capped mRNA in step 1 to compensate for ^{35}S methionine added in step 3, maintaining a final reaction volume of 50 μL.

18. Include a "minus RT" reaction in which the reverse transcriptase is omitted. This provides a control to demonstrate that PCR products are derived from reverse-transcribed RNA, not from sources of contamination such as genomic DNA carried over from the RNA purification procedure.

References

1. Movassagh, M., and Philpott, A. (2008) Cardiac differentiation in Xenopus requires the cyclin-dependent kinase inhibitor, p27Xic1, *Cardiovasc Res 79*, 436–447.
2. Nagao, K., Taniyama, Y., Kietzmann, T., Doi, T., Komuro, I., and Morishita, R. (2008) HIF-1alpha signaling upstream of NKX2.5 is required for cardiac development in Xenopus, *J Biol Chem 283*, 11841–11849.
3. Kumano, G., Ezal, C., and Smith, W. C. (2006) ADMP2 is essential for primitive blood and heart development in Xenopus, *Dev Biol 299*, 411–423.
4. Inui, M., Fukui, A., Ito, Y., and Asashima, M. (2006) Xapelin and Xmsr are required for cardiovascular development in Xenopus laevis, *Dev Biol 298*, 188–200.
5. Zhang, C., Basta, T., and Klymkowsky, M. W. (2005) SOX7 and SOX18 are essential for cardiogenesis in Xenopus, *Dev Dyn 234*, 878–891.
6. Garriock, R. J., D'Agostino, S. L., Pilcher, K. C., and Krieg, P. A. (2005) Wnt11-R, a protein closely related to mammalian Wnt11, is required for heart morphogenesis in Xenopus, *Dev Biol 279*, 179–192.
7. Small, E. M., Warkman, A. S., Wang, D. Z., Sutherland, L. B., Olson, E. N., and Krieg, P. A. (2005) Myocardin is sufficient and necessary for cardiac gene expression in Xenopus, *Development 132*, 987–997.
8. Hilton, E. N., Manson, F. D., Urquhart, J. E., Johnston, J. J., Slavotinek, A. M., Hedera, P., Stattin, E. L., Nordgren, A., Biesecker, L. G., and Black, G. C. (2007) Left-sided embryonic expression of the BCL-6 corepressor, BCOR, is required for vertebrate laterality determination, *Hum Mol Genet 16*, 1773–1782.
9. Bartlett, H. L., and Weeks, D. L. (2008) Lessons from the lily pad: Using Xenopus to understand heart disease, *Drug Discov Today Dis Models 5*, 141–146.
10. Draper, B. W., Morcos, P. A., and Kimmel, C. B. (2001) Inhibition of zebrafish fgf8 pre-mRNA splicing with morpholino oligos: a quantifiable method for gene knockdown, *Genesis 30*, 154–156.
11. Heasman, J., Kofron, M., and Wylie, C. (2000) Beta-catenin signaling activity dissected in the early Xenopus embryo: a novel antisense approach, *Dev Biol 222*, 124–134.
12. Nutt, S. L., Bronchain, O. J., Hartley, K. O., and Amaya, E. (2001) Comparison of morpholino based translational inhibition during the development of Xenopus laevis and Xenopus tropicalis, *Genesis 30*, 110–113.
13. Moulton, J. D. (2007) Using morpholinos to control gene expression, *Curr Protoc Nucleic Acid Chem Chapter 4*, Unit 4 30.
14. Summerton, J. E. (2007) Morpholino, siRNA, and S-DNA compared: impact of structure and mechanism of action on off-target effects and sequence specificity, *Curr Top Med Chem 7*, 651–660.
15. Bill, B. R., Petzold, A. M., Clark, K. J., Schimmenti, L. A., and Ekker, S. C. (2009) A primer for morpholino use in zebrafish, *Zebrafish 6*, 69–77.
16. Eisen, J. S., and Smith, J. C. (2008) Controlling morpholino experiments: don't stop making antisense, *Development 135*, 1735–1743.
17. Morcos, P. A. (2007) Achieving targeted and quantifiable alteration of mRNA splicing with Morpholino oligos, *Biochem Biophys Res Commun 358*, 521–527.
18. Dagle, J. M., and Weeks, D. L. (2001) Oligonucleotide-based strategies to reduce gene expression, *Differentiation 69*, 75-82.
19. Knudsen, H., and Nielsen, P. E. (1996) Antisense properties of duplex- and triplex-forming PNAs, *Nucleic Acids Res 24*, 494–500.
20. Ubbels, G. A., Hara, K., Koster, C. H., and Kirschner, M. W. (1983) Evidence for a functional role of the cytoskeleton in determination of the dorsoventral axis in Xenopus laevis eggs, *J Embryol Exp Morphol 77*, 15–37.

21. Summerton, J. E. (2005) Endo-Porter: a novel reagent for safe, effective delivery of substances into cells, *Ann N Y Acad Sci 1058*, 62–75.
22. Falk, J., Drinjakovic, J., Leung, K. M., Dwivedy, A., Regan, A. G., Piper, M., and Holt, C. E. (2007) Electroporation of cDNA/Morpholinos to targeted areas of embryonic CNS in Xenopus, *BMC Dev Biol 7*, 107.
23. Christine, K. S., and Conlon, F. L. (2008) Vertebrate CASTOR is required for differentiation of cardiac precursor cells at the ventral midline, *Dev Cell 14*, 616–623.
24. Brown, D. D., Martz, S. N., Binder, O., Goetz, S. C., Price, B. M., Smith, J. C., and Conlon, F. L. (2005) Tbx5 and Tbx20 act synergistically to control vertebrate heart morphogenesis, *Development 132*, 553–563.

Chapter 5

Chicken Chorioallantoic Membrane Angiogenesis Model

Domenico Ribatti

Abstract

The chick embryo chorioallantoic membrane (CAM) is an extraembryonic membrane which serves as a gas exchange surface and its function is supported by a dense capillary network. Because of its extensive vascularization and easy accessibility, the CAM has been broadly used to study the morphofunctional aspects of the angiogenesis process in vivo and to investigate the efficacy and mechanisms of action of proangiogenic and antiangiogenic natural and synthetic molecules. The CAM has long been a favored system for the study of tumor angiogenesis and metastasis, because at this stage the chick immunocompetence system is not fully developed and the conditions for rejection have not been established. The CAM may also be used to verify the ability to inhibit the growth of capillaries by implanting tumors onto the CAM and by comparing tumor growth and vascularization with or without the administration of an antiangiogenic molecule. Other studies using the tumor cells/CAM model have focused on the invasion of the chorionic epithelium and the blood vessels by tumor cells. The cells invade the epithelium and the mesenchymal connective tissue below, where they are found in the form of a dense bed of blood vessels, which is a target for intravasation.

Key words: Angiogenesis, Antiangiogenesis, Chorioallantoic membrane

1. Introduction

The chick embryo chorioallantoic membrane (CAM) is an extraembryonic membrane which serves as a gas exchange surface and its function is supported by a dense capillary network (1, 2). Because of its extensive vascularization and easy accessibility, the CAM has been broadly used to study the morphofunctional aspects of the angiogenesis process in vivo and to investigate the efficacy and mechanisms of action of proangiogenic and antiangiogenic natural and synthetic molecules (1, 2). Also, because of the lack of a fully developed immunocompetence system in the chick embryo, the CAM represents a host tissue for tumor engrafting suitable to study

Xu Peng and Marc Antonyak (eds.), *Cardiovascular Development: Methods and Protocols*,
Methods in Molecular Biology, vol. 843, DOI 10.1007/978-1-61779-523-7_5,

various aspects of the angiogenic and metastatic potential that characterizes human malignancies (3).

The allantois of the chick embryo appears at about 3.5 days of incubation as an evagination from the ventral wall of the endodermal hind gut. During the fourth day, it pushes out of the body of the embryo into the extraembryonic coelom. Its proximal portion lies parallel and just caudal to the yolk sac. When the distal portion grows clear of the embryo, it becomes enlarged. The narrow proximal portion is known as the allantoic stalk, the enlarged distal portion as the allantoic vesicle. Fluid accumulation distends the allantois so that its terminal portion resembles a ballon in entire embryos.

The allantoic vesicle enlarges very rapidly from days 4 to 10: an extensive morphometric investigation has shown rapid extension of the CAM surface from 6 cm^2 at day 6 to 65 cm^2 at day 14. In this process, the mesodermal layer of the allantois fuses with the adjacent mesodermal layer of the chorion to form the CAM. An extremely rich vascular network connected to embryonic circulation by the allantoic arteries and veins develops between the two layers. Immature blood vessels scattered in the mesoderm and lacking a complete basal lamina and smooth muscle cells grow very rapidly until day 8, giving rise to a capillary plexus. The plexus associates with the overlaying chorionic epithelium and mediates gas exchange with the outer environment. Capillary proliferation continues rapidly until day 10; then, the endothelial cell mitotic index declines rapidly and the vascular system attains its final arrangement on day 18, just before hatching (4). Besides sprouting angiogenesis that characterizes the early phases of CAM development, late CAM vascularization is supported by intussusceptive microvascular growth in which capillary network increases its complexity and vascular surface by insertion of transcapillary pillars. At day 14, the capillary plexus is located at the surface of the ectoderm adjacent to the shell membrane. This circulation and the position of the allantois immediately adjacent to the porous shell confer a respiratory function on the highly vascularized CAM. In addition to the respiratory interchange of oxygen and carbon dioxide, the allantois also serves as reservoir for the waste products excreted by the embryo—mostly urea at first, and chiefly uric acid later.

The CAM is used to study molecules with angiogenic and antiangiogenic activity following their delivery in ovo (5). Many protocols have been envisaged to deliver macromolecules and low molecular weight compounds onto the CAM by using silostatic rings, methylcellulose discs, silicon rings, filters, and plastic rings. Also, collagen and gelatin sponges treated with stimulators or inhibitors of blood vessel formation have been implanted on growing CAM. The gelatin sponge is also suitable for the delivery of cell suspensions onto the CAM surface and the evaluation of their angiogenic potential. This latter experimental condition allows the slow, continuous delivery of growth factors released by few implanted cells. As compared with the application on the CAM of large amounts of a pure recombinant angiogenic cytokine in a single bolus, implants of cells overexpressing angiogenic cytokines enable the continuous delivery of growth factors, following a more "physiological" mode of interaction with the CAM vasculature.

Besides in ovo experimentation, a number of shell-less culture techniques have been devised, involving cultures of avian embryos with associated yolk and albumin outside of the eggshell. Shell-less cultures facilitate experimental access and continuous observation of the growing embryo. Nevertheless, shell-less culture techniques are expensive, occupy large amounts of space, and long-term viability is low.

Typically, an angiogenic response occurs 72–96 h after stimulation in the form of increased vessel density around the implant, with the vessels radially converging toward the center-like spokes in a wheel. Conversely, when an angiostatic compound is tested, the vessels become less dense around the implant and eventually disappear. Alternatively, the molecules can be directly inoculated into the cavity of the allantoic vesicle so that their activity reaches the whole vascular area in an uniform manner.

Several semiquantitative and quantitative methods are used to evaluate the extent of vasoproliferative response or angiostatic activity at macroscopic and microscopic levels. Quantification of the CAM vasculature has been performed with the use of morphometric point-count methods, radiolabeled proline incorporation to measure collagenous protein synthesis, and fractal analysis of digital images.

Many techniques can be applied within the constraints of paraffin and plastic embedding, including histochemistry and immunohistochemistry. Electron microscopy can also be used in combination with light microscopy. Moreover, unfixed CAM can be utilized for biochemical studies, such as the determination of DNA, protein and collagen content, and for reversal-transcriptase polymerase chain reaction (RT-PCR) analysis of gene expression. Recently, the study of intracellular signaling pathways mediating the angiogenic response to growth factors and cytokines has been successfully performed.

The main advantages of the CAM in vivo assay are its low cost, simplicity, reproducibility, and reliability, which are important determinants for the choice of a method (Table 1). Nevertheless, some limitations characterize this experimental model (Table 1). The major disadvantage is that the CAM already contains a well-developed vascular network and the vasodilatation that follows its manipulation may be hard to distinguish from the effects of the test substance. Moreover, real neovascularization can hardly be distinguished from a falsely vascular density due to the rearrangement of existing vessels that follows contraction of the membrane (6).

Table 1
Advantages and disadvantages of chorioallantoic membrane assay

Advantages
High embryo survival rate
Easy methodology
Sterility is not required
Low cost
Reproducibility
Reliability
Disadvantages
Difficult monitoring
Nonspecific inflammatory reactions
Preexisting vessels

Another limitation is nonspecific inflammatory reactions that may develop as a result of grafting, inducing a secondary vasoproliferative response that cannot be distinguished from direct angiogenic activity of the test material without detailed histological study (7).

It should be emphasized that species-specific differences and the lack of avian-specific reagents (as well as limited genomic information) may represent serious disadvantages. However, in the last few years, retroviral, lentiviral, and adenoviral vectors have been used to infect the CAM (as well as the whole chick embryo), leading to the expression of the viral transgene. This allows the long-lasting presence of the gene product that is expressed directly by CAM cells. This makes feasible the study of the effects of intracellular or membrane-bound proteins as well as of dominant-negative gene products. This approach, together with different developmental models (including Zebrafish and mouse embryos), will shed new lights on the mechanisms of blood vessel formation and inhibition in physiologic and pathologic conditions.

The variety of in vivo bioassays of angiogenesis has enabled investigators to make rapid progress in elucidating the mechanism of action of a variety of angiogenic factors and inhibitors. Cost, simplicity, reproducibility, and reliability are important determinants dictating the choice of methods. Each of the assays has its own advantages and disadvantages, and each one has an application for which it is best suited (Table 2). In choosing a particular assay, the investigator should consider the suitability of different model systems to answer specific questions. Ideally, two different assays should be performed in parallel to confirm the angiogenic or antiangiogenic activities of test substances.

Table 2
Advantages and disadvantages of the other in vivo angiogenesis assays

Corneal micropocket Advantages: new vessels are easily identified; immunologically privileged site; permits noninvasive and long-term monitoring Disadvantages: atypical angiogenesis, as the normal cornea is avascular; technically demanding; traumatic technique; exposure to oxygen via surface can affect angiogenesis; nonspecific inflammatory response with some compounds
Sponge/matrix implant Advantages: technically simple; inexpensive; well tolerated; suitable for study of tumor angiogenesis Disadvantages: encapsulated by granulation tissue; time-consuming; variable retention of test compound within implant; nonspecific inflammatory response
Disc angiogenesis assay (DAS) Advantages: technically simple; assesses wound healing and angiogenesis; quantitative analysis. Disadvantages: encapsulated by granulation tissue
Matrigel plug Advantages: technically simple; suitable for large-scale screening; rapid quantitative analysis Disadvantages: matrigel is not chemically defined; analysis in plugs is time-consuming; expensive
Dorsal skin chamber Advantages: permits long-term monitoring; simple procedure Disadvantages: nonspecific inflammatory response
Rabbit ear chamber Advantages: clearest optical preparation for intravital microscopy; permits long-term monitoring Disadvantages: technically demanding procedure; nonspecific inflammatory response; expensive
Zebrafish Advantages: intact whole animal; allows gene analysis of vessel development; large number of animals available for statistical analysis Disadvantages: nonmammalian; embryonic

2. Materials

2.1. Reagents

1. White chicken egg obtained at day 1–2 postlaying (see Note 1).
2. 70% (vol/vol) ethanol in dH_2O.
3. Sterile routine tissue culture medium (MEM Amino Acid Solution, Sigma).
4. Sterilized gelatin sponges (Gelfoam, Upjohn).
5. Angiogenic molecule (dissolved in 1–3 μL of sterile routine tissue culture medium at doses ranging between 10 and 500 ng

per implant) or tumor cell suspension (from 1×10^4 to 6×10^6 cells per sponge resuspended in 3–4 μL of sterile routine tissue culture medium).

6. Bouin's fluid solution.
7. Standard ethanol solutions for paraffin embedding.
8. Toluene.
9. Embedding paraffin (Tissue-Tek VIP, electron Microscopy Sciences).
10. Toluidine blue 0 (Sigma. use a 0.5% (vol/vol) aqueous solution).

2.2. Equipment

1. Egg incubator (Kemps Koops), 37°C and 60% humidity.
2. 25- or 26-G hypodermic needles and 1-mL syringes.
3. Curved-tip forceps.
4. Small dissecting scissors.
5. Transparent tape or glass coverslip, approximately 10×10 mm.
6. Microtome.
7. Stereomicroscope.
8. Double-headed light microscope (BX51, Olympus, Italia), including a square mesh insert consisting of 12 lines per side for each eyepiece.

3. Methods

3.1. CAM Samples Preparation

1. Sterilize all instruments in 70% ethanol before use.
2. Clean the fertilized white chicken eggs with 70% ethanol and incubated at 37°C and 60% humidity in an egg incubator for 48 h (see Note 2).
3. Aspirate 2–3 mL albumen from the egg using a 25- or 26-G hypodermic needle and 1-mL syringe at the acute pole of the egg on day 3 of incubation (Fig. 1) (see Note 3).
4. After albumen removal, cut a square window into the shell with the aid of small dissecting scissors (Fig. 1) (see Note 4).
5. On day 8 of incubation, open the window under sterile conditions with a laminar-flow hood and implant a 1-mm^3 sterilized gelatin sponge onto the CAM (see Note 5).
6. Pipe the angiogenic molecule onto the sponge. Use a sponge containing vehicle alone as the negative control. Similarly, the gelatin sponge is suitable for the delivery of tumor cell suspensions onto the CAM surface and for the evaluation of their angiogenic potential. The sample may be a mixture of an

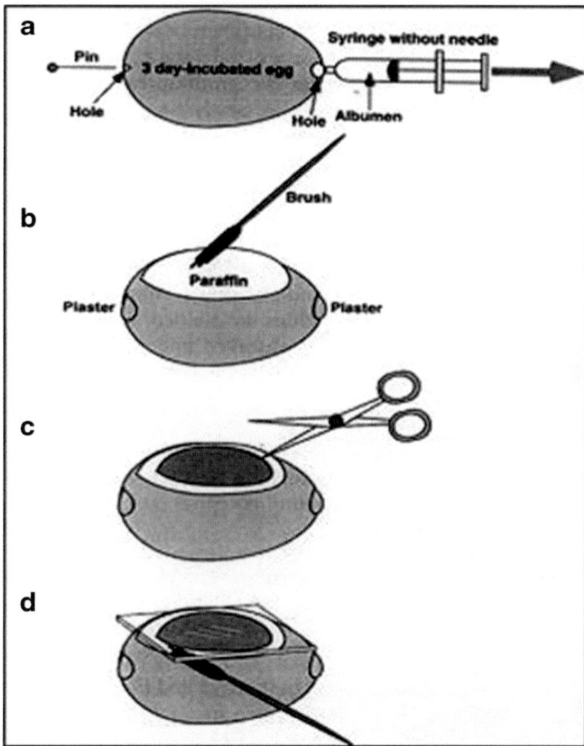

Fig. 1. Preparation of the egg for the CAM assay. On day 3 of incubation, 2–3 mL of albumen are aspirated at the acute pole of the egg (**a**) to detach the developing CAM from the shell; the holes are closed with plaster. The upper surface of the eggs is brushed on with paraffin (**b**) and cut with scissor kept parallel to the surface so as not to damage the embryo (**c**). The window is covered with a glass slide and sealed with paraffin (**d**).

angiogenic molecule and potential antiangiogenic compounds (see Note 6).

7. On day 12, fix the embryos and their membranes in ovo by pipetting 10 μL of Bouin's fluid solution onto the CAM surface and allowing the embryos to fix for 3 h at room temperature.
8. Cut the sponges and the underlying and immediately adjacent CAM portions with curved-tip forceps and transfer each specimen to a culture tube.
9. Dehydrate tissue samples in an ethanol series, clear them in toluene, and immerse them in embedding paraffin for 2 h, according to manufacturer's instructions.
10. Using a microtome, cut 8-μm serial sections from each sample of paraffin-embedded CAMs in parallel to the surface of the membrane and stain the sections with a 0.5% aqueous solution of toluidine blue for 1 min at room temperature.

3.2. Macroscopic Evaluation of the Vasoproliferative Response

On incubation day 12, macroscopic observation shows that the gelatin sponge treated with an angiogenesis stimulator is surrounded by allantoic vessels that develop radially towards the implant in a "spoked-wheel" pattern (see Note 7).

1. Analyzing the convergence of blood vessels toward the graft. For each egg, count the total number of microscopic vessels that converge toward the graft under the stereomicroscope at 10× magnification at different time points after implantation from day 8 to day 12. Express the data for each experimental group as the mean ±1 s.d. and obtain kinetics curves for proangiogenic or antiangiogenic stimuli compared with controls.
2. Analyzing variations in the distribution and density of CAM vessels next to the site of grafting. The intensity of the angiogenic response is scored under a stereomicroscope at regular intervals following the grafting procedure from day 8 to day 12 by means of a 0–5 scale of arbitrary values: 0 describes a condition of the vascular network that is unchanged with respect to the time of grafting; 1 marks a slight increment in vessel density associated to occasional changes in the course of vessels converging towards the grafting site; 2, 3, 4, and 5 correspond to a gradual increase in vessel density associated with increased irregularity in their course; a 5 rating also highlights strong hyperemia. A coefficient describing the degree of angiogenesis can also be derived from the ratio of the calculated value to the highest attainable value; thus, the coefficient's lowest value is equal to 0 and the highest value is 1.
3. Analyzing blood-vessel branching. A vascular index based on blood vessel branching may represent an alternative semiquantitative method to assess the vasoproliferative response. According to this procedure, all the vessels converging toward the implant and contained inside a 1-mm diameter ring superposed to the CAM are enumerated: the ring is drawn around the implant in such a way that it will form an angle of less than 45° with a straight line drawn starting from the implant's center. Vessels branching dichotomically outside the ring are scored as 2, while those branching inside the ring are scored as 1.

3.3. Microscopic Evaluation of the Angiogenic Response

Quantitative evaluation of the angiogenic response, expressed as microvessel density, can be obtained by applying a morphometric method of "point counting" on histological CAM sections. Briefly, two investigators simultaneously identify transversally cut microvessels (diameter ranging from 3 to 10 μm) among the gelatin sponge trabeculae with a double-headed photomicroscope at ×250 magnification. A square mesh consisting of 12 lines per side, giving 144 intersection points, is inserted in the eyepiece. Ten sections are analyzed for each CAM specimen by observing every third section within 30 serial slides. For each section, six randomly chosen microscopic fields are evaluated for the number of intersection points occupied by microvessels. Then, mean values ± 1 standard deviation are determined for each CAM specimen. The microvessel density is expressed as percentage of intersection points occupied by microvessels. Statistically significant differences between the mean values of the intersection points in the experimental CAMs and control ones are determined by Student's *t* test for unpaired data.

At microscopic level, a highly vascularized tissue is recognizable among the trabeculae of the sponges treated with the angiogenesis stimulator. The tissue consists of newly formed blood vessels growing perpendicularly to the plane of the CAM, mainly capillaries with a diameter ranging from 3 to 10 μm within an abundant network of collagen fibers. In contrast, no blood vessels are present among trabeculae of the implants treated with vehicle alone. Otherwise, in the specimens treated with an angiogenesis inhibitor or with vehicle alone, few blood vessels are detectable around the sponge. Also, angiogenesis inhibitor causes the progressive regression of blood vessels distributed at the boundary between sponge and CAM mesenchyme, while they are still detectable in embryos treated with vehicle alone.

4. Notes

1. Chicken embryos from different vendors can vary significantly in their degree of vascularization and developmental status. Thus, consistent use of the same vender can decrease experimental variability.
2. Cleaning the egg shell before incubation remove any debris associated with the outer surface and decrease the risk of infection. The embryo is immunodeficient until just before hatching. The eggs are very susceptible to mixed bacterial infections from feces-derived shell organisms, including *Aspergillus fumigatus*, *Staphylococcus aureus*, and *Pseudomonas aeruginosa*. Furthermore, specific incubation conditions, including constant temperature and humidity, are of critical importance for proper vascularization and embryo survival. It is important to remove only the number of eggs from the incubator that correspond to the investigator's speed, since it is critical that embryos are not left outside the incubator for an extended period of time.
3. This procedure creates a false air sac directly over the CAM, allowing its dissociation from the egg shell membrane. Make sure the needle opening is pointing away from the embryo during albumen aspiration. In addition, regular changes of needle and syringe limit the carryover of infection from egg to egg.

4. This window can be enlarged to approximately 10 × 10 mm. The underlying embryo and CAM vessels are revealed. Seal the window with transparent tape or a glass coverslip of the same dimension, and return the egg to the incubator. This step should be done in an enclosed area such as a laminar-flow hood to minimize the risk of infection. If large pieces of shell fall onto the CAM, it may be possible to remove these using fine forceps. It is probably best to discard eggs where pieces of shell have fallen onto the CAM and have not been removed very easily, as these eggs may develop false positive response due to inflammation.
5. For this purpose, the sponge is cut by hand with a blade and gently placed on top of the growing CAM. Use sterile gloves to minimize the risk of infection. Reject eggs with an excessively humid CAM; otherwise, sponges may float off during the incubation period. The CAM is an expanding membrane with vessels developing over its entire surface. It is preferable to place the sponges between two large vessels and not place outer edges of the CAM.
6. Although most substances are soluble in water, small organic molecules, such as synthetic angiogenesis inhibitors, may require organic solvents. Ethanol, but not DMSO, can be used without adverse effects by soaking the gelatin sponge in the dissolved compound of interest and allowing the solvent to evaporate before implantation onto the CAM.
7. Two operators, preferably blinded to the sample identity, should grade the angiogenic/antiangiogenic response. Different test substances can produce a range of different types of angiogenic response, such as a mixed response of microvascular growth and large vessel deformation/growth towards the point of application. Samples may also induce local bleeding and the presence and severity of these reactions should be noted, as the response may be secondary to the bleeding or inflammation.

Acknowledgments

Supported in part by MIUR (PRIN 2007), Rome, and Fondazione Cassa di Risparmio di Puglia, Bari, Italy.

References

1. Ribatti, D. (2008) Chick embryo chorioallantoic membrane as a useful tool to study angiogenesis, *Int Rev Cell Mol Biol 270*, 181–224.
2. Cimpean, A. M., Ribatti, D., and Raica, M. (2008) The chick embryo chorioallantoic membrane as a model to study tumor metastasis, *Angiogenesis 11*, 311–319.
3. Deryugina, E. I., and Quigley, J. P. (2008) Chick embryo chorioallantoic membrane model systems to study and visualize human tumor cell metastasis, *Histochem Cell Biol 130*, 1119–1130.
4. Ausprunk, D. H., Knighton, D. R., and Folkman, J. (1974) Differentiation of vascular endothelium in the chick chorioallantois: a structural and autoradiographic study, *Dev Biol 38*, 237–248.
5. Ribatti, D. (2010) Different Morphological Techniques and Methods of Quantifying the Angiogenic Response Used in the Study of Vascularization in the Chorioallantoic Membrane, in *The chick embryo chorioallantoic membrane in the study of angiogenesis and metastasis.* (Ribatti, D., Ed) pp 71-74 Springer, New York.
6. Knighton, D. R., Fiegel, V. D., and Phillips, G. D. (1991) The assay of angiogenesis, *Prog Clin Biol Res 365*, 291–299.
7. Jakob, W., Jentzsch, K. D., Mauersberger, B., and Heder, G. (1978) The chick embryo choriallantoic membrane as a bioassay for angiogenesis factors: reactions induced by carrier materials, *Exp Pathol (Jena) 15*, 241–249.

Chapter 6

Visualizing Vascular Networks in Zebrafish: An Introduction to Microangiography

Christopher E. Schmitt, Melinda B. Holland, and Suk-Won Jin

Abstract

Visualizing the circulatory pattern in developing embryos becomes an essential technique for the field of cardiovascular biology. In the zebrafish model system, there are currently several techniques available to visualize the circulatory pattern. Microangiography is a simple technique in which a fluorescent dye is injected directly into the Sinus Venosus and/or the Posterior Cardinal Vein, allowing for the rapid labeling and easy detection of patent vessels. Here, we compare microangiography to other vascular labeling techniques, describe the benefits and potential applications of microangiography, and give step by step instructions for microangiography.

Key words: Microangiography, Zebrafish, Vascular lumen, Cardiovascular development

1. Introduction

In recent years, unique advantages of zebrafish as a model system have facilitated its emergence as one of the most prominent model systems for the study of vascular biology (1–5). For instance, zebrafish embryo develops rapidly and as a result, the cardiovascular system is fully functional within 24 h post-fertilization' (hpf) (3, 6). In addition, the embryo is externally fertilized and optically transparent, which allows easy embryological manipulations such as microangiography.

Microangiography is a relatively simple and versatile technique to rapidly visualize the entire vascular system (1). In this chapter, we provide step-by step-instructions for microangiography, list potential applications of this technique, and discuss advantages as well as disadvantages of microangiography in comparison with other techniques that are conventionally used to visualize the vascular system.

Xu Peng and Marc Antonyak (eds.), *Cardiovascular Development: Methods and Protocols*,
Methods in Molecular Biology, vol. 843, DOI 10.1007/978-1-61779-523-7_6,

1.1. Analysis of Vascular Morphology by Microangiography

The advent of transgenic animals has provided a unique opportunity to expand our current knowledge of vascular development using diverse vertebrate model systems. In the majority of cases, however, the use of transgenic animals is not well situated for assessing the function of vasculature. In zebrafish, multiple transgenic lines which express a specific fluorescent protein under an endothelial specific promoter have been generated (1, 7–12). However, since the majority of transgenic animals express the molecular tag in all endothelial cells, it is extremely difficult to rely on transgenic animals to examine whether a specific vessel is used for circulation. Analyzing circulating red blood cells using high power bright-field or video microscopes is adequate to obtain such information, but requires significant time and effort (13).

Microangiography can offer a simple yet sophisticated alternative to visual observation under high power bright-field microscopes. By labeling all patent vessels used for circulation, microangiography significantly reduces the time required for the observation of the circulatory pattern (1). Furthermore, in combination with various transgenic animals that express fluorescent proteins in a tissue-specific manner, one can carry out more sophisticated analyses of the vascular system by using microangiography.

1.2. Application of Microangiography

Microangiography may be used in any scenario where the vascular system needs to be visualized. For instance, microangiography can be used to determine the patency of developing vessels (1, 14). In addition, it can be readily used to assess the vascular integrity since any vascular leakage leading to extravasation of plasma will be labeled with injected dye (15, 16).

Since microangiography can be used at any developmental period, this technique can be combined with morpholino-injected, chemical-treated, or even surgically altered embryos, in addition to various mutant embryos (17, 18). Once injected into the blood stream, dye can stay within the vasculature for a few days. Therefore, microangiography can either precede or follow these treatments.

However, because the injected dye is passively spread within the vascular lumen, microangiography will not always reveal dynamic morphology of endothelial cells such as filopodial extensions in the migrating tip cell. In addition, microangiography is not an efficient technique to use in mutants without blood flow (19). Even with the limitations, microangiography is an extremely useful technique to rapidly visualize patent vessels.

1.3. Microangiography: General Considerations and Experimental Design

When attempting an experiment using microangiography, it is useful to keep in mind that a number of factors will determine the experimental outcomes. We have enumerated the most important factors to consider before the experimental design.

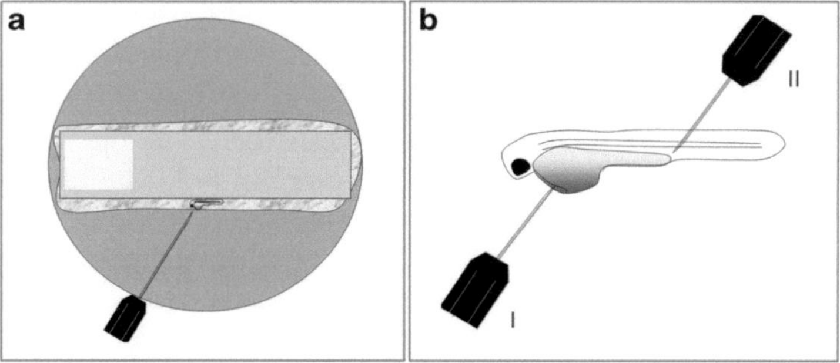

Fig. 1. Schematic drawings of microangiography. (**a**) An anesthetized embryo will be lined up against slide glass within the petri dish. (**b**) Dye can be injected into either the sinus venosus (I) or the posterior cardinal vein (PCV) of the embryo.

1. Developmental Stage of Embryos.
   Dye can be injected into Sinus Venosus (SV) and/or Posterior Cardinal Vein (PCV) (Fig. 1). Depending on the age of the embryo, the method of injection will vary slightly. For the best results, we recommend trying both sites first and determine whether SV or PCV yields better outcomes.
2. Condition of the Embryos.
   Microangiography can be combined with various experimental procedures as aforementioned. However, if microangiography is performed in embryos that are previously treated with small chemicals or morpholino, any developmental delay or morphological abnormality that might potentially impede microangiography should be carefully examined.
3. Intended Method of Observation.
   Embryos that are injected with dye can be analyzed by various methods. If the injected embryos will be analyzed after fixation, sufficient time must be allowed for the dye to completely perfuse the entire vascular system. This can be monitored on a fluorescent microscope. Alternatively, if the embryos are to be observed in vivo, attention should be paid to minimize any interference to the cardiac function.

2. Materials

2.1. Equipment

1. Microinjector.
   A microinjector is used to perfuse the vascular system of the embryos with a defined amount of dye. Based on the mechanism used to deliver the dye into the embryos, there are two main types of microinjectors widely used for the microinjection. Hydraulic microinjectors, such as the Nanoject (from Drummond Scientific) require oil to fill the injection needle.

Pneumatic microinjectors, such as Picospritzer (from Parker) or Femtojet (from Eppendorf) use compressed air, rather than oil, to push out dye into the embryos.

2. Micromanipulator.
   Although one can hold the injection needle with hand, using a micromanipulator to modulate the microinjector provides better control of the delivery of dye. Normally, the micromanipulator can be mounted onto a stand, which allows the microinjector to approach the embryos at a 45° angle. Some stand-alone systems (i.e., Femtojet) do not need an external micromanipulator.
3. Needle Puller.
   The shape of needle is one of the most critical factors that affect the outcome of the microangiography. Traditionally, the needle puller makes the injection needle by heating the glass capillary tube with the Tungsten filament and pulling with a defined force. The parameters that determine the force that applies to the heated needle needs to be empirically determined. The new lines of needle pullers, however, use a CO_2 laser to heat up the glass capillary, providing more precise control.
4. Injection Molds.
   There are several prefabricated plastic molds available, which can create a series of grooves in which the embryos settle if placed on top of melted agarose. These molds allow the injection to large quantity of embryos quickly. Alternatively, by gluing capillary tubes or slide glass to the bottom of a Petri dish and pouring the agarose on top of the tubes, a homemade injection mold can be made. Both work equally well and are reusable (Fig. 1).

2.2. Solutions and Dyes

1. Embryo Medium: 1.0 mL Hank's Stock #1 (8.0 g NaCl, 0.4 g KCl in 100 mL H_2O),0.1 mL Hank's Stock #2 (0.358 g Na_2HPO_4 Anhydrous, 0.60 g KH_2PO_4 in 100 mL H_2O), 1.0 mL Hank's Stock #4 (0.72 g $CaCl_2$ in 50 mL H_2O), 1.0 mL Hank's Stock #5 (1.23 g $MgSO_4 \times 7H_2O$ in 50 mL H_2O), 1.0 mL fresh Hank's Stock #6 (0.35 g $NaHCO_3$ in 10 mL H_2O), and 95.9 mL double distilled water. Alternatively, use 1.5 mL stock salts (i.e., Instant Ocean) added to 1 L distilled water to achieve 60 μg/mL final concentration.
2. HEPES: 10 mM HEPES, pH 7.6 is added to the injection mix (5 mM final concentration). HEPES will buffer the injection mix to physiological pH.
3. Dye: Dextran-conjugated fluorophores are easy to use and effective. Alternatively, fluorescent microspheres such as Quantum dot can be used. Based on the fluorophores, these dyes have a wide range of excitation and emission spectra, allowing the user more flexibility.

4. Ethyl 3-aminobenzoate methanesulfonate salt (40 μL/mL): Ethyl 3-aminobenzoate methanesulfonate salt, commonly known as Tricaine, is used to anesthetize the embryos for injection. Per 1 mL of embryo media, 40 μL of 24× stock solution of Tricaine (500 mg Tricaine, 196 mL dH_2O, and 4.2 mL 1 M Tris pH 9.0) needs to be added. Since an excessive amount of Tricaine can attenuate the cardiac muscle contraction, which eventually stops circulation, the appropriate amount of Tricaine needs to be empirically determined.
5. Methylcellulose: Since the viscosity of 3% methylcellulose in embryo media is sufficient to temporally slow down the movement of embryos without anesthetization, the embryos mounted in the methylcellulose can be positioned in a way allows an easy access to the PCV plexus or the SV. In addition, it provides additional protection for the embryos since it will partially absorb pressure from the injection needle to the embryos.

3. Method

1. Use a pair of forceps to remove the chorion. Alternatively, a short pulse of Pronase treatment can be used to dechorionate large numbers of embryos (20). Removal of the chorion will allow for more efficient penetration of the injection needle into embryos.
2. Prepare the injection mold by adding 3% methylcellulose onto the petri dish. Methylcellulose immobilizes the embryos within the well and allows for easy repositioning, while the well itself acts as a backstop (Fig. 1).
3. Place embryos into wells using a glass Pasteur pipette. Avoid adding excessive embryo medium while transferring the embryos since this will dilute the Tricaine.
4. Add a layer of 40 μL/mL Tricaine in embryo media on top of the 3% methylcellulose. The most critical aspect of zebrafish cardinal vein dye injection is the concentration of Tricaine. Soaking the embryos in a solution of 40 μL/mL Tricaine in embryo medium will allow for the immobilization of the embryo without immediately stopping the heart.
5. Prepare the microinjector. A standard microcapillary tube pulled and cut to 5–10 nm is sufficient for this method. Additional grinding or sharpening of the needles is not necessary. The injection needle should be filled with dye mix. Turn and dial the micromanipulator such that the needle is close to the first embryo (Fig. 2).

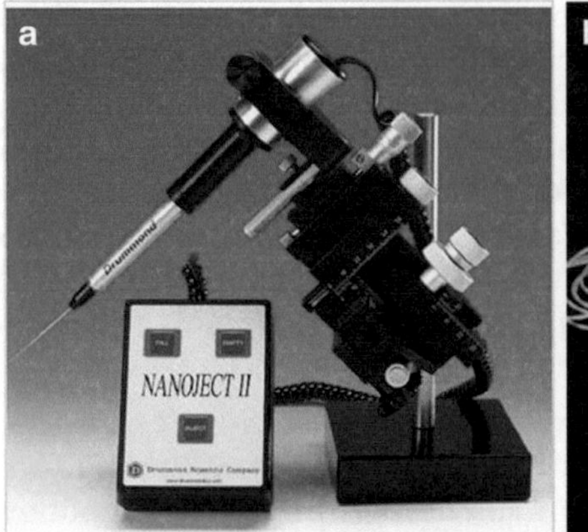

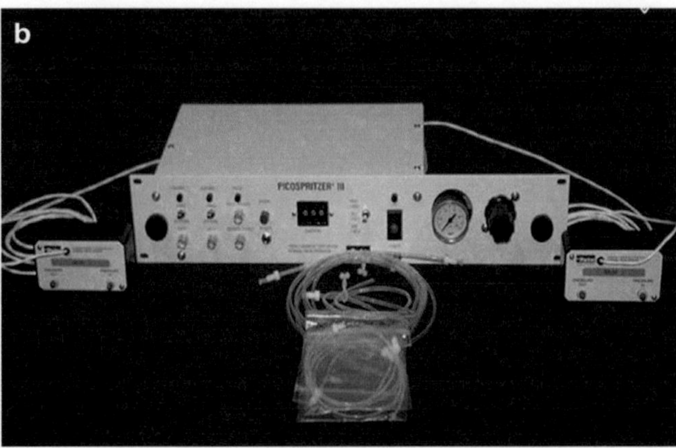

Fig. 2. Commonly used microinjectors for microangiography. Both hydraulic and pneumatic microinjectors can be used to deliver dye into the embryos to visualize vascular network. An example of a hydraulic microinjector (**a**) and a pneumatic microinjector (**b**) are shown.

6. For 24–72 hpf embryos, inject the dye to the PCV plexus. For older embryos, one can inject directly into the SV, through the pericardium. We normally inject 4.6 nL of dye mixture into 24 hpf embryos. Injecting both areas on the same embryo will ensure rapid perfusion of the dye (see Note 1). By gently moving the needle in a circular motion, one can "drill" through external tissues that may be difficult to penetrate (see Note 2).

   If embryos will not be immediately imaged, after injecting ~20 embryos, draw them up using a glass Pasteur pipette and put them into fresh media. If the heart stops, dye will typically take longer to disseminate, thus, washing out the anesthetic with embryo media can speed perfusion. Zebrafish embryos are typically reared at 28.5°C, but we find that recovery and imaging work well, if not better, at room temperature.

7. For imaging the result of microangiography, wait at least 10 min for perfusion to complete. We often inject on a bright-field microscope (see Note 3), but injections may be performed on a fluorescence microscope to determine immediately if the dye has been perfused (see Notes 4 and 5).

8. Alternatively, embryos can be fixed for later observation since Dextran-conjugated probes can be fixed. After injection and perfusion, embryos are washed once with PBS and put into 1 mL of 4% PFA in PBS and incubated overnight at 4°C. Once fixed, embryos can be stored in methanol at for –20°C for several weeks. Either sectioned or whole embryos can be analyzed by confocal microscopy after fixation (see Note 6) (Fig. 3).

9. Concluding Remarks.

   Microangiography is a relatively simple, yet powerful technique to visualize patent vessels. It also provides a powerful way to analyze vascular development and maintenance in combination with the increasing number of available transgenic lines.

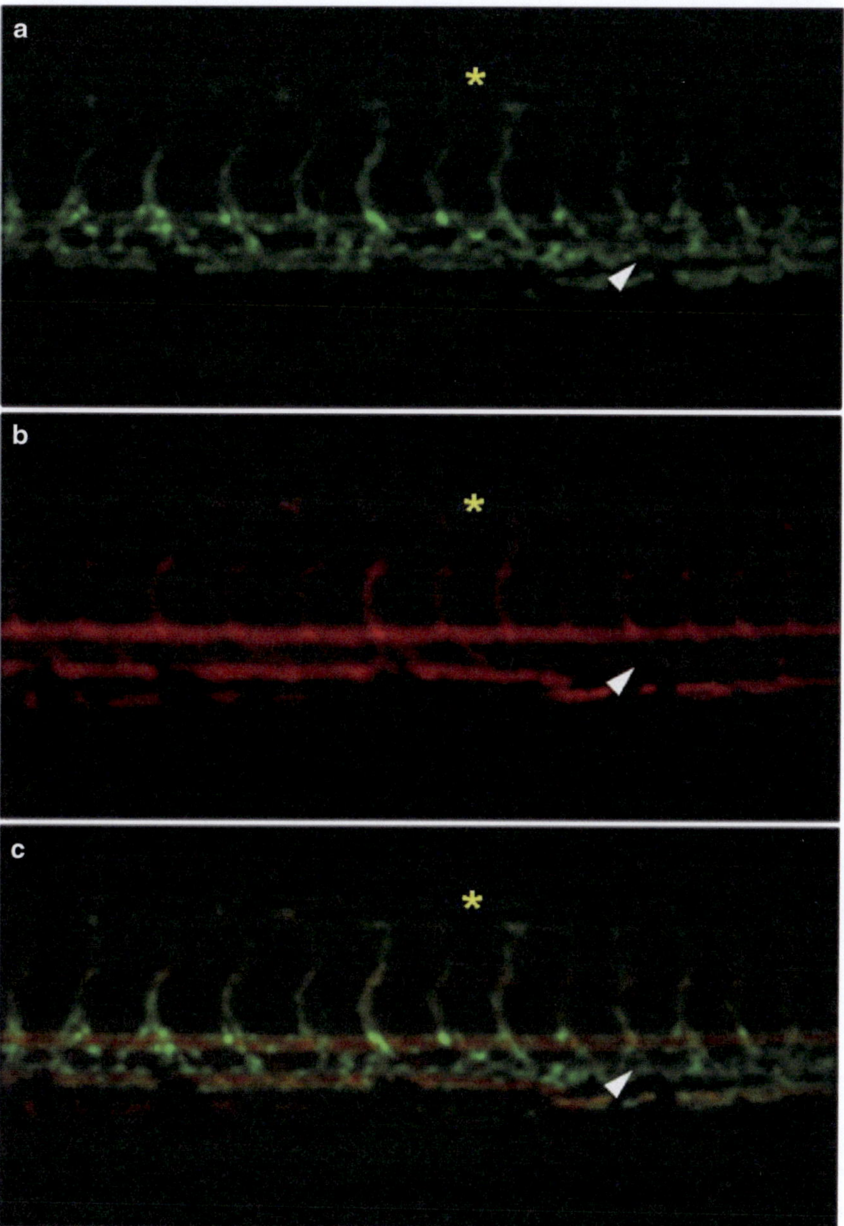

Fig. 3. An exemplary result of microangiography. The trunk region of a 60-hpf embryo after the microangiography. (**a**) All the vascular network is visualized by *Tg(kdrl:EGFP)*, which expresses EGFP under an endothelial specific promoter, *kdrl*. (**b**) Microangiography of the same embryo. (**c**) Merged image. Notice microangiography is only visualizing vessels actively used for circulation. For instance, the dorsal vein (*white arrowhead*) which constricts and shrinks to become the hematopoietic niche, or the dorsal longitudinal anastomotic vessel (*yellow asterisk*) which is not patent yet are not labeled with microangiography.

For instance, using endothelial specific transgenic lines, one can easily distinguish lumenized vessels within the developing vascular network. Furthermore, in combination with transgenic lines that label adjacent tissue, one can analyze the functional relationship between the vascular network and neighboring tissues.

In addition, microangiography can be extremely useful to detect the subtle changes of the circulatory pattern since it can rapidly visualize the patent vessels. By selectively labeling those vessels used for circulation, microangiography can provide information on the functionality of specific vessels, which cannot be achieved by analyzing endothelial specific transgenic lines.

With the advent of chemical biology and powerful imaging techniques, the potential application of microangiography is ever increasing.

4. Notes

1. Embryos may be injected at multiple sites to ensure rapid perfusion of dye.
2. Embryos may also be injected in the Common Cardinal Vein which is located below the Sinus Venosus before 4 days post-fertilization.
3. Dextran-conjugated dyes, particularly Rhodamine, can be detected using the bright-field scope. Therefore, it is possible to monitor the perfusion efficacy immediately after the dye injection.
4. We have observed that embryos may survive a significant and acute puncture wound. Take the time to empirically determine how much trauma the embryos can withstand.
5. Similarly, determine the proper needle diameter: thinner takes less force to penetrate tissues but may flex too much with mature tissues while thicker needles create more trauma.
6. Any unused Dextran-conjugated dye may be frozen at –20°C and reused for longer than 6 months.

References

1. Isogai, S., Horiguchi, M., and Weinstein, B. M. (2001) The vascular anatomy of the developing zebrafish: an atlas of embryonic and early larval development, *Dev Biol 230*, 278–301.
2. Lawson, N. D., and Weinstein, B. M. (2002) Arteries and veins: making a difference with zebrafish, *Nat Rev Genet 3*, 674–682.
3. Lee, R. K., Stainier, D. Y., Weinstein, B. M., and Fishman, M. C. (1994) Cardiovascular development in the zebrafish. II. Endocardial progenitors are sequestered within the heart field, *Development 120*, 3361–3366.
4. Stainier, D. Y., Fouquet, B., Chen, J. N., Warren, K. S., Weinstein, B. M., Meiler, S. E., Mohideen, M. A., Neuhauss, S. C., Solnica-Krezel, L., Schier, A. F., Zwartkruis, F., Stemple, D. L., Malicki, J., Driever, W., and Fishman, M. C. (1996) Mutations affecting the formation and function of the cardiovascular system in the zebrafish embryo, *Development 123*, 285–292.
5. Swift, M. R., and Weinstein, B. M. (2009) Arterial-venous specification during development, *Circ Res 104*, 576–588.
6. Stainier, D. Y., Lee, R. K., and Fishman, M. C. (1993) Cardiovascular development in the zebrafish. I. Myocardial fate map and heart tube formation, *Development 119*, 31–40.

7. Chi, N. C., Shaw, R. M., Jungblut, B., Huisken, J., Ferrer, T., Arnaout, R., Scott, I., Beis, D., Xiao, T., Baier, H., Jan, L. Y., Tristani-Firouzi, M., and Stainier, D. Y. (2008) Genetic and physiologic dissection of the vertebrate cardiac conduction system, *PLoS Biol 6*, e109.
8. Choi, J., Dong, L., Ahn, J., Dao, D., Hammerschmidt, M., and Chen, J. N. (2007) FoxH1 negatively modulates flk1 gene expression and vascular formation in zebrafish, *Dev Biol 304*, 735–744.
9. Jin, S. W., Beis, D., Mitchell, T., Chen, J. N., and Stainier, D. Y. (2005) Cellular and molecular analyses of vascular tube and lumen formation in zebrafish, *Development 132*, 5199–5209.
10. Lawson, N. D., and Weinstein, B. M. (2002) In vivo imaging of embryonic vascular development using transgenic zebrafish, *Dev Biol 248*, 307–318.
11. Motoike, T., Loughna, S., Perens, E., Roman, B. L., Liao, W., Chau, T. C., Richardson, C. D., Kawate, T., Kuno, J., Weinstein, B. M., Stainier, D. Y., and Sato, T. N. (2000) Universal GFP reporter for the study of vascular development, *Genesis 28*, 75–81.
12. Roman, B. L., Pham, V. N., Lawson, N. D., Kulik, M., Childs, S., Lekven, A. C., Garrity, D. M., Moon, R. T., Fishman, M. C., Lechleider, R. J., and Weinstein, B. M. (2002) Disruption of acvrl1 increases endothelial cell number in zebrafish cranial vessels, *Development 129*, 3009–3019.
13. Schwerte, T., Uberbacher, D., and Pelster, B. (2003) Non-invasive imaging of blood cell concentration and blood distribution in zebrafish Danio rerio incubated in hypoxic conditions in vivo, *J Exp Biol 206*, 1299–1307.
14. Kamei, M., Saunders, W. B., Bayless, K. J., Dye, L., Davis, G. E., and Weinstein, B. M. (2006) Endothelial tubes assemble from intracellular vacuoles in vivo, *Nature 442*, 453–456.
15. Buchner, D. A., Su, F., Yamaoka, J. S., Kamei, M., Shavit, J. A., Barthel, L. K., McGee, B., Amigo, J. D., Kim, S., Hanosh, A. W., Jagadeeswaran, P., Goldman, D., Lawson, N. D., Raymond, P. A., Weinstein, B. M., Ginsburg, D., and Lyons, S. E. (2007) pak2a mutations cause cerebral hemorrhage in redhead zebrafish, *Proc Natl Acad Sci U S A 104*, 13996–14001.
16. Liu, J., Fraser, S. D., Faloon, P. W., Rollins, E. L., Vom Berg, J., Starovic-Subota, O., Laliberte, A. L., Chen, J. N., Serluca, F. C., and Childs, S. J. (2007) A betaPix Pak2a signaling pathway regulates cerebral vascular stability in zebrafish, *Proc Natl Acad Sci U S A 104*, 13990–13995.
17. Hogan, B. M., Bos, F. L., Bussmann, J., Witte, M., Chi, N. C., Duckers, H. J., and Schulte-Merker, S. (2009) Ccbe1 is required for embryonic lymphangiogenesis and venous sprouting, *Nat Genet 41*, 396–398.
18. Nicoli, S., Standley, C., Walker, P., Hurlstone, A., Fogarty, K. E., and Lawson, N. D. (2010) MicroRNA-mediated integration of haemodynamics and Vegf signalling during angiogenesis, *Nature 464*, 1196–1200.
19. Zhong, T. P., Rosenberg, M., Mohideen, M. A., Weinstein, B., and Fishman, M. C. (2000) gridlock, an HLH gene required for assembly of the aorta in zebrafish, *Science 287*, 1820–1824.
20. Westerfield, M. (2000) *The zebrafish book*, A Guide for the laboratory use of zebrafish (Danio rerio), 4th Ed. University of Oregon Press, Eugene.

Chapter 7

Whole-Mount Confocal Microscopy for Vascular Branching Morphogenesis

Yoh-suke Mukouyama, Jennifer James, Joseph Nam, and Yutaka Uchida

Abstract

We introduce a whole-mount immunohistochemistry method for analyzing intricate vascular network formation in mouse embryonic tissues. Laser scanning confocal microscopy with multiple labeling allows for robust imaging of blood and lymphatic vessel branching morphogenesis with excellent resolution.

Key words: Confocal microscopy, Whole-mount immunohistochemistry, Mouse embryo, Blood vessel, Lymphatic vessel, Fluorescence, Antibody, Patterning

1. Introduction

The circulatory system is crucial for organ development during embryogenesis, as well as for organ maintenance and reproductive function in the adult. The specific pattern of blood vessel branching in each organ is achieved by a complex process, termed angiogenesis, in which a preexisting primitive capillary plexus is reorganized into a hierarchically branched vascular network. Emerging evidence in mouse genetics demonstrates that a variety of intercellular signaling systems are implicated in patterning the vascular network.

Whole-mount immunohistochemical analysis for imaging the entire vasculature is pivotal for understanding the cellular mechanisms of branching morphogenesis. The confocal microscope is a powerful tool to visualize intact blood vessels as well as their cellular components including endothelial cells, pericytes, and smooth muscle cells, using specific fluorescent markers. This chapter describes a simple and robust protocol to stain intact blood vessels with vascular-specific antibodies and fluorescent secondary

Xu Peng and Marc Antonyak (eds.), *Cardiovascular Development: Methods and Protocols*,
Methods in Molecular Biology, vol. 843, DOI 10.1007/978-1-61779-523-7_7,

antibodies, which is applicable for vascularized embryonic organs where we are able to follow the process of vascular development. We will provide examples from embryonic limb skin (1) and heart (*manuscript in preparation*) for whole-mount multiple imuuno-fluorescence confocal microscopy (see Note 1).

2 Materials

2.1. Tissues

E13.5~E17.5 mouse embryos for harvesting limb skin and heart specimen

2.1.1. Antibodies for Vascular Markers

see Table 1.

2.2.2. Antibodies for Reporter Genes (GFP and lacZ)

see Table 2.

2.2. Solutions

1. 70% Ethanol (EtOH) in Water.
2. Hanks' Balanced Salt Solution (HBSS).
3. Phosphate Buffer Saline (PBS).
4. Triton X-100 (TX100).
5. Goat Serum (heat inactivation in 56°C for 30 min).
6. Donkey Serum.
7. 4% (w/v) Paraformaldehyde in PBS (PFA) (freshly prepare from 16% stock).
8. PBT (PBS+0.2%TX100): add 0.2 mL of Triton X-100 to 100 mL of PBS.
9. 75%, 50%, 25%Methanol (MeOH)/PBT.
10. Blocking buffer for goat secondary antibodies: 10%HIGS (Heat Inactivated Goat Serum)/PBS+0.2%TX100 (keep at 4°C for 2 weeks).
11. Washing buffer for goat secondary antibodies: 2%HIGS/PBS+0.2%TX100 (keep at 4°C for 2 weeks).
12. Blocking buffer for donkey secondary antibodies: 10%DS (Donkey Serum)/PBS+0.2% TX100 (keep at 4°C for 2 weeks).
13. Washing buffer for donkey secondary antibodies: 2%DS/PBS+0.2%TX100 (keep at 4°C for 2 weeks).
14. Nuclear counterstaining solution: To-Pro-3 1:3,000 dilution.

Table 1
Summary of vascular-specific antibodies for whole-mount staining of mouse tissues

Antibody	Species	Company	Working condition
Pan-endothelial cell marker			
PECAM-1	Armenian hamster (M)	Chemicon (MAB1398Z)	1:100 dilution[a]
PECAM-1	Rat (M)	BD Pharmingen (553369)	1:300 dilution
VEGFR2	Rat (M)	eBioscience (14-5821-82)	1:200 dilution
CD34	Rat (M)	eBioscience (13-0341)	1:300 dilution
Collagen IV	Rabbit (P)	AbD Serotec (2150-1470)	1:300 dilution[b]
Arterial endothelial cell marker			
Neuropilin-1	Rabbit (P)	The Alex Kolodkin lab[c]	1:3,000 dilution
Unc5H2	Goat (P)	R&D (AF1006)	1:200 dilution
Venous endothelial cell marker			
EphB4	Goat (P)	R&D (AF446)	1:100 dilution
Lymphatic endothelial cell marker			
LYVE-1[d]	Rabbit (P)	Abcam (ab14917)	1:200 dilution
LYVE-1[d]	Rat (M)	MBL (D225-3)	1:300 dilution
Prox-1	Rabbit (P)	Chemicon (AB5475)	1:1,000 dilution
Prox-1	Goat (P)	R&D (AF2727)	1:50 dilution
Neuropilin-2	Rabbit (P)	Cell signaling (3366)	1:100 dilution
Podoplanin	Syrian hamster (M)	Hybridoma bank (8.1.1)	1:200 dilution
Smooth muscle cell/pericyte marker			
αSMA-Cy3	Mouse (M)[e]	Sigma (c-6198)	1:500 dilution[f]
NG2	Rabbit (P)	Chemicon (AB5320)	1:200 dilution
SM22α	Rabbit (P)	Abcam (ab14106)	1:200 dilution

P polyclonal antibody; *M* monoclonal antibody

[a]Goat anti-Armenian hamster-Cy3 (Jackson ImmunoResearch 127-165-160) antibody should be used as a secondary antibody

[b]The collagen IV antibody can be used to detect blood vessels after in situ hybridization

[c]The neuropilin-1 antibody was kindly provided by the Alex Kolodkin lab in the Johns Hopkins University

[d]The LYVE-1 antibodies also detect a subset of macrophages in the embryonic skin and heart

[e]The anti-αSMA antibody is mouse IgG2a monoclonal antibody

[f]The Cy3-donjugated αSMA antibody is incubated for 1 h at room temperature together with secondary antibodies for other primary antibodies

2.3. Dissection Tools

1. Microdissecting forceps.
2. Microdissecting scissors.
3. Microdissecting fine tweezers (Inox #5).
4. Ring forceps.

2.4. Supplies for Dissection and Staining

1. Bench paper.
2. Paper towel.
3. 100 × 15-mm Petri dish.

Table 2
Summary of antibodies for reporter genes (*GFP* and *lacZ*)

Antibody	Species	Company	Working condition
GFP reporter			
GFP	Rabbit (P)	Invitrogen (A11122)	1:300 dilution
GFP	Rat (M)	Nacalai tesque (04404-84)	1:1,000 dilution
GFP	Chick (P)	Chemicon (P42212)	1:300 dilution
LacZ reporter			
β-gal	Rabbit (P)	MP biomedical (55976)	1:5,000 dilution
β-gal	Goat (P)	AbD Serotec (4600-1409)	1:500 dilution
β-gal	Chick (P)	Abcam (ab9361)	1:200 dilution

P polyclonal antibody; *M* monoclonal antibody

4. 35 × 10-mm Petri dish.
5. 24-well plate cell culture plate.
6. 5-mL Polypropylene round-bottom tube.
7. 2-mL Conical screw-cap microcentrifuge tube.
8. 0.22-μm PVDF membrane syringe filters.

2.5. Supplies for Mounting

1. Anti-fade mounting media (Prolong Gold, Invitrogen).
2. Spacer for mounting (Secure-Seal™ spacer, 9 mm diameter, 0.12 mm deep, Invitrogen).
3. Microscopic slides with adhesive coating (Matsunami MAS-GP, EverMark Select EMS200W⁺).
4. Cover glass 25 × 25 mm.
5. Kimwipe.

2.6. Equipment

1. Dissecting stereomicroscope.
2. Fiber optic illumination system for reflected light.
3. Gentle shaker.

3. Methods

3.1. Collecting Specimen

1. Euthanize plugged females by approved procedure.
2. Lay the euthanized animal on an absorbent paper towel and soak it thoroughly in 70% EtOH/H_2O from a squeeze bottle.

3. Dissect the uterus intact and place it in a 100 × 15-mm Petri dish containing ice-cold HBSS to wash out blood.
4. Separate and dissect the embryo. Remove the very thin amnion from the embryo.
5. (Option) Dissect a single embryo in a 35 × 10-mm Petri dish if each embryo needs to be genotyped.
6. Cut off the forelimbs of embryo and dissect the heart from the embryo under the microscope.
7. Transfer these tissues (forelimbs and hearts) by a ring forceps into 24-well plate containing 2 mL of ice-cold fresh 4%PFA in PBS.
8. Fix the tissues with gentle mixing on the Nutator Mixer at 4°C overnight.
9. On the following day, remove the PFA and wash the tissues three times for 5 min in 2 mL of PBS with gentle mixing on the Nutator Mixer at room temperature.
10. Stock the tissues in 100% MeOH at –20°C enzyme freezer (the freezer with critical temperature control and without automatic defrost function) (see Note 2). Primary antibodies listed in Tables work after the 100% MeOH treatment.
11. (Forelimb skin) Peel off skin from the forelimb using fine tweezers in 100% MeOH (see the details in Fig. 1).

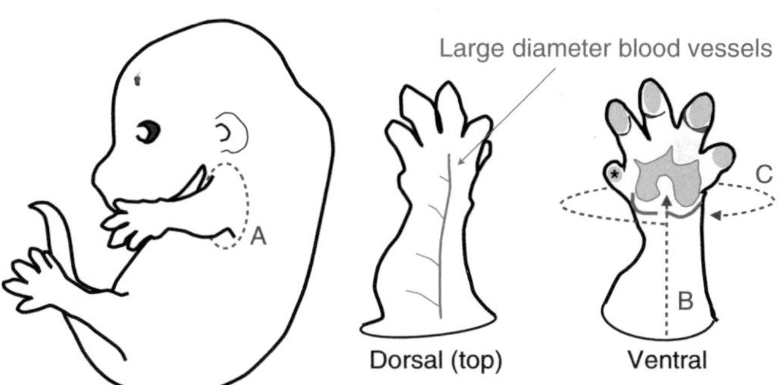

Fig. 1. Limbs can be dissected postmethanol dehydration in a small dish containing methanol, respectively. Carefully pull apart skin at the base of the limb with tweezers, following the *blue dashed line* (**a**). Snip through muscle and bone completely. Large diameter vessels may be visible on the dorsal surface of the limb as depicted. The dissection of limb skin must be performed on MeOH-dehydrated limbs in a dish containing 100% methanol. Limb skin separates easily from the limb skin when dehydrated in this manner. To avoid dissecting through the branched vessel plexus on the dorsal surface of the limb, invert the limb so that the ventral side faces up. Using fine tweezers, dissect through skin near the base of the limb toward the paw in a straight line (**b**). Next dissect around the entire limb, peeling the limb skin off gently as you turn the limb (**c**). Note: dissect in opposite directions for the right and left limbs, and toward the digit labeled with an *asterisk* in the diagram.

3.2. Staining of Whole-Mount Tissues

1. Rehydrate the tissues in 5-mL polypropylene round-bottom tube with graded series of MeOH/PBT (75, 50, and 25%) for 5 min each and then wash twice for 5 min in PBT with gentle mixing on the Nutator Mixer at room temperature.
2. (Heart) Cut the heart to divide dorsal and ventral potions (see the details in Fig. 2).
3. Block the tissues with either 10%HIGS/PBS + 0.2%TX100 for goat secondary antibodies or 10%DS/PBS + 0.2%TX100 for donkey secondary antibodies for 2 h with gentle mixing on the Nutator Mixer at room temperature.
4. Place the tissues on a 35 × 10-mm Petri dish and transfer by a ring forceps into 2-mL microcentrifuge tube with 800 μL of primary antibodies (appropriate dilution as listed in Tables) in the blocking buffer (either 10%HIGS/PBS + 0.2%TX100 or 10%DS/PBS + 0.2%TX100) (see Note 3).
5. Incubate the tissues with gentle mixing on the Nutator Mixer at 4°C overnight.
6. Place the tissues on a 35 × 10-mm Petri dish and transfer by a ring forceps into 5-mL polypropylene round-bottom tube with 4 mL of the washing buffer (either 2%HIGS/PBS + 0.2%TX100 or 2%DS/PBS + 0.2%TX100). Wash five times for 15 min with gentle mixing on the Nutator Mixer at room temperature.
7. Place the tissues on a 35 × 10-mm Petri dish and transfer by a ring forceps into 2-mL microcentrifuge tube with 800 μL of

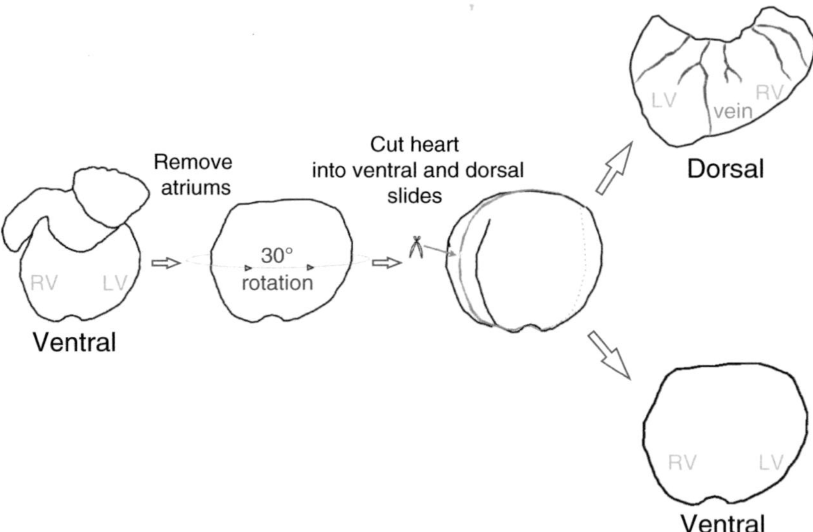

Fig. 2. The ventral side of heart is facing the upward and dorsal side facing the downward. The heart is oriented this way to minimize the damage on the dorsal surface of heart under the stereomicroscope with low illumination to avoid extensive bleaching. The atriums are removed carefully from the heart. Rotate the heart about 30° and use microdissecting scissors to divide the heart into the ventral and dorsal side.

secondary antibodies in the blocking buffer (either 10%HIGS/PBS+0.2%TX100 or 10%DS/PBS+0.2%TX100). Filter the secondary antibody solution using 0.22-µm PVDF membrane syringe filters to remove aggregated particles of the secondary antibodies (see Note 3).

8. Incubate the tissues in the dark or wrapped with aluminum foil for 1 h with gentle mixing on the Nutator Mixer at room temperature.
9. Place the tissues on a 35 × 10-mm Petri dish and transfer by a ring forceps into 5-mL polypropylene round-bottom tube with 4 mL of the washing buffer (either 2%HIGS/PBS + 0.2%TX100 or 2%DS/PBS + 0.2%TX100). Wash five times for 15 min in the dark or wrapped with aluminum foil with gentle mixing on the Nutator Mixer at room temperature.
10. (Option for counterstaining against nucleus) Incubate the tissues with 4 mL of the washing buffer (either 2%HIGS/PBS + 0.2%TX100 or 2%DS/PBS + 0.2%TX100) with To-Pro-3 in the dark or wrapped with aluminum foil for 10 min with gentle mixing on the Nutator Mixer at room temperature (see Note 4). Then, wash three times for 5 min with 4 mL of the washing buffer (either 2%HIGS/PBS + 0.2%TX100 or 2%DS/PBS + 0.2%TX100) in the dark or wrapped by aluminum foil with gentle mixing on the Nutator Mixer at room temperature.

3.3. Mounting Limb Skin on Slide

1. Place the limb skins on a 35 × 10-mm Petri dish. Remove dusts, crystals, and fibers from the inner layer of the skins using fine tweezers under the stereomicroscope with low illumination to avoid extensive photo bleaching.
2. Transfer the limb skins to adhesive microscopic slide by a ring forceps. Place the skins with the inner layer lying upward on the slide (i.e., towards coverslip). Flatten the skins carefully using fine tweezers and remove carry-over washing buffer by Kimwipe.
3. Mount in anti-fade mounting media without air bubbles.
4. Cure on a flat surface in the dark (e.g., the samples mounted using ProLong Gold reagent are placed overnight in the dark at room temperature before viewing). For long-term storage, seal the coverslip to the slide and store at 4°C.

3.4. Mounting Heart on Slide

1. Place the hearts on a 35 × 10-mm Petri dish. Clean up the hearts using fine tweezers under the stereomicroscope with low illumination to avoid extensive bleaching.
2. Place 1 ~ 2 layers of Secure-Seal™ spacer (9 mm diameter, 0.12 mm deep) on adhesive microscopic slide.

3. Transfer the hearts to the slide by a ring forceps. Place the hearts with the outer surface lying upward on the slide (i.e., towards coverslip) to image coronary vasculature. Remove carry-over washing buffer by Kimwipe.
4. Mount in anti-fade mounting media without dirt and air bubbles.
5. Cure on a flat surface in the dark (e.g., The samples mounted using ProLong Gold reagent are placed for overnight in the dark at room temperature before viewing). For long-term storage, seal the coverslip to the slide and store at 4°C.

3.5. Confocal Microscopy

1. Set up appropriate lasers for fluorophores. We use Leica TCS SP5 confocal microscope with three laser sources including Argon 488 nm (for Alexa Fluor 488 and GFP), DPSS 561 nm (for Alexa Fluor 568 and Cy3), and HeNe 633 nm (for Alexa Fluor 633, Cy5 and To-Pro-3).
2. Use sequential scan tool to avoid or reduce cross talk in which all dyes in double or triple-stained samples will be excited at the same time. In the sequential scan mode, images will be recorded in a sequential order.
3. More general information about fluorescent dyes and lasers for excitation may be founded in "Confocal Microscopy for Biologists" by Hibbs (2004) (2).

4. Notes

1. General comment.
   Whole-mount confocal microscopy with multiple labeling by vascular markers permitted us to image blood and lymphatic endothelial cells and their neighbors including smooth muscle cells and pericytes in the tissues. In addition to the vascular marker antibodies, antibodies for reporter gene products (β-galactosidase, β-gal, and green fluorescent protein, GFP, Table 2) that recapitulate the expression pattern of endogenous genes of your interest can be used. Figure 3 shows forelimb skin and heart from embryos carrying *lacZ* reporter targeted to the *ephrinB2* (3) or *EphB4* locus (4), which provides a histochemical indicator of *ephrinB2* or *EphB4*. EphrinB2, a transmembrane ligand, is expressed by arteries but not veins, whereas its receptor, the tyrosine kinase EphB4, is preferentially expressed by veins (3). Whole-mount double-label confocal immnofluorescence microscopy with antibodies to β-galactosidase (Fig. 3 red) and the pan-endothelial marker PECAM-1 (Fig. 3 green) revealed a characteristic branching

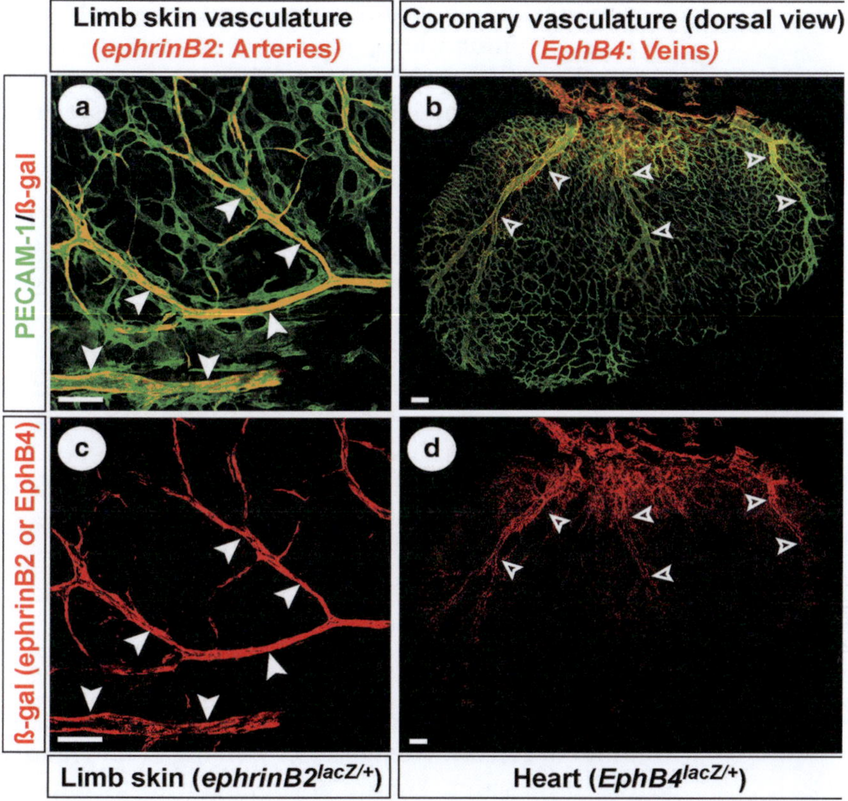

Fig. 3. (**a–b**) Double-labeled confocal microscopy with anti-β-gal (*red*) and PECAM-1 (*green*) antibodies revealed that ephrinB2^{+} arterial branching (*white arrowheads*) is seen in the limb skin of *ephrinB2*$^{lacZ/+}$ embryos at E15.5. The images were taken by 20× objective lens with confocal Z-series. Scale bar, 100 μm. (**c–d**) Double-labeling showed larger diameter EphB4^{+} coronary veins (*open arrowheads*) on the dorsal cardiac surface of *EphB4*$^{lacZ/+}$ embryos at E15.5. The images were taken by 20× objective lens with confocal Z-series and tiling. Scale bar, 100 μm.

pattern of ephrinB2^{+} arteries in the limb skin vasculature (Fig. 3a, b) and a stereotypic pattern of EphB4^{+} veins in the coronary vasculature (Fig. 3c, d).

The study of different stages of these vascular systems reveals the cellular dynamics of angiogenesis including vascular branching, arterial/venous differentiation, lymphatic vessel development, and smooth muscle/pericyte coverage in the developing limb skin (1) and heart (*manuscript in preparation*).

2. Tissue storage in 100% methanol.
   Limb skin separates easily from the limb when dehydrated. After overnight storage at –20°C, limb skin can be dissected out. According to our staining experiences, heart without MeOH-dehydration gives you a better immunostaining.
3. Primary and secondary antibodies combination.

Multiple primary antibodies derived from different species (e.g., rat monoclonal antibody+rabbit polyclonal antibody) can be used simultaneously. Different fluorescent-conjugated secondary antibodies derived from different species can be also used simultaneously.

4. To-pro-3 for nuclear counterstaining.
   For a nuclear counterstaining, DAPI (4′, 6-Diamidino-2-phenylindole) is widely used because of its high specificity for nuclear DNA. DAPI shows a blue fluorescence under ultraviolet (UV 364 nm); however, it is not suitable for a regular confocal microscope equipped with Argon-laser (488 nm excitation), DPSS-laser (561 nm excitation), and HeNe-laser (633 nm excitation) illumination system. The optimal counterstaining with DAPI needs a UV-laser. To-pro-3 is an alternative to DAPI, which provides strong and specific staining for nuclei in a specific emission (HeNe 633 nm excitation).

Acknowledgments

Work supported by Intramural Research Program of National Institutes of Health. We thank Dr. Wenling Li for critical comments on this manuscript. We are also grateful to Heesuk Zang, John Hatch, and Izumi Onitsuka for their contributions to this whole-mount immunohistochemistry method.

References

1. Mukouyama, Y.S., Shin, D., Britsch, S., Taniguchi, M., Anderson, D.J. (2002) Sensory nerves determine the pattern of arterial differentiation and blood vessel branching in the skin. Cell. **109**, 693–705.
2. Hibbs, A.R. (2004) Confocal Microscopy for Biologist. Springer
3. Wang, H.U., Chen, Z.F., Anderson, D.J. (1998) Molecular distinction and angiogenic interaction between embryonic arteries and veins revealed by ephrin-B2 and its receptor Eph-B4. Cell. **93**, 741–53.
4. Gerety, S.S., Wang, H.U., Chen, Z.F., Anderson, D.J. (1999) Symmetrical mutant phenotypes of the receptor EphB4 and its specific transmembrane ligand ephrin-B2 in cardiovascular development. Mol Cell. **4**, 403–14.

Chapter 8

Visualization of Mouse Embryo Angiogenesis by Fluorescence-Based Staining

Yang Liu, Marc Antonyak, and Xu Peng

Abstract

The establishment of a blood vessel network is fundamental to embryonic development and plays a critical role in many diseases including coronary heart disease and cancer. Vascular endothelial cells are central players in blood vessel formation and line the inside of the entire blood vessel system. PECAM-1 is expressed in all types of endothelial cells and is therefore a useful marker for the detection of blood vessels. In this manuscript, we describe PECAM-1 staining in whole-mount and sectioned tissues in mouse embryos.

Key words: Angiogenesis, Vascular endothelial cells, Whole-mount staining, Immunofluorescence staining

1. Introduction

Blood vessel formation is essential for embryonic development and plays an important role in the pathogenesis of many diseases including coronary heart disease, diabetes, and cancer. Angiogenesis is a process in which the growth of new capillaries sprouts from the preexisting vasculature (1). Owing to the importance of angiogenesis for many diseases, several clinical trails targeting therapeutic angiogenesis are ongoing, but preliminary results suggest that the benefits of these methods are condition-dependent and limited. The major obstacle for improving the efficiency of treatment is that we sill have a large knowledge gap in complete understanding of the mechanisms of blood vessel formation.

Present angiogenesis studies are largely dependant on various in vitro and in vivo models (2, 3). An in vitro angiogenesis model, such as endothelial cell tube formation on Matrigel, is a relatively quick method and can be used for screening a large number of drugs

Xu Peng and Marc Antonyak (eds.), *Cardiovascular Development: Methods and Protocols*, Methods in Molecular Biology, vol. 843, DOI 10.1007/978-1-61779-523-7_8,

or chemicals at the same time, but these results need to be validated and confirmed in vivo. Even though several in vivo analysis tools have been developed (4), the use of genetically modified mice is absolutely the ideal model in investigating the molecular mechanism underlying angiogenesis in vivo. Genes of interest that have potential roles in angiogenesis can be either up- or down-regulated in genetically modified mice. The embryo and extra-embryonic tissues including the yolk sac can be obtained for study at certain developmental stages. In the earlier embryonic development stage (before E11.5), whole-mount staining is useful to visualize a full 3-dimentional picture of blood vessel networks. After E12.5, the developed embryonic skin prevents the penetration of antibodies, which makes it difficult for whole-mount staining. Thus, embryos need to be sectioned and then stained with markers for blood vessels.

Vascular endothelial cells line the inside of the entire circulation system and are good markers for visualization of blood vessel network. Platelet endothelial cell adhesion molecule-1 (PECAM-1), also referred to as CD31, is a cell adhesion molecule that belongs to the immunoglobulin superfamily (5). It is a transmembrane glycoprotein which is constantly expressed on the surface of all vascular endothelial cells. PECAM-1 has provided a useful immunohistochemical marker of blood vessels, and here we will introduce the protocols for PECAM-1 immunofluorescence staining using whole embryo (or yolk sac) and cryostat tissue sections.

2. Materials

2.1. Whole-Mount Embryo Immunofluorescence Staining

1. 1× Phosphate-Buffered Saline (PBS): 137 mM NaCl, 2.7 mM KCl, 10 mM Ha_2HPO_4, 2 mM KH_2PO_4. Adjust the pH to 7.4 with HCl and store the buffer at room temperature.
2. Plastic transfer pipettes.
3. 4% Paraformaldehyde in PBS.
4. Shaker.
5. PBT: 0.2% BSA, 0.1% Triton X-100 in PBS.
6. Methanol.
7. 5% hydrogen peroxide in methanol.
8. PBST: 0.5%Triton X-100 in PBS.
9. PBSMT: 3% instant skim milk, 0.1% triton X-100 in PBS.
10. PECAM-1 primary antibody (BD Pharmingen). Make 1:100 dilution in PBSMT.
11. Immunofluorescence-labeled secondary antibody (Invitrogen). Make 1:100 dilution of secondary antibody in PBSMT.
12. Glass slides (VWR).

13. Cover slide (Corning labware & Equipment).
14. Anti-fade medium(Invitrogen, Component A: Anti-fade reagent in glycerol/PBS).

2.2. Immuno-fluorescence Staining for Section Embryo Tissue

1. 1× PBS.
2. Serum blocking solution (Santa Cruz Biotechnology).
3. 37°C incubator.
4. Shaker.
5. Humid box (see Note 1).
6. PECAM-1 primary antibody (BD Pharmingen). Make 1:100 dilution in PBS or serum blocking solution.
7. Immunofluorescence-labeled secondary antibody (Invitrogen). Make 1:100 dilution of secondary antibody in PBS.
8. Hoechst33258 for nucleus staining. Make 1:5,000 or 1:10,000 Hoechst dilution with water depending on signal.
9. Aluminum Foil.
10. Cover slide (Corning labware & Equipment).
11. Nail polish.
12. Anti-fade medium (Invitrogen, Component A: Anti-fade reagent in glycerol/PBS).

3. Methods

3.1. Harvest Mouse Embryos from Time-Crossed Pregnant Female Mice

1. Euthanize pregnant female by CO_2 asphyxiation according to Institutional Animal Care and Use Committee (IACUC) protocol.
2. Make a small horizontal incision in the skin near the base of lower abdomen. Expose the abdomen by pinching the skin above and below the incision and pulling it apart in opposite directions.
3. Make a "⊥" shape cut in peritoneum to expose the abdominal cavity. Move away intestine to expose reproductive organs. The uterine horns with embryos will resemble a beaded necklace.
4. Remove the uterus by lifting one uterine horn and cut it away along the mesometrium. Place the dissected uterus in a petri dish with PBS. Rinse uterus twice in PBS to wash away blood cells.
5. Remove each embryo from uterus by cutting the uterus between implantation sites under surgical microscope using a pair of fine tip forceps and scissors.

6. Use a pair of fine tip forceps to hold an embryo at the cutting site. Gently peel the surrounding uterine muscular tissue off to expose the sponge-like decidua.
7. Tear apart the decidua at the apex carefully. Gently remove the decidua that surrounds the embryo. Disconnect the Reichert's membrane from the decidua and visceral yolk sac from the actual embryo.
8. Carefully transfer embryos into a 1.5-mL Eppendorf tube or 24-well plate using a plastic transfer pipette. Cut 1 cm off of the pipette tip to make sure the embryos will go through. Rinse embryos twice with PBS to remove blood cells.

3.2. Whole-Mount Embryo Immuno-fluorescence Staining for PECAM-1

1. Fix embryos in 4% paraformaldehyde in PBS at 4°C overnight (see Note 2).
2. Wash embryos in PBS twice with gently shaking, each for 5 min.
3. Dehydrate embryos at room temperature as follows:
   - 25% Methanol in PBT for 5 min with gentle shaking.
   - 50% Methanol in PBT for 5 min with gentle shaking.
   - 75% Methanol in PBT for 5 min with gentle shaking.
   - 100% Methanol twice, each for 5 min with gentle shaking (see Note 3).
4. Bleach embryos with 5% hydrogen peroxide in methanol for 4–5 h at room temperature. Shake gently.
5. Rehydrate embryos at room temperature as follow:
   - 100% Methanol twice, each for 5 min with gentle shaking (see Note 4).
   - 75% Methanol in PBST for 5 min with gentle shaking.
   - 50% Methanol in PBST for 5 min with gentle shaking.
   - 25% Methanol in PBST for 5 min with gentle shaking.
6. Wash embryos in PBST three times, each for 5 min. Shake gently.
7. Block embryos in PBSMT at room temperature twice, each for 1 h. Shake gently.
8. Incubate embryos with PECAM-1 antibody at 4°C for 2 days with gentle shaking (see Note 5). Use 1:100 dilution of PECAM-1 antibody in PBSMT.
9. Wash embryos in PBSMT five times, 1 h each at 4°C with gentle shaking.
10. Incubate embryos with immunofluorescence-labeled secondary antibody at 4°C for one overnight with gentle shaking. Use 1:500 dilution of secondary antibody in PBSMT (see Note 6).
11. Wash embryos in PBSMT five times, 1 h each at 4°C with gentle shaking.

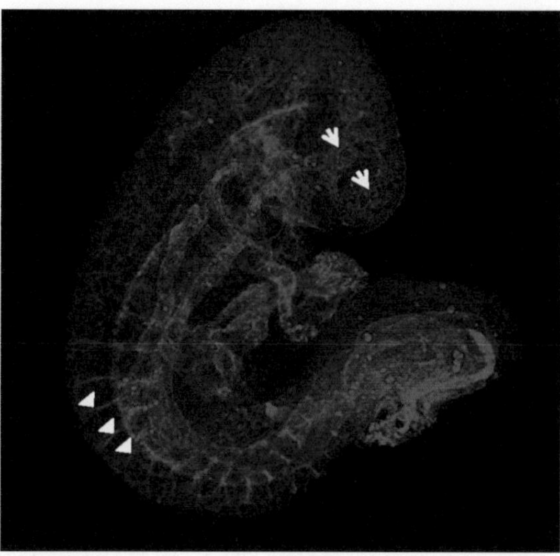

Fig. 1. PECAM-1 whole-mount staining on E9.5 embryo. The branched blood vessels (*arrows*) were presented in the head region, and intersomitic blood vessels were well organized (*arrow heads*).

12. Transfer each embryo to a glass slide using plastic transfer pipette. Remove excess PBSMT around the embryos using a piece of Kimwipes® tissue.
13. Mount embryos with anti-fade medium.
14. Gently apply a cover slide on the top of embryos. Do not push on the cover slide, as the embryos could be damaged.
15. Cover the slide with embryos with Aluminum Foil. Visualize the staining by fluorescence or confocal microscopy immediately (Fig. 1).

3.3. Immunofluorescence Staining of Cryostat Tissue Sections for PECAM-1

1. Thaw frozen tissue sections at room temperature for at least 20 min.
2. Rehydrate the tissue sections in 1× PBS for 20 min with *gentle* shaking.
3. Wipe off excess PBS on slide using Kimwipes®. Make a hydrophobic barrier around the section tissue with a wax-pen.
4. Add few drops of serum blocking solution on top of the section tissue. Incubate slide in serum blocking solution for 30 min at 37°C in a humidity chamber (see Note7 and 8).
5. Wash slide in 1× PBS twice for 5 min with gentle shaking. Use fresh PBS for each wash.
6. Incubate slide with PECAM-1 primary antibody for 1 h at 37°C in humidity chamber (see Note 9).
7. Wash slide in 1× PBS three times for 3 min with gentle shaking. Use fresh PBS for each wash.

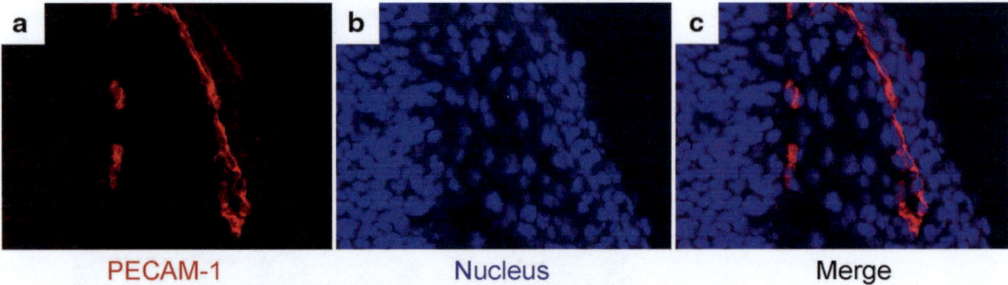

Fig. 2. PECAM-1 and Hoechst 33258 staining on the section of E9.5 embryo. (**a**) PECAM-1 staining on E9.5 embryonic brain section and showed well-developed blood vessels. (**b**) Hoechst 33258 staining of nuclei and (**c**) is a merged picture.

8. Incubate slide with immunofluorescence secondary antibody for 1 h at 37°C in a humidity chamber. Make 1:100 dilution of secondary antibody in PBS. Keep samples in the dark hereafter.
9. Wash slide in 1× PBS three times for 3 min. Use fresh PBS for each wash.
10. Counterstain with Hoechst 33342 for 1 min.
11. Wash slide in 1× PBS twice for 2 min.
12. Add several drops of anti-fade medium to cover the tissue.
13. Put a cover slide on top of tissue section and seal the edge of cover slide with nail polish.
14. Cover the slide with Aluminum Foil and visualize the staining by fluorescence microscopy immediately (Fig. 2).

4. Notes

1. The humidity chamber can be made using a plastic container with a lid. Put a small tube rack or a block inside the plastic container. Apply few layers of towel tissue over the rack. Wet the tissue with water and close the lid.
2. 4% Paraformaldehyde should be made fresh every time. Alternatively, you can make a batch and then aliquot smaller volumes and store at −20°C. The volume of 4% Paraformaldehyde should be 10× the volume of the embryos for proper fixation.
3. Samples can be stored at −20°C for prolonged periods (>1 year) in 100% Methanol.
4. The staining process can be stopped at this step if desirable. Leave embryos at −20°C in 100% Methanol.
5. We have tried PECAM-1 antibodies from different companies and found anti-mouse PECAM (CD31) from BD Pharmingen (Cat: 553370) to work the best.

6. After adding the immunofluorescence-labeled secondary antibody, the following steps should be handled under low light intensity to avoid loss of fluorescence signals due to irreversible photobleaching processes.
7. It is recommended to use serum from the same species as that which the secondary antibody was produced from (in order to block nonspecific binding). For example, if the secondary antibody is anti-mouse antibody, the first choice of serum blocking solution should be mouse serum. Otherwise, donkey or goat serum is an option. Make sure the tissue section is completely covered by serum blocking solution.
8. From this point on, it is very important to prevent the tissue from drying out at any point during the whole staining process. Check the humidity of the humidity chamber each time before putting the slide in. Add enough water in the humidity chamber to make sure the towel tissue will not dry out during incubation. Carefully put the slide on top of the wet towel tissue and cover the plastic box with foil after adding the immunofluorescence-labeled secondary antibody.
9. Make fresh antibody dilutions for each experiment. Make 1:100 dilution with 1× PBS or serum blocking solution that was used in step 4. If serum blocking solution has been used to make the primary antibody dilution, step 5 washing can be skipped. That means, after step 4, aspirate the serum blocking solution and then add serum-diluted primary antibody directly to the tissue section. If the fluorescence signal is weak after staining, try incubating with primary antibody overnight at 4°C in the humidity chamber.

Acknowledgment

This work was supported by American Heart Association Scientist Development Grant and Texas A&M Health Science Center Startup Grant to Xu Peng.

References

1. Beck, L., Jr., and D'Amore, P. A. (1997) Vascular development: cellular and molecular regulation, *FASEB J 11*, 365–373.
2. Jain, R. K., Schlenger, K., Hockel, M., and Yuan, F. (1997) Quantitative angiogenesis assays: progress and problems, *Nat Med 3*, 1203–1208.
3. Auerbach, R., Lewis, R., Shinners, B., Kubai, L., and Akhtar, N. (2003) Angiogenesis assays: a critical overview, *Clin Chem 49*, 32–40.
4. Staton, C. A., Reed, M. W., and Brown, N. J. (2009) A critical analysis of current in vitro and in vivo angiogenesis assays, *Int J Exp Pathol 90*, 195–221.
5. Gordon, M. S., Mendelson, D. S., and Kato, G. Tumor angiogenesis and novel antiangiogenic strategies, *Int J Cancer 126*, 1777–1787.

Chapter 9

Miniaturized Assays of Angiogenesis In Vitro

May J. Reed and Robert B. Vernon

Abstract

Assays of angiogenesis in vitro provide insights into vascular development and are useful in studies of agents that modulate blood vessel formation. This chapter describes techniques to induce angiogenesis-like sprouting from aortic and microvascular explants cultured in 3-dimensional native collagen gels. The chapter focuses on explants derived from mice and use of a miniaturized format that permits efficient utilization of reagents, ease of processing, rapid analysis, and conventional imaging.

Key words: Mice, Fat, Microvessels, Aorta, Rings, Angiogenesis, 3D, Collagen

1. Introduction

Angiogenesis, which is the generation of new vasculature from preexisting blood vessels, is a critical component of normal reparative processes such as wound healing and pathological processes that include diabetes, scleroderma, and cancer. Models of angiogenesis in vitro have proven useful in studies of vascular morphogenesis and age-related changes in neovascularization, and also as assays to screen compounds for therapeutic regulation of blood vessel growth. The generation of blood vessel (capillary)-like structures in vitro occurs best in 3-dimensional (3D) extracellular matrix (ECM) gels comprised of collagen, fibrin, or basement membrane material that simulate the connective tissue environment in vivo. Typical models utilize either isolated, cultured endothelial cells (ECs) or vascular explants as starting material. The latter are comprised of segments of macro- or microvessels that contain an endothelium and associated supportive (mural) cells.

3D ECM-based models utilizing isolated ECs can generate credible vascular structures. For example, human umbilical vein

Xu Peng and Marc Antonyak (eds.), *Cardiovascular Development: Methods and Protocols*, Methods in Molecular Biology, vol. 843, DOI 10.1007/978-1-61779-523-7_9,

ECs (HUVECs) dispersed in type I collagen gels can be reliably induced to develop tubes with wide, patent lumens that closely resemble capillaries in vivo (1, 2). Like HUVECs, adult human microvascular ECs, under specific conditions of stimulus, can also develop into tubular structures with patent lumens (3). Models that incorporate isolated ECs are used widely, but have been criticized on the basis that their genesis of capillary-like structures is more representative of early embryonic vasculogenesis rather than true angiogenesis, which requires a "parent" blood vessel as the source of new sprouts. This potential shortcoming has been addressed by the development of 3D ECM-based models that induce sprout formation from explanted vascular segments. Substantial success has been achieved using explants of adipose tissue-derived microvessels and aortae from rats (4–11). However, the multiplicity of powerful genetic tools developed for mice has provided a strong incentive to devise models of angiogenesis that use aortae and microvasculature explanted from mice (12–15).

Vascular explants, by virtue of their shape and volume, require a 3D ECM gel in which to sprout. A form of ECM used frequently for in vitro culture systems is native type I collagen extracted from bovine dermis or the tail tendons of rats (16–18). In addition to these sources of type I collagen (which are available commercially and are relatively affordable), a growing interest in studying angiogenesis in mice has led to the use of 3D gels of mouse type I collagen as supports for mouse ECs or vascular explants. Although commercial sources of murine collagen exist, it is currently more cost-effective for the investigator to prepare their own extracts. Therefore, methods for extraction of native type I collagen from mouse tails are outlined in Subheading 3.3.

In addition to considerations regarding the sources of cellular starting material and ECM, there exists the ever-present problem of scarcity and/or expense of bioactive compounds selected for study, which has created the need for angiogenesis assays in miniaturized formats. To address this issue, an EC-based angiogenesis assay was developed in 1999 that utilized rings of nylon mesh to support lenticular collagen gels that were small enough to fit in a standard 96-well assay plate (19). This miniaturized approach was subsequently adapted for use with murine microvascular explants and aortic explants (14), which are the focus of this chapter.

2. Materials

2.1. Murine Microvascular Explants

1. Epididymal fat pads from 3 to 5 mice (6–10 fat pads).
2. 60-mm diameter cell culture dishes.
3. Small dissecting scissors.

4. Dulbecco's Modified Eagle Medium (DMEM) supplemented with antibiotics (100 U/mL penicillin, 100 μg/mL streptomycin, and 0.25 μg/mL amphotericin).
5. Bovine serum albumin.
6. Type II collagenase.
7. Fetal bovine serum.
8. 50-mL Erlenmeyer flask.
9. Disposable plastic syringes (one 10 mL and two 20 mL).
10. Two Swinnex® filter holders (25 mm diameter) (Millipore Corp., Billerica, MA).
11. 30-μm mesh nylon screen (Sefar America, Inc.).
12. 300-μm mesh nylon screen (Millipore Corp.).
13. 18-gauge needles.
14. Centrifuge, rotary incubator/shaker.

2.2. Murine Aortic Explants

1. Mouse aortae, removed surgically.
2. 60-mm diameter cell culture dishes.
3. MCDB 131 medium (Gibco/Invitrogen) supplemented with antibiotics (100 U/mL penicillin, 100 μg/mL streptomycin, and 0.25 μg/mL amphotericin).
4. #20 scalpel blade on a size #4 handle.
5. Coarse-tipped (#1) and fine-tipped (#3, or #5) watchmaker's tweezers.
6. Small dissecting scissors.

2.3. Extraction of Mouse Tail Collagen

1. Isolated, skinned mouse tails (3–5 per preparation).
2. Strong tweezers or hemostat.
3. #10 scalpel blade on a size #3 handle.
4. Small dissecting scissors.
5. 50 mM Tris-buffered saline, pH 7.4–7.6 (TBS).
6. Acetone.
7. 70% isopropanol.
8. 0.05 N acetic acid.
9. Sircol™ Soluble Collagen Assay (Accurate Chemical and Scientific Corp., Westbury, NY).

2.4. Preparation of Collagen Solution for 3D Gels

1. Collagen extract (Subheading 3.3).
2. 10-strength Medium 199 (Gibco/Invitrogen).
3. Dulbecco's Modified Eagle Medium.
4. Fetal bovine serum.
5. 0.1 N HCl or NaOH (for adjustment of pH).

2.5. Fabrication of 3D Collagen Gel Assemblies and Culture of Explants

1. Cold-stamped rings made from nylon (Nitex) mesh (Sefar type 03-100/44) with inner and outer diameters of 3 and 5.6 mm, respectively (Sefar America, Inc.).
2. 60-mm diameter plastic cell culture dishes.
3. Parafilm M™ (for lining the plastic culture dishes) (Pechiney Plastic Packaging, Chicago, IL).
4. Human vascular endothelial growth factor 165 ($VEGF_{165}$) (PeproTech, Rocky Hill, NJ) 10 ng/mL in phosphate-buffered saline (PBS).
5. Filter paper.
6. Mouse tail collagen solution (Subheading 3.4).
7. 96-well cell culture plates.
8. MCDB 131 medium with antibiotics.
9. Fetal bovine serum.

3. Methods

3.1. Murine Microvascular Explants

Typically, murine microvasculature for explants is obtained from masses of highly vascularized fat, such as that surrounding the epididymis (4, 5, 15, 20). Sprout development from these explants is considered to be representative of angiogenesis insofar as there are parent microvessels comprised of ECs and mural cells from which the sprouts emanate. The model is characterized by spontaneous growth in defined media with minimal serum, clear evidence of lumen formation, and an easily quantified sprouting response.

1. To isolate microvessels, epididymal fat pads from 3 to 5 male mice are pooled, gently cut with small dissecting scissors into cubes 1–2 mm on each side, and placed in 20 mL of DMEM containing 2 mg/mL of fatty acid free, low endotoxin, cell culture tested bovine serum albumin, and 2 mg/mL of Type II collagenase prewarmed to 37°C.
2. The suspended fat is placed in a 50-mL Erlenmeyer flask and agitated at 37°C in a rotary incubator/shaker at 120–160 rpm until the fat is digested into a slurry (digestion requires approximately 20–30 min).
3. Blood vessels are separated from adipocytes by centrifuging the mixture at 1,000 × *g* for 5 min (the adipocytes float to the top while the vasculature is pelleted).
4. The vascular pellet is washed by gentle resuspension in 8 mL of DMEM supplemented with 10% fetal bovine serum (FBS) and antibiotics followed by 3 min of centrifugation at 1,000 × *g*. Washing is performed twice.

5. The pellet is then resuspended in 8 mL of DMEM/10% FBS/antibiotics and poured through a 20-mL syringe body fitted with a 25-mm diameter Swinnex filter holder containing a 300-μm mesh nylon screen in order to remove tissue fragments and pieces of large-caliber vasculature.
6. The filtrate, consisting primarily of microvascular segments and single cells, is then passed through a 20-mL syringe body fitted with a 25-mm diameter Swinnex holder containing a 30-μm mesh nylon screen which traps the microvascular segments, but allows single cells to pass through.
7. Subsequently, the microvascular segments are washed from the 30-μm mesh screen into a 60-mm diameter cell culture dish by jets of DMEM/10% FBS/antibiotics delivered from a 10-mL syringe fitted with an 18-gauge needle.
8. Typical isolates consist of 20–40 microvascular segments with lengths of 30–150 μm. The isolated segments are suspended in 3D collagen gels within 30 min, as described in Subheading 3.5 (see Note 1).

3.2. Murine Aortic Explants

Previous studies have shown that explanted segments of rat aortae placed in 3D ECM gels will give rise to arborizing, capillary-like sprouts with an endothelial lining (6–11). Coincident with the use of microvascular explants derived from murine adipose tissue, an ongoing interest in studying genetically modified mice has led to the use of mouse aortic segments as an alternative to rat segments. Under permissive conditions in vitro, mouse aortic segments will generate microvascular sprouts similar to sprouts formed by rat segments (12–14).

1. To obtain aortic segments from mice, the aorta is identified by its location with respect to the heart. The aorta is more easily obtained from the posterior wall of the thoracic cavity after careful removal of the lungs.
2. The aorta is cut at the arch and at its junction with the diaphragm and transferred to a sterile 60-mm diameter cell culture dish containing 5 mL of MCDB 131 medium supplemented with antibiotics.
3. Isolated aortae are rinsed twice with this medium to remove extravasated blood and then are gently cleaned of loose perivascular connective tissue. A complete removal of this connective tissue minimizes fibroblast contamination of the explant.
4. The cleaned aortae are cut transversely with a scalpel (fitted with a #20 blade) into segments 1 mm in length. The cut is made by moving the curved edge of the scalpel blade through the tissue with a single rocking motion, which minimizes damage to the endothelial lining.

5. Subsequently, the aortic segments are rinsed in the MCDB 131 medium and, within 30 min, are placed into 3D collagen gels, as described in Subheading 3.5 (see Note 2).

3.3. Extraction of Collagen from Mouse Tails

Although a variety of ECM hydrogels (type I collagen, fibrin, basement membrane matrix) support vascular sprout formation in vitro, we and others have found that type I collagen extracted from mouse tail tendons is an effective, relatively inexpensive support. Notably, mouse tail collagen permits experimentation in an "all-mouse" system in which the ECM support and vascular explant can be matched syngeneically (21).

1. To prepare collagen extracts, tendons are peeled from the skinned tails of 3–5 mice by pulling the tendons away from the vertebral bodies with a strong tweezers or hemostat while cutting the tendons' connections to the vertebrae with #10 scalpel blade fitted to a #3 handle. More than 3 mice are needed if the animals are greater than 18 months of age.
2. The isolated tendons are pooled, minced with small dissecting scissors, and immersed for sequential, 5-min periods in 50 mM TBS, acetone, and 70% isopropanol.
3. Type I collagen is extracted by stirring the tendons overnight in 50 mL of 0.05 N acetic acid at 4°C.
4. The resulting viscous solution is centrifuged at 4,000 × *g* for 15 min at 4°C to remove insoluble material.
5. Collagen content (which is typically between 1.5 and 2.5 mg/mL) is quantified by the Sircol™ Soluble Collagen Assay. The Sircol assay is specific for collagen and does not detect proteoglycans, elastin, or other ECM components.
6. Collagen extracts should be stored under refrigeration at 4°C, but never frozen.

3.4. Preparation of Collagen Solution for 3D Gels

1. 3D collagen gels are prepared by combining 1 volume of collagen extract (Subheading 3.3), 1/9 volume of 10-strength Medium 199, and sufficient DMEM and FBS to yield a solution with final collagen and FBS concentrations of 1.5 mg/mL and 2.5%, respectively. If necessary, the pH of the collagen solution is adjusted to 7.0–7.2 with 0.1 N HCl or NaOH.
2. The collagen solution is kept on ice prior to dispensing it over ring-shaped supports of nylon mesh, as described in Subheading 3.5.
3. To provide additional buffering capacity, the 10-strength Medium 199 can be supplemented with powdered $NaHCO_3$, added to saturation.

3.5. Fabrication of 3D Gel Assemblies and Culture of Explants

Although there is consensus that 3D ECM gels are optimal for support of angiogenesis in vitro, the fragility of these gels can make analyses (i.e., staining, imaging) problematic. Moreover, gels of relatively large size, which are typically easier to handle and image, are wasteful of scarce and expensive reagents. We have found that explants of murine microvasculature and aortae can be embedded within low-volume (30 μL) 3D collagen gels supported at the edges by rings of nylon mesh. This approach combines the extensive capabilities of the mouse experimental system with a culture method that optimizes specimen handling, staining, and economical use of reagents. Of note, the clear lenticular gels can be imaged by conventional, wide-field microscopy in addition to confocal microscopy.

Assemblies comprised of nylon mesh rings, 3D collagen gels, and vascular explants are prepared as follows:

1. Custom-made, cold-stamped nylon (Nitex) mesh rings (mesh type 03-100/44) with inner and outer diameters of 3 and 5.6 mm, respectively, are placed on 60-mm diameter plastic cell culture dishes lined with UV-sterilized sheets of Parafilm M™ to create a hydrophobic surface.
2. The rings are then flooded with 10 μL of the mouse tail collagen solution described in Subheading 3.4 and the dishes covered with their plastic tops, which are lined with moist filter paper.
3. After 30 min in a tissue culture incubator at 37°C/5%CO_2/100% humidity to gel the collagen, 3–5 microvessels (suspended in a small volume of culture medium) or single aortic segments are placed on the collagen gel, carefully overlaid with an additional 20 μL of the collagen solution, and returned to the incubator for 30 min to gel the collagen overlay.
4. The assemblies are then transferred to 96-well cell culture plates filled with 50 μL (per well) of MCDB 131 medium supplemented with 0–2.5% FBS, and antibiotics. $VEGF_{165}$ added at 10 ng/mL serves as a positive control for induction of vascular growth.
5. After 3–10 days of culture (with media changed every 2 days), the assemblies are rinsed in PBS, fixed 20 min in 10% neutral-buffered formalin (NBF), and stored in PBS prior to analysis (Subheading 3.6).

3.6. Analyses of Sprouts Produced by Microvascular and Aortic Explants

1. Embedded microvascular explants (Fig. 1) give rise to multicellular sprouts after 2–4 days. Emergent single cells are excluded from analysis.
2. Typically, multicellular sprouts grow from embedded aortic segments after 4 days (14) (Fig. 2).
3. After fixation in NBF, the nuclei of sprouts can be labeled with conventional nucleic acid dyes such as DAPI, propidium iodide, or TO-PRO®-3 iodide and their cytoplasm labeled with fluorescent (e.g., Alexa-fluor®)-conjugated phalloidin, which binds to f-actin.

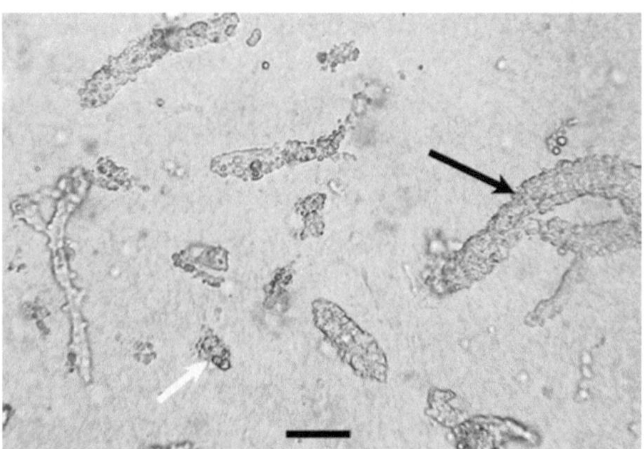

Fig. 1. Murine microvascular segments embedded in a type I collagen gel. This preparation includes segments representing the largest (*black arrow*) and smallest (*white arrow*) examples within the typical range of segment sizes. Scale bar = 50 μm.

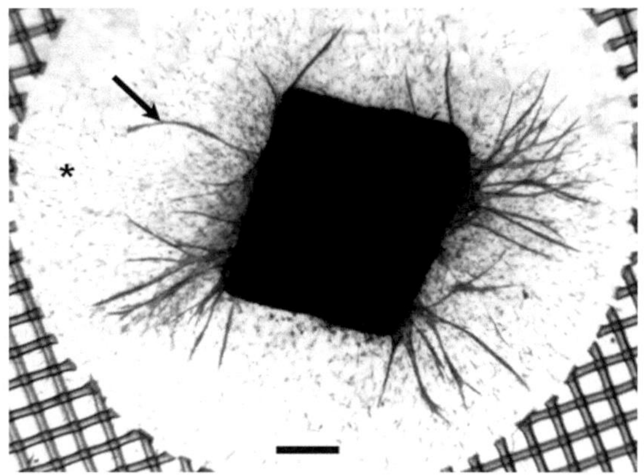

Fig. 2. A murine aortic segment cultured in a type I collagen gel for 7 days has produced a large number of sprouts (e.g., *arrow*). A field of single cells that have migrated from the segment is indicated by the *asterisk*. The supportive ring of nylon mesh can be seen at the periphery of the image. Scale bar = 200 μm.

4. After labeling, the 3D gel assemblies are mounted on slides and coverslipped using a photo-bleach resistive mountant, such as Vecta-Shield®.
5. The nylon mesh rings of the assemblies act as spacers that allow the collagen gels to be flattened slightly between the slide and coverslip, but not crushed. Consequently, the assemblies remain intact and can be demounted from the slides (several times, if necessary for washing and restaining) by immersing the slides on edge in PBS until the coverslips slide off.
6. As an alternative to imaging by fluorescence, fixed sprout preparations can be visualized by staining with a general protein stain,

such as 2% crystal violet for 10 min followed by multiple washes in PBS or TBS until the collagen gels became transparent.

7. Sprout formation from labeled preparations can be quantified by use of MetaMorph® (Molecular Devices, Sunnyvale, CA) or other image analysis software according to parameters of cell number, lumen diameter, and the number and length of primary, secondary, tertiary, and quaternary branches.
8. Measurements can be made using wide-field microscopy; however, greater discrimination, particularly with respect to luminal morphology, can be achieved by measurement of z-stacked images taken with a confocal microscope.
9. ECs can be distinguished from mural cells by uptake of DiI-acetylated low-density lipoprotein or by immunofluorescence with anti-CD31/PECAM antibodies.
10. Mural cells can be identified by their negativity for endothelial markers or by positive immunofluorescence for alpha smooth muscle actin.

3.7. Summary

In vitro models of angiogenesis within miniaturized, 3D ECM supports permit efficient visualization and measurement of vascular growth. Explanted microvessels or aortic segments obtained from mice of different ages or genetic backgrounds can act as parent blood vessels for angiogenesis-like sprout formation. 3D angiogenic models can be used to evaluate a multiplicity of factors that could regulate sprouting, including: (1) specific gene products expressed by ECs and/or mural cells, (2) the composition and physical characteristics of the surrounding ECM, and (3) exogenously added drugs, biological agents, or other chemical compounds with the potential to promote or inhibit angiogenesis.

4. Notes

1. *Murine microvascular explants*: Successful isolation of microvascular explants (Subheading 3.1) involves a number of factors, which include the initial size range of the cubed epididymal fat, specific activity of the Type II collagenase, and the time, temperature, and degree of agitation during digestion. Microvessels will not be released from under-digested fat, whereas over-digestion will result in fragile microvessels that will disintegrate during the washing and filtration steps. Even if isolation is successful, over-digested microvessels may die in culture. Establishing the optimal conditions for digestion that result in collection of viable microvessels requires a certain amount of trial and error.

2. *Murine aortic explants*: As mentioned in Subheading 3.2, the freshly isolated aortae should be gently cleaned of loose perivascular connective tissue prior to being cut into short segments for embedment in collagen. Removal of connective tissue can be accomplished by a combination of two techniques, which involve (1) holding the aorta at one end with a relatively coarse-tipped (e.g., a #1) watchmaker's tweezer and pulling the tags of connective tissue away with a fine-tipped (e.g., #3 or #5) tweezer held in the opposite hand, and (2) holding the aorta at one end with the coarse-tipped tweezer and using a small dissecting scissors to trim the connective tissue away. Scissors with the blades set at an angle to the handle are particularly useful, as the angle allows the blades to be brought parallel to the aorta for a close cut that removes superficial tissue without penetrating the aortic wall. After the aorta is cleaned of connective tissue, the portion of the aorta held by the coarse tweezer (which is usually crushed) can be trimmed away and discarded.

3. *Preparation of collagen solution for 3D gels*: Collagen extracts of mouse tail tendons (Subheading 3.3) and similar, commercial extracts of rat tail tendons or bovine dermis are comprised primarily of native collagen monomers. Adjustment of these extracts to physiological ionic strength and pH, followed by heating to 37°C (Subheadings 3.4, steps 1 and 3.5, step 3), causes the monomers to assemble spontaneously into long, banded fibrils 70–100 nm in diameter. Collectively, these fibrils form a meshwork with the physical properties of a malleable but dimensionally stable hydrogel. To avoid premature polymerization, it is important to chill all of the components of the collagen solution on ice prior to combining them and to keep the resultant mixture on ice prior to dispensing it onto the nylon mesh supports. Best results are obtained when the DMEM, 10-strength Medium 199, and FBS are combined first and the acidic collagen extract added last. All components should be combined in a centrifuge tube and mixed slowly by hand by rocking the tube end-over-end 5–8 times. Vortexers or magnetic stir bar-type mixers should be avoided, as energetic mixing can cause the collagen monomers to quickly precipitate into a whitish, amorphous mass. In addition, overmixing—even gently—can cause the collagen to polymerize rapidly into clumps of short fibrils, resulting in a weak, paste-like gel of diminished clarity. The tendency for premature polymerization, precipitation, and clumping of collagen fibrils is increased in solutions that are excessively basic; therefore, it is important to adjust the pH to no higher than 7.2.

4. *Fabrication of nylon mesh rings*: As mentioned in Subheading 3.5, small rings of nylon mesh are used to support the collagen gel. Custom-made rings are prepared commercially either by

cold-stamping with a sharp-edged punch or by laser-cutting. In our experience, we prefer cold-stamped rings to laser-cut rings, as the former have clean, incised edges, whereas the latter have melted edges of greater irregularity. Commercially made rings are relatively expensive, but provide a highly uniform product and save the investigator the time required for fabrication by hand. However, to limit expense, rings can be cut out of bulk nylon mesh (available from Sefar America or McMaster-Carr, Inc., Santa Fe Springs, CA) using disposable 3- and 6-mm biopsy punches (Thermo Fisher Scientific, Inc., Waltham, MA) for the inner and outer diameters, respectively. Alternatively, small rectangular frames can be cut out from bulk mesh using hobby knives or #11 scalpel blades and printed paper templates generated with Microsoft PowerPoint or Adobe Photoshop.

Acknowledgments

We thank Mamatha Damodarasamy, MS for assistance with the manuscript. We also acknowledge the following grant support: NIH grants R01 AG015837 and R21 AG024458 (MJR) and R21 EB005652 (RBV).

References

1. Davis, G.E., and Camarillo, C.W. (1996) An alpha 2 beta 1 integrin-dependent pinocytic mechanism involving intracellular vacuole formation and coalescence regulates capillary lumen and tube formation in three-dimensional collagen matrix. Exp Cell Res 224: 39–51.
2. Montesano, R., Kumar, S., Orci, L., and Pepper, M.S. (1996) Synergistic effect of hyaluronan oligosaccharides and vascular endothelial growth factor on angiogenesis in vitro. Lab Invest 75: 249–262.
3. Koike, T., Vernon, R.B., Gooden, M.D., Sadoun, E., and Reed, M.J. (2003) Inhibited angiogenesis in aging: a role for TIMP-2. J Gerontol A Biol Sci Med Sci 58: B798–805.
4. Wagner, R.C., and Matthews, M.A. (1975) The isolation and culture of capillary endothelium from epididymal fat. Microvasc Res 10: 286–297.
5. Hoying, J.B., Boswell, C.A., and Williams, S.K. (1996) Angiogenic potential of microvessel fragments established in three-dimensional collagen gels. In Vitro Cell Dev Biol Anim 32: 409–419.
6. Nicosia, R.F., Chao, R., and Leighton, J. (1982) Histotypic angiogenesis in vitro: light microscopic, ultrastructural, and radioautographic studies. In Vitro 18: 538–549.
7. Mori, M., Sadahira, Y., Kawasaki, S., Hayashi, T., Notohara, K., and Awai, M. (1988) Capillary growth from reversed rat aortic segments cultured in collagen gel. Acta Pathol Jpn, 38: 1503–1512.
8. Diglio, C.A., Grammas, P., Giacomelli, F., Wiener, J. (1989) Angiogenesis in rat aorta ring explant cultures. Lab Invest 60: 523–531.
9. Nicosia, R.F., and Ottinetti, A. (1990) Growth of microvessels in serum-free matrix culture of rat aorta. A quantitative assay of angiogenesis in vitro. Lab Invest, 63: 115–122.
10. Nicosia, R.F., Bonanno, E., and Villaschi, S. Large-vessel endothelium switches to a microvascular phenotype during angiogenesis in collagen gel culture of rat aorta (1992). Atherosclerosis 95: 191–199.
11. Zhu, W.H., and Nicosia, R.F. (2002) The thin prep rat aortic ring assay: a modified method for the characterization of angiogenesis in whole mounts. Angiogenesis 5: 81–86.
12. Masson, V.V., Devy, L., Grignet-Debrus, C., Bernt, S., Bajou, K., Blacher, S., Roland, G., Chang, Y., Fong, T., Carmeliet, P., Foidart,

J.M., and Noe, A. (2002) Mouse Aortic Ring Assay: A New Approach of the Molecular Genetics of Angiogenesis. Biol Proced Online 4: 24–31.

13. Zhu, W.H., Iurlaro, M., MacIntyre, A. Fogel, E., and Nicosia, R.F. (2003) The mouse aorta model: influence of genetic background and aging on bFGF- and VEGF-induced angiogenic sprouting. Angiogenesis 6: 193–199.
14. Reed, M.J., Karres, N., Eyman, D., and Vernon, R.B. (2007) Culture of murine aortic explants in 3-dimensional extracellular matrix: A novel, miniaturized assay of angiogenesis in vitro. Microvasc Res.73:248–252
15. Nunes, S.S., Greer, K.A., Stiening, C.M., Chen, H.Y., Kidd, K.R., Schwartz, M.A., Sullivan, C.J., Rekapally, H., and Hoying, J.B. (2010) Implanted microvessels progress through distinct neovascularization phenotypes. Microvasc Res 79: 10–20.
16. Chandrakasan, G., Torchia, D.A., Piez, and K.A. (1976) Preparation of intact monomeric collagen from rat tail tendon and skin and the structure of the nonhelical ends in solution. J Biol Chem 251: 6062–6067.
17. Abrass, C.K., and Berfield, A.K. (1995) Phenotypic modulation of rat glomerular visceral epithelial cells by culture substratum. J Am Soc Nephrol 5: 1591–1599.
18. Rajan, N., Habermehl, J., Cote, M.F., Doillon, C.J., and Mantovani, D. (2006) Preparation of ready-to-use, storable and reconstituted type I collagen from rat tail tendon for tissue engineering applications. Nat Protoc 1: 2753–2758.
19. Vernon, R.B., and Sage, E.H. (1999) A novel, quantitative model for study of endothelial cell migration and sprout formation within three-dimensional collagen matrices. Microvasc Res 57: 118–133.
20. Krishnan, L., and Hoying, J.B. Nguyen H Song H Weiss JA (2007) Interaction of angiogenic microvessels with the extracellular matrix. Am J Physiol Heart Circ Physiol 293: H3650–3658.
21. Damodarasamy, M., Vernon, R.B., Karres, N., Chang, C.H., and Bianchi-Frias, D., Nelson, P.S., and Reed, M.J. (2010) Collagen extracts derived from young and aged mice demonstrate different structural properties and cellular effects in three-dimensional gels. J Gerontol A Biol Sci Med Sci 65: 209–218.

Part II

Cell and Molecular Biology Methods

Chapter 10

Analysis of the Endocardial-to-Mesenchymal Transformation of Heart Valve Development by Collagen Gel Culture Assay

Yiqin Xiong, Bin Zhou, and Ching-Pin Chang

Abstract

Malformations of heart valves are one of the most common serious congenital defects. Heart valves are developed from endocardial cushions of the heart. The endocardial cushion in early heart development consists of two cell layers: an outer myocardial cell layer and an inner endocardial cell layer with abundant extracellular matrix (cardiac jelly) in between. Endocardial cells of the cushion, triggered by signals from myocardial cells, delaminate from the surface of the endocardial cushion and undergo transdifferentiation into mesenchymal cells. This process of endocardial-to-mesenchymal transformation (EMT) begins in the atrioventricular canal at embryonic day 9 (E9) and in the cardiac outflow tract at E10 of mouse development. Once formed by the EMT, the mesenchymal cells invade the cardiac jelly, proliferate, and populate the endocardial cushion. The cellularized endocardial cushion then undergoes morphological remodeling; it lengthens and matures into a thin elongated valve leaflet. Here we describe a method to culture endocardial cushions and measure EMT ex vivo. EMT can thus be analyzed independent of other concurrent developmental defects in mice. This culture method also enables ex vivo manipulations of signaling or gene function during EMT to delineate molecular pathways essential for heart valve development.

Key words: Heart valve, Endocardial-to-mesenchymal transformation, Endocardial cushion, Heart development, Atrioventricular canal, Cardiac outflow tract

1. Introduction

Heart valve malformations occur in at least 2–3% of the population (6). Severe valve anomalies cause serious illness in infants and children. Milder forms of valve defects do not produce disease until adulthood, when they generate significant morbidity and mortality. Studies of heart valve development are thus important in

Xu Peng and Marc Antonyak (eds.), *Cardiovascular Development: Methods and Protocols*, Methods in Molecular Biology, vol. 843, DOI 10.1007/978-1-61779-523-7_10,

understanding congenital valve diseases that are prevalent in both the pediatric and adult population.

Endocardial cushions in the developing heart are where prospective valves are formed. Endocardial cushions also regulate the septation of atrioventricular (AV) canal and cardiac outflow tract (OFT). Therefore, cushion malformations can cause heart valve abnormalities, AV septal defects, and cardiac OFT anomalies. These cushion defects are characteristic of Trisomy 21 or Down syndrome, the leading cause of congenital heart disease (7). Cellularization of the endocardial cushion initiates heart valve morphogenesis and occurs in early embryogenesis through endocardial-to-mesenchymal transformation (EMT) (1–5). This EMT process can be studied by an ex vivo assay, where endocardial cushions are cultured on collagen gels that provide the extracellular matrix for EMT and subsequent mesenchymal cell growth and invasion. This collagen gel culture assay consists of four major steps: collagen gel preparation, harvest of embryos at the appropriate age, explantation and culture of endocardial cushions, and quantitation of EMT.

2. Materials

2.1. Instruments/Equipment

1. Dissecting microscope.
2. Dissecting forceps.
3. Plastic pipettes.
4. Petri dishes.
5. MutiDish 4 well, Nunclon Sterile or other 96-well tissue culture plates.
6. Tissue culture incubator.

2.2. Media and Reagents

1. Dissecting medium: 1× OptiMEM-I medium (Gibco Invitrogen, Carlsbad, CA), kept at 4°C or on ice.
2. Culture medium: 1× OptiMEM-I medium, 1% of fetal calf serum, 100 U/mL of penicillin, and 100 μg/mL of streptomycin, kept at 4°C.
3. Collagen Type I (Rat Tail)(BD Biosciences, Bedford, MA), stored at 4°C. It is stable for at least 3 months or longer.
4. NaOH: 1 N stock, kept in a glass container at 4°C.
5. Phosphate buffered saline (PBS), kept at room temperature.

3. Methods

3.1. Collagen Gel Preparation

1. The type I rat-tail collagen stock (approximately 4 mg/mL, see Note 1) is diluted with 1× PBS and buffered with 1 N NaOH to a final concentration of 1 mg/mL collagen with 2 mM NaOH in PBS. For 8 wells of Nucleon plates, prepare a 5-mL solution containing 3.75 mL of PBS, 1.25 mL of liquid rat-tail collagen (4 mg/mL), and 10 μL of 1 N NaOH (see Note 2) at room temperature in the tissue culture hood.
2. Dispense 600 μL of the collagen solution to each well of the Nuclon plate, and incubate in 5% CO_2 at 37°C for 1–3 h for the liquid collagen to solidify.
3. After the collagen gel forms at 37°C, gently pipette off the residual solution on top of the gel and rinse the gel once with prewarmed or room-temperature OptiMEM-I (see Note 3).
4. Rinse the well by gently filling with 300–500 μL of OptiMEM-I and then pipette off the media.
5. Soak the gel with the culture media by filling the well with 300–500 μL of prewarmed or room-temperature culture media (see Note 3), and then incubate the gel at 37°C. After 2–4 h of incubation, the collagen gel is ready for use (see Note 4).
6. Remove the culture media from the gel by pipetting before harvesting the embryos or explanting the endocardial cushion (see Note 5). The gel should be dried as much as possible so that explanted cushions can adhere to the gel without floating.

3.2. Harvest of Embryos

For AV cushion studies, E9.0-E9.5 embryos with 15–25 pairs of somites are harvested from the deciduas in cold PBS. For OFT cushion studies, E10.5 embryos with approximately 35 pairs of somites are harvested. After the harvesting, all embryos are transferred to a petri dish containing cold OptiMEM-I and placed on ice, while endocardial cushions of the embryos are explanted one by one. The cover lid of the petri dish can be used for dissecting the endocardial cushions (see below).

3.3. Explantation and Culture of the Atrioventricular Cushion

Endocardial cushions are explanted by a method that we designed and termed "drop dissection" technique, where the embryos and the hearts are dissected within a drop of water (or media) (Fig. 1). The surface tension of water molecules in the small drop helps to anchor the embryos and hearts to facilitate the dissection of AV or OFT cushions.

1. Transfer the embryo from the petri dish above by a plastic pipette along with a drop of cold OptiMEM-1 on to a dry cover lid of a petri dish (see Note 6).
2. Dissect the embryo within the medium drop with two pairs of forceps.

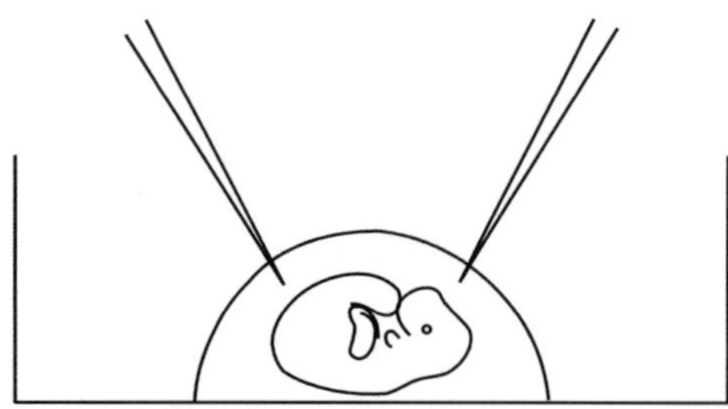

Fig. 1. Schematic illustration of the drop dissection technique.

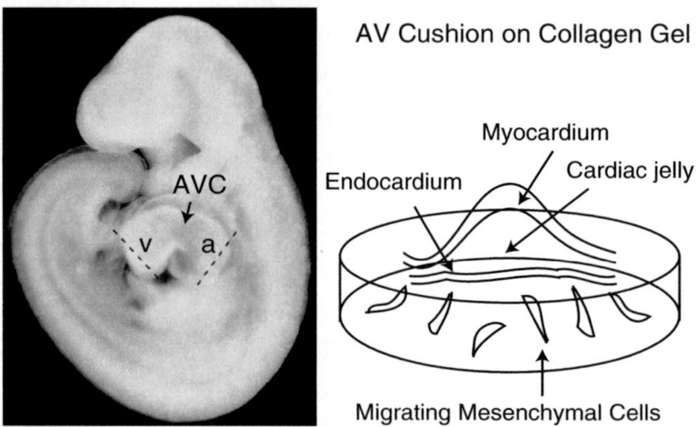

Fig. 2. Lateral view of an E9.5 mouse embryo and the collagen gel culture assay. The *dash lines* indicate the dissection planes at the atrial and ventricular sides of the atrioventricular canal (AVC). *a* atrium; *v* ventricle. The *right* panel illustrates an AV cushion cultured on the collagen gel and the formation of mesenchymal cells.

3. Remove the pericardial sac.
4. Cut the heart with the forceps at two points to release the AV canal from the heart—one at the mid left ventricular level, and the other at mid-atrial or atrial-sinus venosus junction (Fig. 2, dash lines) (see Note 7).
5. Trim the heart explant at the mid-atrial level with the forceps in the same drop of medium (see Note 8). Keep the atrial and ventricular stumps of the explant to protect the endocardial cushion from damage.
6. Gently slice the AV canal with one arm of the forceps along the fissure between the two halves of the endocardial cushion (see Note 9). This fissure is visible under the dissecting microscope. The slicing should extend gently from the ventricular to the atrial side of the AV canal without touching the endocardial cushion.
7. Use the forceps to grasp the ventricular stump of the AV canal and gently pull the explant from the medium drop.

8. Transfer the explant onto the collagen gel surface (see Note 10). Place 3–5 cushion explants in each well of the Nucleon plate.
9. Place the endocardial side of the AV cushion in direct contact with the collagen gel surface. If necessary, flip the AV canal to place the endocardial side onto the gel (see Note 11).
10. Allow the cushion explant to "adhere" to the gel for 1–3 h in incubation at 37°C before adding the media or any pharmacologic agent.
11. Add 60 μL of culture media (prewarmed or at room temperature) to each well of collagen gel (see Note 12). For pharmacologic treatment, add 60 μL of the drug prepared at 10× concentration in the culture media to each well. Since each well contains 600 μL of collagen gel, the drug concentration becomes 1× after equilibration within the porous gel.
12. Incubate the cushion explants in 5% CO_2 at 37°C for 24–48 h. EMT generally takes place within that time window.

3.4. Explantation and Culture of the OFT Cushion

1. Cut the heart with forceps at two points—one at the junction of OFT and the ventricle; the other at an anatomic bend in mid-OFT that separates the distal (truncus) from the proximal (conus) OFT (Fig. 3)—to release the proximal OFT cushion where EMT takes place (see Note 13).
2. Gently slice the proximal OFT cushion with the forceps along the fissure between two adjacent halves of the cushion.
3. Use the forceps to grab the ventricular stump of the explant, pull the explant from the medium drop, and place it onto the collagen gel with the endocardium facing down. Four cushion explants can be plated in each well of the Nucleon for incubation.

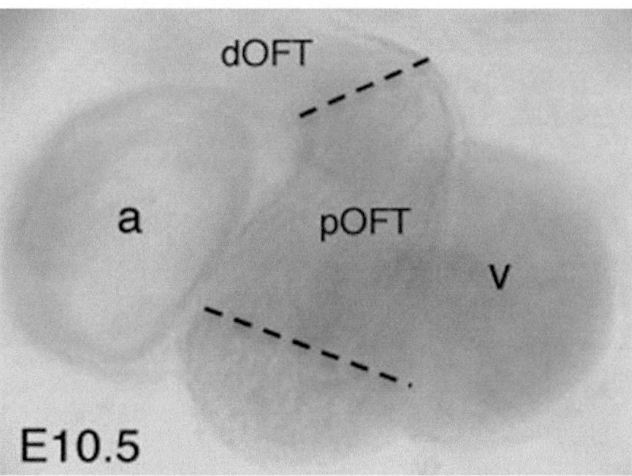

Fig. 3. Frontal view of an E10.5 heart. The *dash lines* indicates the dissection planes for the isolation of proximal cardiac outflow tract (pOFT) or conus. *a* atrium; *v* ventricle; *dOFT* distal outflow tract or truncus.

4. Incubate the explants in 5% CO_2 at 37°C for 24–48 h. EMT generally takes place within that time window.

3.5. Quantitation of the EMT

After 24–48 h of incubation, mesenchymal cells migrating from the endocardial cushions are counted using an inverted microscope that allows focusing on the mesenchymal cells present on different planes of the collagen gel (Fig. 4). Mesenchymal cells are identified by their elongated or spindle-shaped morphology, distinct from the round endocardial cells (3) (Fig. 4). A single cushion explant gives rise to approximately 40–80 (AV cushion) or 10–30 (OFT cushion) mesenchymal cells within 24 h. The number of mesenchymal cells usually doubles every 24 h in the first 2–3 days of culture (see Note 14), but the mesenchymal cell number could vary by up to twofolds among the control explants, depending on the exact age of embryos harvested and the consistency of the explantation technique.

Wild-type littermate cushion explants are used for internal control in the EMT assay. The mean number of mesenchymal cells of all explants in the control group (N > 3–5) is set to represent a 100% degree of EMT. The degree of EMT of given explant is then defined by the explant's mesenchymal cell number relative to the mean in the control group. For example, if an explant gives 40 mesenchymal cells, and the control group has a mean of 80 cells, this explant has 50% EMT (40 divided by 80). Each explant in the control and study group will therefore have a number representing the degree of its EMT. Variations of the EMT among different cushion explants

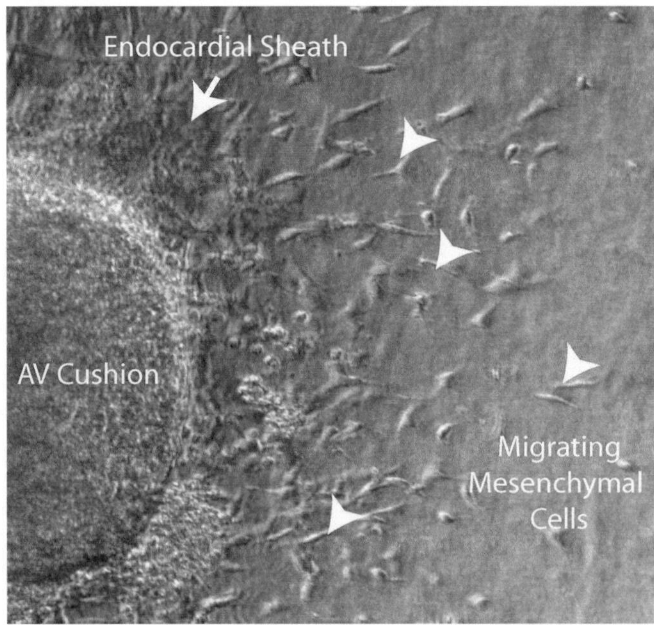

Fig. 4. Atrioventricular cushion (AV cushion) 24–30 h after collagen gel culture. An endocardial cell sheath is formed (*arrow*) around the endocardial cushion, and spindle-shaped mesenchymal cells (*arrowheads*) migrate from the AV cushion into the collagen gel.

within the control or study group are then measured by the standard deviation of the degree of EMT of these explants. Statistical analysis, such as Student's *t*-test, can be applied to compare the difference in the degree of EMT between the control and study group.

4. Notes

1. Each lot of rat tail collagen has different concentrations. Prepare your collagen solution to a final concentration of 1 mg/mL. However, if the collagen does not solidify well or if the gel is fragile, you can increase the collagen concentration or adjust the pH for the gel preparation.
2. When preparing the 5 mL collagen solution, we add 10 μL of NaOH (1 N) to the side of 15-mL falconer tube, followed by 3.75 mL of PBS and then 1.25 mL of liquid collagen. Mix the solution by gently swirling the falconer tube. The stock of NaOH, which erodes plastic containers, should be kept in a glass bottle.
3. Gently add the media to the side of the well to fill the well. Dropping media directly on the gel will break the gel. Cold media may dissolve the gel.
4. We usually prepare the collagen gel one day before the experiment and leave the gel soaked with the culture media in the tissue culture incubator at 37°C overnight. Collagen gels soaked with culture media can be kept at 37°C in the incubator for 2–4 weeks. However, we generally use freshly prepared or up to 3–4-day-old collagen gels for EMT assays.

   Alternatively, gel can be prepared as follows: The type I rat tail collagen maintains as liquid due to its acidic pH. To make a 10-mL solid collagen gel (1 mg/mL, final concentration), 3 mL of liquid collagen (3.33 mg/mL) is first mixed with 1 mL of 10× OptiMEM-I medium, 0.1 mL of 100% fetal calf serum, and 0.1 mL of 100× penicillin & streptomycin on ice. The acidic collagen mixture is then neutralized with 0.3 mL of 2.2% $NaHCO_3$ (1/10 of original gel volume) and immediately dispense to 4-well Nucleon plates (300 μL/well). The plates are then let sit in the culture hood without disturbing. This step allows solidification of the collagen gel in 20–30 min. Afterwards, the gel is preincubated with culture media containing 1× OptiMEM-I medium, 1% fetal calf serum, and 1× penicillin & streptomycin in 5% CO_2 at 37°C for 1 h before use.
5. When removing the excess media, slant the Nucleon plate slightly in one direction to pool the media to the side of the well and then pipette off the media against the side. This avoids breaking the soft collagen gel. Repeat this procedure a few times by slanting the plate in different directions and then pipetting off the residual fluid.

6. Plastic pipettes are cut at the mouth by a pair of scissors to create an opening large enough for transferring an E9.5 or E10.5 embryo. Also, each cover lid of a petri dish is good for the dissection of multiple embryos as long as the medium drops are separate from each other. One lid is usually sufficient for dissecting one litter of embryos.
7. During the dissection, it is important not to damage the endocardial cushion. The best way is not to touch the endocardial cushion at all. Use two pairs of forceps to separate the AV canal from the heart at the mid-atrial and mid-ventricular level. The inclusion of flanking atrial and ventricular tissues in the explants ensures that the entire endocardial cushion is isolated intact without damage.
8. Too much residual atrial tissue hinders the transfer of AV canal out of the media drop since the surface tension of water molecules pulls the floppy atria back to the media. This may break the AV canal. However, too little atrial tissue renders the AV canal “unprotected” because the canal will be directly pulled by the surface tension and the forceps in opposite directions.
9. When slicing the AV canal, use one forceps to anchor the explant by pressing its ventricular stump against the lid (keep this hand stationery), and then use one arm of the other forceps as a knife to slice along the fissure in the AV canal. This opens up the AV canal and exposes the endocardial cushion. Try not to touch the cushion.
10. After pulling the explant out of the media drop, wait for a few seconds and let the excess media on the forceps to drip before placing the explant onto the gel. This avoids wetting the gel. If the gel becomes too wet, remove the excess media by pipetting (see Note 5); otherwise, the explant may float in the media without adhering to the gel. In an experienced hand, the entire procedure—from embryo harvest, cushion explantation to explant placement on the gel—can be completed within an hour for one litter of embryos.
11. A small hole can be dug in the gel with a pair of forceps. The hole can hold parts of the explant and serve as a fulcrum to facilitate the flipping of the endocardial cushion. After flipping, nudge the cushion to the smoother part of the gel surface for culturing.
12. When adding the media to the well, do not flush the cushions. Add the media dropwise at multiple points adjacent to the cushion explants or along the side wall of the well.
13. The mesenchyme of the proximal OFT (conal cushion) arises from EMT, whereas that of the distal OFT (truncal cushion) is derived from neural crest cells. It is therefore critical to separate the proximal from the distal OFT, and only use the

proximal OFT for EMT assays. EMT assays using the entire OFT will be confounded by migratory neural crest cells.

14. After 48 h of incubation, mesenchymal cells invade deeper into the gel, are present at many different planes, and their number may increase to several hundreds, making an accurate determination of the mesenchymal cell number challenging. Also, the longer mesenchymal cells are cultured on the gel, the more their number depends on the proliferation of mesenchymal cells rather than the EMT process alone. Therefore, quantitation of EMT should be performed within the first 24–48 h after explantation.

Acknowledgments

C.P.C. is supported by funds from National Institute of Health (NIH), March of Dimes Foundation, Children's Heart Foundation, Office of the University of California (TRDRP), American Heart Association (AHA), California Institute of Regenerative Medicine, Kaiser Foundation, Baxter Foundation, Oak Foundation, and Stanford Cardiovascular Institute; Y.X. by fellowships from the Oak foundation, AHA, and the Lucile Packard Pediatric Research Fund Award; B.Z. by NIH and AHA.

References

1. Eisenberg, L. M., and Markwald, R. R. (1995) Molecular regulation of atrioventricular valvuloseptal morphogenesis. *Circ Res 77*, 1–6.
2. Zhou, B., Wu, B., Tompkins, K. L., Boyer, K. L., Grindley, J. C., and Baldwin, H. S. (2005) Characterization of Nfatc1 regulation identifies an enhancer required for gene expression that is specific to pro-valve endocardial cells in the developing heart. *Development 132*, 1137–46.
3. Chang, C. P., Neilson, J. R., Bayle, J. H., Gestwicki, J. E., Kuo, A., Stankunas, K., Graef, I. A., and Crabtree, G. R. (2004) A field of myocardial-endocardial NFAT signaling underlies heart valve morphogenesis. *Cell 118*, 649–63.
4. Mjaatvedt, C. H., and Markwald, R. R. (1989) Induction of an epithelial-mesenchymal transition by an in vivo adheron-like complex. *Dev Biol 136*, 118–28.
5. Lakkis, M. M., and Epstein, J. A. (1998) Neurofibromin modulation of ras activity is required for normal endocardial-mesenchymal transformation in the developing heart. *Development 125*, 4359–67.
6. Brickner, M. E., Hillis, L. D., and Lange, R. A. (2000) Congenital heart disease in adults. Second of two parts. *N Engl J Med 342*, 334–42.
7. Ferencz, C., Neill, C. A., Boughman, J. A., Rubin, J. D., Brenner, J. I., and Perry, L. W. (1989) Congenital cardiovascular malformations associated with chromosome abnormalities: an epidemiologic study. *J Pediatr 114*, 79–86.

Chapter 11

Quantification of Myocyte Chemotaxis: A Role for FAK in Regulating Directional Motility

Britni Zajac, Zeenat S. Hakim, Morgan V. Cameron, Oliver Smithies, and Joan M. Taylor

Abstract

Formation of a fully functional four-chambered heart involves an intricate and complex series of events that includes precise spatial–temporal regulation of cell specification, proliferation, and migration. The formation of the ventricular septum during mid-gestation ensures the unidirectional flow of blood, and is necessary for postnatal viability. Notably, a majority of all congenital malformations of the cardiovascular system in humans involve septal abnormalities which afflict 1 out of 100 newborn children in the United States. Thus, a clear understanding of the precise mechanisms involved in this morphogenetic event will undoubtedly reveal important therapeutic targets. The final step in valvuloseptal morphogenesis occurs, in part, by directed movement of flanking myocytes into the cushion mesenchyme. In order to identify the molecular mechanisms that regulate this critical myocyte function, we have developed two in vitro methodologies; a transwell assay to assess population changes in motility and a single-cell tracking assay to identify signals that drive the coordinated movement of these cells. These methods have proven effective to identify focal adhesion kinase (FAK) as an intracellular component that is critical for myocyte chemotaxis.

Key words: Congenital heart disease, Ventricular septation, Cardiomyocytes, Chemotaxis, Motility, Directional persistence, FAK

1. Introduction

Chemotaxis requires a series of dramatic and coordinated changes in the actin cytoskeleton that enables the cell to polarize toward a chemoattractant, protrude a stable leading edge lamellipodium, and generate the tension required to translocate the remaining cell body (1). One can imagine that this process is even more complex in cardiomyocytes, in which the actin cytoskeleton is aligned in a rigid fashion best suited for isotonic contraction. However, it is

Xu Peng and Marc Antonyak (eds.), *Cardiovascular Development: Methods and Protocols*, Methods in Molecular Biology, vol. 843, DOI 10.1007/978-1-61779-523-7_11,

becoming clear that cardiomyocyte motility does occur in vivo, particularly during muscularization of the proximal outflow tract (OFT) septum between E11.4 and E15.5 in mice (2, 3). During this developmental window, a subset of cardiomyocytes that flank the cushion mesenchyme dissociates from their existing cell–cell interactions and protrudes into the cushion mesenchyme. Though myocyte chemotaxis is thought to be critical for proper cardiac septation and for alignment of the heart with the great vessels, surprisingly little is known regarding the molecular mechanisms that control this process.

Recent genetic evidence indicates that the integrin class of fibronectin-binding adhesion receptors ($\alpha_5\beta_1$ and others) can regulate both the form and function of the heart (4–10). One of the central proteins involved in the integrin intracellular signaling cascade is the 125 kDa non-receptor protein tyrosine kinase, FAK, which is strongly and rapidly activated by various growth factors and by ligation of two-thirds of the known integrin receptors (11). FAK is expressed at relatively high levels in the mouse myocardium from E8 onward, and we recently generated a line of mice with conditional deletion of myocardial FAK by crossing fak$^{flox/flox}$ mice with an *nkx*2.5^{Cre} line that directs recombination in cardiac primordia (termed FAK^{nk} mice). We reported that FAK^{nk} mice died shortly after birth and that FAK was essential for appropriate ventricular septation and OFT alignment (12). Interestingly, the defects we observed in the FAK^{nk} hearts resemble some of the most common congenital malformations in humans that involve inappropriate muscularization of the conus (such as DiGeorge Syndrome and Tetralogy of Fallot). Interestingly, we showed that a large number of MF20-positive cardiomyocytes were present in the septal and parietal conal ridges of control, but not FAK^{nk} hearts by E13.5. To determine whether the septal abnormality was a result of impaired myocyte chemotaxis, we developed an in vitro system to monitor the motility of isolated embryonic cardiomyocytes. Herein, we describe in detail two methods to evaluate myocyte chemotaxis in vitro: a transwell migration assay and a single-cell tracking analysis from cardiac explants.

2. Materials

2.1. Cardiomyocyte Cell Isolation

1. Phosphate buffered saline (PBS): Add 8.0 g of NaCl, 0.2 g of KCl, 1.15 g $Na_2HPO_4{\cdot}7\ H_2O$, 0.2 g of KH_2PO_4 in 1 L distilled water, adjust to pH 7.4 with NaOH and sterilize by autoclaving.
2. Penicillin/streptomycin (PS) stock solution (10,000 U/mL Penicillin, 10,000 μg/mL Streptomycin).

3. Ice cold PBS + PS (0.5%).
4. Trypsin stock solution: Dissolve 0.25 g porcine trypsin in PBS.
5. Trypsin digestion buffer: Add 2 μL of trypsin stock to 998 μL PBS.
6. Dulbecco's minimum essential media (DMEM) containing 4.5 g/L D-Glucose, L-Glutamine, and 110 mg/mL sodium pyruvate.
7. Media 199 (M199) with Earle salts and L-Glutamine.
8. Prepare DMEM:M199 [4:1] containing PS (0.5%) with or without 15% fetal bovine serum (FBS).
9. Fibronectin (1 mg/mL solution).
10. Sterile 1.5-mL polypropylene tubes.
11. Sterile 100-mL petri dishes.
12. Sterile dissection tools (razor blades, Dumont #5 and #7 fine forceps, large scissors).
13. Wide bore sterile plastic transfer pipettes.
14. Cell strainers (70 μm Nylon).

2.2. Transwell Assay (with Isolated Cardiomyocytes)

1. Control transwell inserts (8 μm pore; 24-well plate). Coat the evening before myocyte isolation with fibronectin by applying 300 μL of 10 μg/mL of fibronectin diluted in PBS per well (see Note 1) and placing chamber on a rocker overnight at 4°C.
2. PBS (see step 1, Subheading 2.1 above).
3. DMEM:M199 [4:1] containing PS (0.5%) with or without 15% FBS.
4. Paraformaldehyde (EM grade): Prepare a 4% (w/v) of solution in PBS (see Note 2).
5. Cotton-tipped wooden applicators.
6. Inverted microscope with fluorescent capacity.

2.3. Single-Cell Tracking Analysis from Cardiac Explants

1. 12-well tissue culture plate. Coat the evening before myocyte isolation with fibronectin by applying 1 mL of 10 μg/mL of fibronectin diluted in PBS per well. Rock gently at 4°C overnight.
2. Inverted fluorescent microscope with temperature, humidity, and CO_2 control that is equipped with a motorized programmable *x–y* stage.
3. Digital CCD camera and image collection software. Details provided herein for use of OpenLab software (PerkinElmer).

2.4. Quantification of Cell Speed and Directional Persistence

Cell tracking image analysis software. Details provided herein for use of IMARIS imaging software (ANDOR Technology).

3. Methods

Our initial experiments using either isolated cells or cardiac explants from FAK^{nk} and genetic control hearts proved problematic in distinguishing myocytes from non-myocytes in three-dimensional migration assays. To overcome this hurdle, we crossed the *fak*$^{flox/flox}$ and *nkx2-5*^{Cre} mice to a novel line of mice in which nucleus-targeted GFP is expressed under the control of a truncated β-MHC promoter (hereafter referred to as β-GFP mice). FAK-containing and FAK-null cardiomyocytes isolated from these mice were easily identified by nuclear GFP expression, and these cells exhibited comparable well-defined sarcomeric actin organizations (12) (see Figs. 1 and 2). Importantly, nuclear GFP was not observed in non-myocyte cells that frequently contaminate these cultures.

We next utilized these GFP-targeted cells to examine cardiomyocyte migration in vitro using a Boyden transwell system (see Fig. 1a). Using methods described in detail below, we found that 15% serum-containing media stimulated a robust chemotactic response in cardiomyocytes isolated from genetic control^{gfp} hearts, while chemotaxis was dramatically reduced in FAK$^{nk/gfp}$ cardiomyocytes (12) (see Fig. 1b).

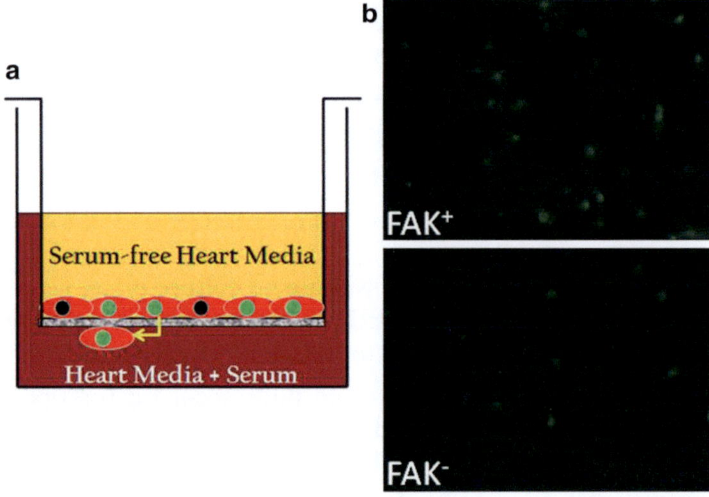

Fig. 1. FAK depletion impairs cardiomyocyte motility. (**a**) Schematic depicting the method for determining chemotactic responses using a Transwell assay. (**b**) Cells isolated from E13.5 β-GFP genetic control and βGFP/FAK^{nk} hearts were plated on transwell chambers pre-coated with fibronectin (10 μg/mL) as described in Subheading 3.2. Representative images of FAK-containing (FAK$^+$) and FAK-null (FAK$^-$) GFP-positive cells that migrated to the undersurface of the insert are shown (10× magnification). Note significant reduction in numbers of migrated FAK$^-$ cells in comparison to controls.

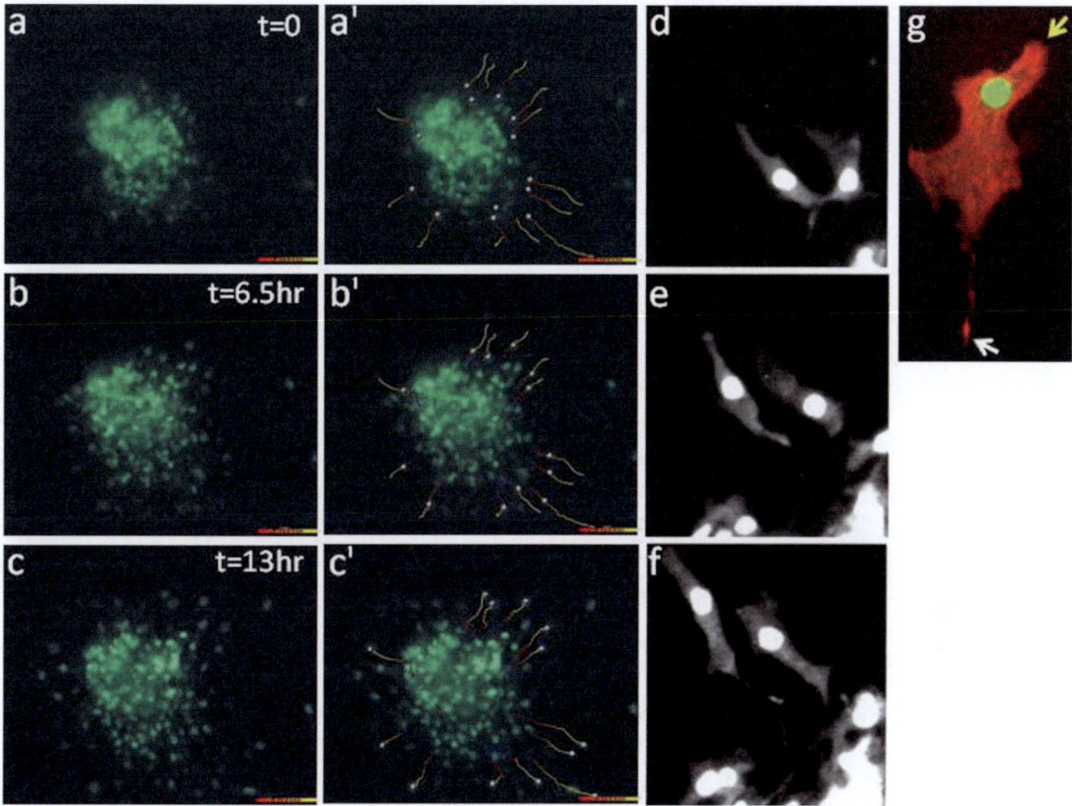

Fig. 2. Assessment of cardiomyocyte motility in cardiac explant cultures. (**a**–**c**) Time-lapse imaging was performed on cardiac explants from E14.5 βGFP mice at 10× magnification. Individual cell tracks were determined using the Imaris program (as described in Subheadings 3.3 and 3.4) and are shown for each time-point in frames (**a′**–**c′**). (**d**–**g**) High-power images of motile myocytes at 20 (**d**–**f**) and 40× (**g**) magnification reveal directional and polarized cardiomyocyte motility. Cell in (**g**) was stained with phalloidin (*red*) to detect polymerized actin. *Arrows* demarcate the leading (*yellow*) and trailing edges (*white*).

3.1. Cardiomyoctye Isolation

1. Prepare the trypsin digestion buffer, heart medium, and chilled PBS containing PS, before starting.
2. Place pregnant dame at embryonic day 13.5 of gestation in isoflurane chamber for 3–4 min or until mouse stops breathing. Euthanize by cervical dislocation.
3. Wash lower abdomen with 70% ethanol. Using forceps and a large scissor make an incision through the skin of the carcass at the base of the abdomen and then peel back the skin with forceps to the level of the sternum (to expose the underlying membrane).
4. Wash exposed membrane with small amount of 70% ethanol (to remove any hair). Cut through membrane and move aside intestines and fat to expose uterus. Grab leftmost end of uterus with forceps and remove entire string while trimming away

attached muscle, fat, and blood vessels. Place uterus in 50-mL beaker with 20 mL of chilled PBS + PS and swirl to remove excess blood.

5. Prepare sufficient number of collection tubes containing chilled PBS + PS for harvested hearts.

6. Transfer uterus to a petri dish filled with chilled PBS + PS and place under dissecting scope (with 1.25× magnification).

7. Using Dumont #3 and #7 forceps, remove uterine muscle from embryonic string and separate embryos from yolk sac.

8. Transfer one embryo at a time to a separate petri dish (containing chilled PBS + PS). Isolate heart using 2× magnification. First, remove head of embryo, then while immobilizing embryo with #3 forceps positioned on either side of heart, gently peel away chest membrane with #7 forceps. Move forceps to the base of the heart (under the atria) and pinch off the ventricles.

9. Transfer ventricles to sterile 6-well plate(s) on ice (containing chilled PBS + PS) and repeat step 8 for remaining embryos.

10. All remaining steps should be performed under a Laminar Flow Hood. Mince ventricles with a sterile razor blade or fine scissors. Transfer minced tissue (using wide bore transfer pipette) to 1.5-mL microfuge tube containing 500 μL chilled PBS.

11. Wash minced tissue by brief centrifugation (2 min at 500 × *g*). Carefully aspirate PBS and repeat. Next, add 200 μL of trypsin digestion buffer (increase to 500 μL if using late embryonic or neonatal hearts) and incubate (while rocking) at 37°C. The incubation time should be 10 min to obtain cardiac explants for single-cell tracking (see Subheading 3.3) or 20 min to obtain single-cell suspensions suitable for Transwell assays (see Subheading 3.2).

12. Gently titrate cell suspension using a 200-μL pipette approximately ten times to disaggregate tissue. Add 500 μL of serum-containing heart media to each tube and mix by inverting tube five to six times. If obtaining cardiac explants, proceed to step 14.

13. If performing Transwell assay, samples can be pooled if embryos are syngeneic. Triturate cell suspension using a 1-mL pipette an additional ten times to obtain a single-cell suspension. Pass cell suspension through a 70-μm nylon cell strainer into a sterile 50 mL conical to remove tissue residue. Proceed with Transwell assay (see Subheading 3.2).

14. For cardiac explants, the dispersed extract is plated directly onto a 12-well tissue culture plastic dish pre-coated with fibronectin (see Subheading 2.3). The plate is then placed in a CO_2 incubator and left undisturbed for at least 18 h. Proceed with Subheading 3.3.

3.2. Transwell Assay (with Isolated Cardiomyocytes)

1. Count isolated cardiomyocytes using a hemocytometer and inverted fluorescent microscope and resuspend 10–30,000 GFP-positive cells in 300 μL heat medium containing 15% FBS.
2. Plate cell solution on the upper surface of fibronectin-coated insert and add 1 mL of heart medium containing 15% FBS into the lower chamber. Place transwell in a 37°C incubator with an atmosphere of 5% CO_2. Do not disturb for 24 h.
3. After 24 h, gently rinse the top and bottom chambers three times with PBS. Add 300 μL of serum-free heart media to the top chamber and add 1 mL of heart medium containing 15% FBS to the bottom chamber (to provide a chemo-attractant gradient). Prior to returning to the incubator, count the number of GFP-positive cardiomyocytes attached to the insert using an inverted fluorescent microscope with a 10× objective (see Note 3).
4. Place transwell in a 37°C incubator in an atmosphere of 5% CO_2 for 24 h.
5. Aspirate media from both chambers, rinse three times with PBS and fix cells by adding 1 mL of 4% paraformaldehyde to the lower chamber for 20 min at room temperature.
6. Remove nonmigrated cells from the upper surface of the insert with the cotton-tipped applicator (swab in circular fashion while applying pressure for approximately 15 s/insert, rinse with PBS and repeat).
7. Count the number of GFP-positive cardiomyocytes attached to the bottom of the insert using an inverted fluorescent microscope with a 10× objective.
8. Normalize the number of migrating cells to the number attached prior to the induction of chemotaxis.

3.3. Single-Cell Tracking Analysis from Cardiac Explants

While the Boyden transwell system is useful for population studies, the value of this approach is limited with respect to defining molecular mechanisms that drive chemotaxis, since primary cultured cardiomyocytes are particularly difficult to transfect. To overcome this limitation, we have recently developed a single-cell tracking assay from cardiac explants in which myocyte chemotaxis can be tracked via time-lapse imaging. The aforementioned β-GFP mice are pivotal to the analysis of migration in these explants as tracking of nuclear GFP in real time provides a direct measure of cardiomyocyte migration without the confounding effects of proliferation that could not be ruled out in past studies.

The wind-rose plots in Fig. 2 depict the change in individual cell tracks of wild-type GFP-tagged cardiomyocytes from explant cultures over a 13-h period. The high power images in panels d–g reveal that motile myocytes (marked by nuclear GFP and positive for cardiac troponin T) exhibit a polarized cell phenotype with identifiable leading and trailing edges. Subsequent kymographic analysis (described in detail below) was used to define the parameters of cardiomyocyte chemokinesis (i.e., the speed and directional persistence of these cells). For these experiments, data obtained from individual cardiomyocytes at the periphery of the explants were chosen. These studies revealed that in the presence of serum, embryonic myocytes move at a rate of 11.4 ± 1.2 nm/s. This speed is slightly lower than the "basal" speed of approximately 15–20 nm/s that we and others have found for mammalian fibroblasts or smooth muscle cells, which contain a less rigid cyto-architecture. As is apparent from the highlighted cell tracks, the outward movement of myocytes from the periphery of the explants is quite persistent (i.e., relatively few changes in direction are observed). Indeed, on a scale of 0–1 (with 1 being a straight line), the directional persistence for these cells was 0.76. Note, the cell explants can be transfected with various m-Cherry-tagged cDNA constructs using the Amaxa Nucleofector electroporation system and/or treated with pharmacological inhibitors (see Note 4) prior to imaging to identify molecules that regulate myocyte speed and directional persistence.

As noted above, an inverted fluorescent microscope with temperature, humidity, and CO_2 control that is equipped with a motorized programmable *x–y* stage, a digital CCD camera, and cell tracking image analysis software are all necessary for this technique. We use an Olympus IX70 inverted microscope encased in Plexiglas housing to control the internal environment (37°C, 5% CO_2, and a relative humidity of 60%) that is equipped with a programmable DeltaT motorized *x–y* stage. Our image collection is performed using OpenLab software, and our image analysis is performed using Imaris (described below in Subheading 3.4).

The following protocol enables simultaneous quantification of the speed and directional persistence of large numbers of migrating cells (typically >400 cells corresponding to approximately 50 cells/condition).

1. Continuing from step 14 in Subheading 3.1, secure 12-well plate containing attached explants in place on the microscope stage, and initiate CO_2 at a rate of 80–90 PCO_2.
2. Use the joystick to identify the center of each well. In the *X–Y* stage click on: Add → New Point. Label Well 1, Well 2, etc. Once this is completed, it is simpler to go through and tell the program to "go to" Well 1, Well 2, etc., without having to remove the covering of the chamber each time.
3. View plate with a 10× fluorescent objective (using a suitable FITC/EGFP filter cube) and scan the wells, using the joystick, to identify the locations of up to 24 well-spread colonies containing 25–100 GFP positive cardiomyocytes. Record an appropriate exposure time, gain, and offset to visualize individual cells within each colony. Also, record the focus value in the

corresponding MoveTo [ ] variable array position (the focus value will appear inside the brackets). This is located in the Variables Window under the View menu. This is important to do before running the automation because it records the focus value you choose for each colony.

4. After appropriate adjustments are made and the image is as clear as possible, click on Add→ New Point, and number colonies sequentially from 1 to 24. This is done for each well, moving to Well 2, Well 3, etc. Once all the points are set and all the parameters are adjusted, Select "GoTo Well 1." View each colony and readjust the exposure time, gain, offset, and focus as necessary.
5. Program automation: Set the delay between loops and total number of loops to be collected. For monitoring cell motility over a 24-h window a 5–10 min delay is best. For monitoring lamellipodial dynamics (usually performed at 40×), a 15–30 s delay is more appropriate. However, it is important to note that the cycle time cannot be shorter than the time it takes the stage to visit each preidentified locale. Thus, the total number of cells or colonies imaged may need to be limited to accommodate the chosen interval.
6. Run the automation: Initiate a test run and review images after completion of one full cycle. If the images need additional focusing and adjustment, stop the automation, close the image windows, and adjust the parameters that need correcting. When satisfied with the program constraints, proceed with automation.
7. After completing the time-lapse imaging, close the image windows, and save files. When using IMARIS software for subsequent analysis, save images as "256 grays" Liff files (note that Tiff files are too large to process in IMARIS but may be suitable for other image analysis software). For viewing purposes, save the files as QuickTime movies.

3.4. Quantification of Cell Speed and Persistence Using IMARIS Programming

1. Open the IMARIS program. Navigate to the folder where all images are saved. Select your first point of interest and click Open. This may take a few minutes; especially if the interval chosen between loops was short.
2. Select Edit→ Image Properties. A window will appear with the Voxel Size, Min, and Max, for each X, Y, and Z variable. Since the Live Cell Imaging was performed in 2-dimensions, the Z variable will be used for the Time dimension (see step 3). The Voxel size should be entered in each dimension (this is a standard value, use 0.9803 for a 10× objective). Enter 0 for all viable minimums. Pressing tab will fill in the rest of the information, as the maximum coordinates are specific for each point and determined by each file.

3. Next, change the Z variable to Time. To this end, first go to the Main Menu and Select→ Image Processing, then Select→Swap Time and Z. This is important because the IMARIS program defaults to a 3-dimension program and this step changes the reference frame to a 2-dimensional image.
4. Record the image interval used for the Live Cell Imaging (i.e., 5 or 10 min). In the main menu, Select Edit→Image Properties and chose All Equidistant. This will open a window denoted Set Equidistant Time Points. There will be four boxes where information can be entered. For the purpose of these experiments, it is only necessary to enter the appropriate value in the Time Interval box (see Note 5).
5. Select color channel and adjust contrast. In the main menu, select File→ Open. Choose the first file you wish to process and click Open. Select the Display Adjustment Box and check the color channel (i.e., green for GFP). The background, Spot and image intensity can be adjusted accordingly in this window. Note the image intensity (the far right toggle) should remain as dim as possible so that individual nuclei can be appropriately identified.
6. In the Main Menu Select fourth box from the left in the nine-box series (the orange-spotted box) to initiate a Wizard that includes a series of six steps for focusing, aligning, and tracking cell migration. It is recommended that data be saved after each step. To move between steps, click on the forward or reverse blue arrow below the work area.

   Step 1: *Algorithm*: There are three settings to choose from:

   i. *Segment Only a Region of Interest*: this allows you to choose a particular region of the image to analyze. For these experiments, leave unchecked. A box will appear below this choice stating that the entire image will be processed.

   ii. *Different Spot Sizes (Region Growing)*: this will implement spheres over each fluorescent cell in the image. There is a separate process for adjusting the parameters of these spheres if necessary. Note: the size of the sphere will be defined below.

   iii. *Track Spots (over Time)*: This box needs to be checked to perform single-tracking analysis.

   Step 2: *Source Channel*: This step indicates the Channel being used (i.e., fluorescent, phase, or both) and allows you to define the source of interest (termed "Spot"). For these experiments, the GFP-labeled nucleus is the Spot. Thus, the size of the nucleus needs to be defined in this window. To this end, click on the Slice function located below the Main Menu. On the left side of the screen under *Measure*, make sure *Line* is highlighted. Next, click on the far right edge of the nucleus. A plus sign will appear. This marks the right edge of the Spot. Click on the far left side of the nucleus. Another plus sign will appear that marks the left side, and a line will form connecting the two marks (which is a rough estimate of the diameter of the nucleus). Record the length of this line (displayed in the Measure box) and repeat this step on several nuclei to obtain an average diameter. Switch back to *Surpass* mode to define Spot size. In the box next to *Estimated Diameter*, enter in a rough average of the values you obtained in *Slice* mode (this is a rough estimate and it is best to error on the low end). When finished, save and proceed to the next page.

Step 3: *Classify Spots*: This step allows for filtering and classifying Spots based on their size, diameter, quality, etc. Several different filters can be used to modify the Spots identified via usage of the aforementioned parameters. Using the *Spherical* mode, we adjust the *Quality* to ensure that a reasonable number of nuclei are demarcated in each explant. Addition or/and deletion of specific nuclei (Spots) can be accomplished in the next step.

Step 4: *Edit Spots*: This step allows you to view the Spots chosen by the program (as per the classifications defined above) and to manually select those you want to track. To this end, under *Create* (on the left side of the screen), select Add/ Delete, and choose "All Visible Channels." Next, switch from the *Navigate* mode to the *Select* mode (the cursor will now appear as a small square). To delete a Spot, move the cursor over the Spot of interest, hold down the shift key and left click on the mouse. To add a Spot, move the cursor over the fluorescing nucleus you wish to identify as a Spot, hold down the shift key and left click on the mouse.

Step 5: *Tracking*: This step allows you to identify the algorithm you wish to utilize to analyze cell movements. For these experiments Autoregressive Motion was chosen in order to obtain the speed and track straightness (i.e., directional persistence) of individual cells. Next set the tracking Parameters. *Max Distance* is the maximum distance each Spot is expected to travel. This number should be estimated high. Once again, *Slice* mode can be used to estimate the average distance traveled over the course of the experiment for a few Spots. Max Gap size is the separation desired between Spots. This value can be set to deselect cells from the analysis due to their close proximity with other cells (i.e., to avoid affects of cell–cell interaction on rates of motility).

Step 6: *Classify Tracks*: This feature allows the tracking of paths based on certain variables. These variables can be turned on and off in the Edit→Preferences tab. For these experiments, *Total Displacement Length* was chosen.

7. Clicking the double right green arrows will exit the Wizard and initiate the single-cell tracking analysis.
8. Data can next be exported to Excel for further analysis. Data can be exported for the entire experiment, or from individual points. To choose individual points, highlight the *Graphing symbol* icon and click *Detailed* to view all statistics collected from all points. Click on any of the listings in this view to export.

4. Notes

1. The effect of extracellular matrix on cellular motility is a bell-shaped curve. Too little matrix will not support nascent attachments at the leading edge of cells, while too much matrix will impede lamellipodial dynamics. It is best to start with a range of 1–100 μg/mL to determine the most efficacious concentration. We have found that the optimal concentrations vary between cardiomyocytes isolated from different staged embryos.
2. Paraformaldehyde: This solution should be carefully prepared in a fume hood. For a 100 mL solution: heat 90 mL of ddH_2O in a glass flask in the microwave for 1 min. Transfer to a preheated hot plate in the fume hood. Add 4 g of Paraformaldehyde and one drop of 1 M NaOH and bring to a boil. Remove and cool in hood. Add 10 mL of 10× PBS, qs to 100 mL with ddH_2O and pH to 7.4.
3. Instead of counting all of the cells attached to the filter, we find that it is generally sufficient to count the number of cells in four random fields at 10× in both the upper and lower chambers (as long as this process gives a value of at least 200 cells).
4. Use of pharmacological inhibitors: Pathway inhibitors can be added to determine the effect of particular enzymes on the chemotactic response. For best results, let the automation run for at least 4 h before adding the inhibitor, so that initial rates can be compared to the rates obtained following treatment. To this end, dilute the appropriate amount of the inhibitor into 1 mL of warm heart media. Upon completion of a scanning cycle, carefully remove the Plexiglass lid and top of cell culture dish, add the media containing the inhibitor to the side of the well and gently resuspend, being careful not to move the plate. When finished, replace the cover and allow the automation to proceed. It is important to complete this step before initiation of the next cycle (i.e., within the 5–10 min delay).
5. It is very important to change the Image Properties and then change how the image is processed, in this order. If this is done in the reverse order, the IMARIS program will take on too much file information too fast and will stall.

Acknowledgments

The authors would like to thank Matthew Medlin and the UNC Microscopy Services Laboratory (including Bob Bagnell and Steven Ray) for excellent technical assistance with image collection and utilization of the OpenLab and Imaris imaging software. This work was supported, in part, by National Heart, Lung, and Blood Institute grants HL-081844 (to J.M.T.) and HL-071054 (to J.M.T.), and American Heart Association Grants 0355776U (to J.M.T.).

References

1. Ridley, A. J., Schwartz, M. A., Burridge, K., Firtel, R. A., Ginsberg, M. H., Borisy, G., Parsons, J. T., and Horwitz, A. R. (2003) Cell migration: integrating signals from front to back. *Science 302*, 1704–9.
2. van den Hoff, M. J., Moorman, A. F., Ruijter, J. M., Lamers, W. H., Bennington, R. W., Markwald, R. R., and Wessels, A. (1999) Myocardialization of the cardiac outflow tract. *Dev Biol 212*, 477–90.
3. Moralez, I., Phelps, A., Riley, B., Raines, M., Wirrig, E., Snarr, B., Jin, J. P., Van Den Hoff, M., Hoffman, S., and Wessels, A. (2006) Muscularizing tissues in the endocardial cushions of the avian heart are characterized by the expression of h1-calponin. *Dev Dyn 235*, 1648–58.
4. Shai, S. Y., Harpf, A. E., Babbitt, C. J., Jordan, M. C., Fishbein, M. C., Chen, J., Omura, M., Leil, T. A., Becker, K. D., Jiang, M., Smith, D. J., Cherry, S. R., Loftus, J. C., and Ross, R. S. (2002) Cardiac myocyte-specific excision of the beta1 integrin gene results in myocardial fibrosis and cardiac failure. *Circ Res 90*, 458–64.
5. Schroeder, J. A., Jackson, L. F., Lee, D. C., and Camenisch, T. D. (2003) Form and function of developing heart valves: coordination by extracellular matrix and growth factor signaling. *J Mol Med 81*, 392–403.
6. Shubeita, H. E., Thorburn, J., and Chien, K. R. (1992) Microinjection of antibodies and expression vectors into living myocardial cells. Development of a novel approach to identify candidate genes that regulate cardiac growth and hypertrophy. *Circulation 85*, 2236–46.
7. Brancaccio, M., Fratta, L., Notte, A., Hirsch, E., Poulet, R., Guazzone, S., De Acetis, M., Vecchione, C., Marino, G., Altruda, F., Silengo, L., Tarone, G., and Lembo, G. (2003) Melusin, a muscle-specific integrin beta1-interacting protein, is required to prevent cardiac failure in response to chronic pressure overload. *Nat Med 9*, 68–75.
8. Hescheler, J., and Fleischmann, B. K. (2000) Integrins and cell structure: powerful determinants of heart development and heart function. *Cardiovasc Res 47*, 645–7.
9. Yang, J. T., Bader, B. L., Kreidberg, J. A., Ullman-Cullere, M., Trevithick, J. E., and Hynes, R. O. (1999) Overlapping and independent functions of fibronectin receptor integrins in early mesodermal development. *Dev Biol 215*, 264–77.
10. Valencik, M. L., Keller, R. S., Loftus, J. C., and McDonald, J. A. (2002) A lethal perinatal cardiac phenotype resulting from altered integrin function in cardiomyocytes. *J Card Fail 8*, 262–72.
11. Parsons, J. T. (2003) Focal adhesion kinase: the first ten years. *J Cell Sci 116*, 1409–16.
12. Hakim, Z. S., Dimichele, L. A., Doherty, J. T., Homeister, J. W., Beggs, H. E., Reichardt, L. F., Schwartz, R. J., Brackhan, J., Smithies, O., Mack, C. P., and Taylor, J. M. (2007) Conditional Deletion of Focal Adhesion Kinase Leads to Defects in Ventricular Septation and Outflow Tract Alignment. *Mol Cell Biol.* **27**, 5352–64.

Chapter 12

Analysis of Neural Crest Cell Fate During Cardiovascular Development Using Cre-Activated *lacZ*/β-Galactosidase Staining

Yanping Zhang and L. Bruno Ruest

Abstract

It is important to identify the mechanisms regulating cardiovascular development. However, complex genetic tools are often required, including transgenic animals that express the *lacZ* transgene encoding the β-galactosidase enzyme under the control of a specific promoter or following recombination with the Cre recombinase. The latter can be useful for identifying specific cell populations of the developing cardiovascular system, including neural crest cells. The tracking of these cells can help clarify their fate in mutant embryos and elucidate the etiology of some congenital cardiovascular birth defects. This chapter highlights the methods used to stain embryonic tissues in whole mount or sections to detect the expression of the *lacZ* transgene with a focus on tracking cardiac neural crest cells using the *Wnt1-Cre* and *R26R* mouse lines. We also provide a protocol using fluorescence-activated cell sorting for collecting neural crest cells for further analysis. These protocols can be used with any embryos expressing *Cre* and *lacZ*.

Key words: Cardiovascular development, Neural crest cell, *lacZ*, β-galactosidase, Fate mapping analysis, Cre recombinase, R26R, Flow cytometry, Cell sorting

1. Introduction

Congenital heart anomalies are the most common birth defects, affecting about 1 out of every 110 children and accounting for the most noninfectious mortalities in children (1, 2). It is imperative to understand the mechanisms regulating cardiovascular development in order to identify avenues that would help reduce the high prevalence of these defects or provide better treatments. However, cardiovascular development is quite complex, requiring the activation of numerous genes and the involvement of various cell types (3–8). Further, the development of this biological pump goes through several structural modifications, thus complicating our

Xu Peng and Marc Antonyak (eds.), *Cardiovascular Development: Methods and Protocols*,
Methods in Molecular Biology, vol. 843, DOI 10.1007/978-1-61779-523-7_12,

understanding of its regulatory mechanisms (3–6, 9, 10). In its early stages, heart development can be recognized as the formation of a mesodermal cardiac crescent soon after gastrulation. This crescent is transformed into a contracting linear tube that eventually loops and is then remodeled to form the ventricles and atria. In addition, the valves and a conduction system also develop. The growth of the developing heart is ensured by the proliferation of the cardiomyocytes originating from the cardiac crescent and the addition to the arterial pole of cardiomyocytes originating from the anterior or secondary heart field (9–12). Septation of the arterial pole requires the involvement of the neural crest cells, not only for the induction of the anterior heart field cardiomyocytes, but also for the proper septation of the outflow tract (7–12).

Neural crest cells are a distinct cell population that delaminate from the neural fold at the junction between the surface ectoderm and neural epithelium (7, 13–18). Following an epithelial to mesenchymal transition in the embryos, they migrate ventrally and develop into various anatomical structures. Several populations of neural crest cells, including cephalic, cardiac (circumpharyngeal), vagal, trunk, and sacral neural crest cells, have been identified. However, the distinctions between populations of neural crest cells are often not clear, and some of the populations may need to be further subdivided based on their gene expression profile and function. Cardiac neural crest cells migrate from the posterior hindbrain into the third, fourth, and sixth pharyngeal arches where they participate in the asymmetric remodeling of the pharyngeal arch arteries (PAA) into the great arteries and form the vascular smooth muscle layer of these vessels (7–9, 19–22). The third PAA are remodeled into the common carotids, the right fourth PAA joins the right subclavian to the right common carotid, the left fourth PAA becomes part of the aortic arch, and the left sixth PAA forms the ductus arteriosus, which eventually regresses (23, 24). A subpopulation of cardiac neural crest cells also migrates into the cardiac outflow tract, where they participate in the septation of this tract into the pulmonary and aortic (ascending) outflows (10, 12, 19, 25).

Numerous tools are needed to study cardiovascular development, including the generation of transgenic mice, some of which may carry a transgene such as *lacZ*, in order to follow the spatial and temporal expression of a specific gene or to track a specific cell population for a short period of time. The *Cre-loxP* system is more suited to characterization using spatial and temporal gene expression and also fate mapping of the cells that previously express a gene with the *Cre* recombinase expression regulated by a specific promoter (26). The latter system is particularly useful for tracking neural crest cells used in conjunction with *Rosa26R* (*R26R*) mice (27) but at the expense of faithfully recapitulating the gene expression. In the *R26R* mice, the *Cre* expression results in the removal of a *loxP*-flanked DNA segment containing stop codons that prevent the expression of the *lacZ* gene. This gene encodes for the enzyme β-galactosidase (β-gal), and the enzymatic activity can be traced with numerous substrates, including X-gal, which produces a blue precipitate once it is cleaved. When crossed with a *Cre* transgenic strain, *lacZ* is irreversibly expressed in the cells/tissues where *Cre* is or was expressed, thus allowing cell fate mapping of daughter cells. While several *Cre* lines can be used to study cardiovascular development [for example, *Nkx2.5-Cre* (28), *αMHC-Cre* (29), *Tbx18-Cre* (30), *Tie2-Cre* (31), *Isl1-Cre* (32), *Ap2α-Cre* (33), and *Hand2-Cre* (34)], the *Wnt1-Cre* (35) and *Pax3-Cre* (36) lines are appropriate to trace cells of neural crest origin. In 2000, Jiang and colleagues published a seminal study about the mapping of cardiac neural crest cells in the mouse using the *Wnt1-Cre* line (22). Further, fate mapping can be useful in conjunction with other mutations, helping to define the etiology of some birth defects (for examples, see ref. 37–41).

In this chapter, we present proven protocols (13, 22, 34, 37, 38) for mapping the fate of cardiac neural crest cells during embryonic development using *lacZ*/β-gal staining with *Wnt1-Cre;R26R* mice. These protocols can be used with any other *Cre* lines or simply staining for the expression of the *lacZ* transgene. They can also be modified for other transgenes. We provide protocols for whole mount or sectional staining, sectioning of whole mount-stained embryos, and counterstaining with either eosin or Nuclear Fast Red. We also provide a protocol to collect isolated neural crest cells with flow cytometry for investigations such as gene microarray analysis.

2. Materials

The protocols described below are fairly simple and generally employ materials commonly available in most laboratories. Common products such as ethanol and xylene are not listed in each section. The preparation of the different solutions is described only once, based on their first appearance in the Subheading 3, although these solutions or products may be used in more than one described protocol.

2.1. Embryo Collection

1. *Wnt1-Cre*, *Rosa26R* (*R26R*), and *R26R-eYFP* mouse transgenic lines (Jackson Laboratory) (stock no. 003829, 003474, and 006148, respectively). *R26R-eYFP* mouse line can be used to observe neural crest cells in live embryos or sections using an appropriately fitted fluorescent microscope or to collect individualized cells using fluorescence-activated cell sorting (FACS). Other transgenic lines are available from other investigators and can be used to track neural crest cell development and fate or other cell populations or to conditionally inactivate a gene.

2. Phosphate buffered saline (PBS): 137 mM sodium chloride, 2.7 mM potassium chloride, 8 mM dibasic sodium phosphate heptahydrate ($Na_2HPO_4 \cdot 7H_2O$), and 2 mM monobasic potassium phosphate (KH_2PO_4). Adjust pH to 7.4 and autoclave. Can be prepared as a 10× stock solution. Commercial PBS are also available.
3. Surgical instruments such as scissors and forceps. For the collection of smaller embryos, #5 needle forceps are recommended.
4. Sterile bacterial culture plate (100 mm) for dissecting the embryos in PBS.
5. Stereomicroscope for the dissection of small embryos.
6. P1000 pipette and tips for embryo transfer. Cut the end of the tip so that the hole is slightly larger than the embryos.
7. OCT (Optimal cutting temperature, Tissue Tek 4583).
8. Round bottom tubes (15 mL).
9. Glass scintillation vials (20 mL) for larger embryos.
10. Polypropylene molds (Polysciences Peel-A-Way, different sizes or shapes).

2.2. Whole Mount Staining of E8.5–E11.5 Embryos

1. 4% paraformaldehyde: 4 g in 100 mL of PBS. Add a few drops of 10 N sodium hydroxide. Heat to 60°C and agitate manually (easier to control the temperature in a water bath) or with a magnetic stirring bar on a heating plate (more difficult to control the temperature). After dissolving, check pH and adjust to 7.3–7.5, if necessary. Filter with a 0.22 μm bottle-top vacuum filtration system. Keep refrigerated for a few weeks.
2. 2 M stock solution of magnesium chloride.
3. 10% stock solution of Nonidet P40 detergent (NP40, Calbiochem/EMD).
4. 10% stock solution of sodium deoxycholate.
5. lacZ/β-gal rinse buffer: 0.2 M sodium phosphate, pH 7.3–7.4 [5.52 g of monobasic sodium phosphate monohydrate ($NaH_2PO_4 \cdot H_2O$) and 42.9 g dibasic sodium phosphate heptahydrate [$Na_2HPO_4 \cdot 7H_2O$) in 1 L of water], 2 mM magnesium chloride (1 mL of stock solution), 0.02% NP40 (2 mL of stock solution), and 0.01% sodium deoxycholate (1 mL of stock solution).
6. X-gal (5-bromo-4-chloro-3-indoxyl-β-D-galactopyranoside): 2% (20 mg/mL) stock solution in dimethyl formamide (DMF). As an alternative, Salmon-gal (6-chloro-3-indolyl-β-D-galactopyranoside) can be used in the same manner [available from Gold Biotechnology (SALGAL), Lab Scientific] and under the name Red-gal [Research Organics].
7. 500 mM stock solution of potassium ferrocyanide [$K_3Fe(CN)_6$].

8. 500 mM stock solution of potassium ferricyanide [potassium hexacyanoferrate trihydrate $K_4Fe(CN)_6 \cdot 3H_2O$].
9. lacZ/β-gal staining buffer: For each 10 mL of lacZ/β-gal rinse buffer, add 50 μL of potassium "ferry" and "ferro" cyanide stocks (2.5 mM each final concentration) and 300 μL of X-gal stock (0.6 mg/mL). The amount of X-gal per 10 mL of staining solution can be reduced to 200 μL (0.4 mg/mL) if the background is high or the β-gal enzymatic activity is strong. Based on our experience, we no longer add the native potassium cyanide chemicals directly to the staining solution in order to reduce the amount of crystal precipitate on the embryos. Reducing the final concentration of these compounds from 5 mM [as often seen in other protocols (13, 22)] to 2.5 mM and reducing the final concentration of X-gal from 1 mg/mL to 0.6 mg/mL helps minimize the precipitate formation without affecting the final results.
10. Glas-Col rotator with the appropriate clips to hold tubes or vials (available from Thermo-Fisher and VWR).
11. 10% neutral buffered formalin.

2.3. Staining of E12.4–E18.5 Embryo Sections

1. Positively charged slides (plus-coated).
2. Cryostat.
3. 0.5% glutaraldehyde in PBS.
4. Slide racks and staining jars or dishes. You will need about 150–200 mL of staining buffer for each container, depending of the number of slides generated. In some racks, it is possible to place the slides back-to-back, reducing the volume of staining buffer needed.

2.4. Embedding and Sectioning of Whole Mount-Stained Embryos

1. Cedarwood oil (Polysciences).
2. Histology cassettes or scintillation vials.
3. Vacuum chamber.
4. Paraplast paraffin.
5. Molds.
6. Microtome.
7. Histological staining dishes and racks.

2.5. Counterstaining with Eosin

1. Eosin. To prepare a stock solution, dissolve 10 g in 200 mL of distilled water and 800 mL of 95% ethanol.
2. Working eosin preparation: mix 150 mL of eosin stock with 450 mL of 80% ethanol (380 mL of 95% and 70 mL of distilled water) and 3 mL of glacial acetic acid.
3. Mounting medium.
4. Coverslips.

2.6. Counterstaining with Nuclear Fast Red

1. Nuclear Fast Red.
2. Preparation of Nuclear Fast Red: Dissolve 5 g of aluminum sulfate in 100 mL of distilled water and add 0.1 g of Nuclear Fast Red. Slowly heat to boil, cool and filter. You can add a grain of thymol as a preservative. May precipiate with time.

2.7. Isolation of Neural Crest Cells by FACS

1. 0.25% Trypsin/2.21 mM EDTA in Hank's buffered salt solution.
2. 37°C incubator.
3. 100-mm plates with the bottom covered with solidified 2% agarose in water.
4. 1.5-mL microcentrifuge tubes.
5. PBS supplemented with 10% FBS.
6. 30-gauge needles (with syringe) or tungsten needles (with handle).
7. FACS with cell analysis and cell collecting capacities.
8. Sheath fluid.

3. Methods

3.1. Embryo Collection

1. Breeding is arranged so that one parental line provides the *Wnt1-Cre* allele, and the other provides the *R26R* mutant allele carrying the *lacZ* gene. When analyzing the fate or the presence of neural crest cells in mutant embryos, each parent should also carry a copy of the studied gene mutant allele to obtain homozygous embryos. Embryonic day (E) 0.5 is defined as noon of the day that a vaginal plug is observed.
2. E8.5–E15.5 embryos are collected in PBS using fine forceps, taking care to preserve the embryonic membranes to extract DNA for genotyping. Older embryos can be collected by cutting the uterus and amniotic membranes with scissors, and a small tail biopsy can be used for genotyping.
3. Gently transfer the E8.5–E11.5 embryos with a cut P1000 pipette tip into a round bottom 15-mL tube or a glass scintillation vial. Proceed with Subheading 3.2.
4. E12.5–E15.5 embryos are gently transferred by grasping the umbilical cord with fine forceps. Older embryos can be transferred by gripping the hind legs or tail with a forceps. Embryos are either directly embedded in OCT or fixed prior to embedding (see Note 1), as described below.
5. Fix the embryos in 0.2% glutaraldehyde in PBS for 30 min at room temperature.
6. Incubate by rotating the embryos in 10% sucrose in PBS for 30 min at 4°C.

7. Transfer the embryos to a solution of 2 mM $MgCl_2$, 30% sucrose, and 50% OCT in PBS and rotate for 2 h at 4°C.
8. Transfer the embryos to polypropylene molds and cover them with OCT, taking care to avoid air bubbles. Gently remove the bubbles with a forceps, pipette tip, or needle.
9. Gently position each embryo with a forceps or pipette tip so that it is appropriate for the chosen cutting angle. For transverse sections, we recommend positioning the embryo on its head.
10. Gently transfer the molds to a 95% ethanol/dry ice bath to freeze the OCT, taking care to maintain the position of the embryo (see Note 2). You can gently nudge the embryo to ensure the proper positioning before the OCT begins solidifying.
11. Once the OCT is fully solidified, dry the molds by wiping them and label them.
12. Keep the embryos frozen at –80°C until sectioning and staining (see Subheading 3.3).

3.2. Whole Mount Staining of E8.5–E11.5 Embryos

For whole tissues, see Note 3.

1. Fix the embryos in 4% paraformaldehyde in PBS for 30–60 min on ice (4°C), starting with 30 min for the E8.5 embryos and adding 10 min for each additional day.
2. Rinse the embryos three times for 10 min in *lacZ*/β-gal rinse buffer at room temperature.
3. Incubate the embryos overnight in *lacZ*/β-gal staining solution at room temperature or at 37°C (see Note 4). Gentle agitation is recommended, such as on a Glas-Col rotator with the carousel almost horizontally positioned.
4. The following day, rinse the embryos three times in PBS for 10 min each. Photographs can be captured at this step or at later stages (see Fig. 1a, c).
5. Fix the embryos overnight in 10% neutral buffered formalin.
6. Rinse the embryos a few times in PBS and proceed with paraffin embedding or store in 70% ethanol.

3.3. Staining of E12.5–E18.5 Embryo Sections

1. Warm the OCT-embedded embryo for 30 min to the cutting temperature, usually between –15 and –22°C.
2. Cut the embryo in a cryostat and collect 8- to 12-μm sections on positively charged "Plus-coated" microscope slides.
3. Briefly warm the sections at room temperature to melt the OCT and attach the tissue to the slide. Keep the sections frozen until ready to stain.
4. Dry the sections at room temperature.
5. Fix the sections in 0.5% glutaraldehyde in PBS for 30 min.

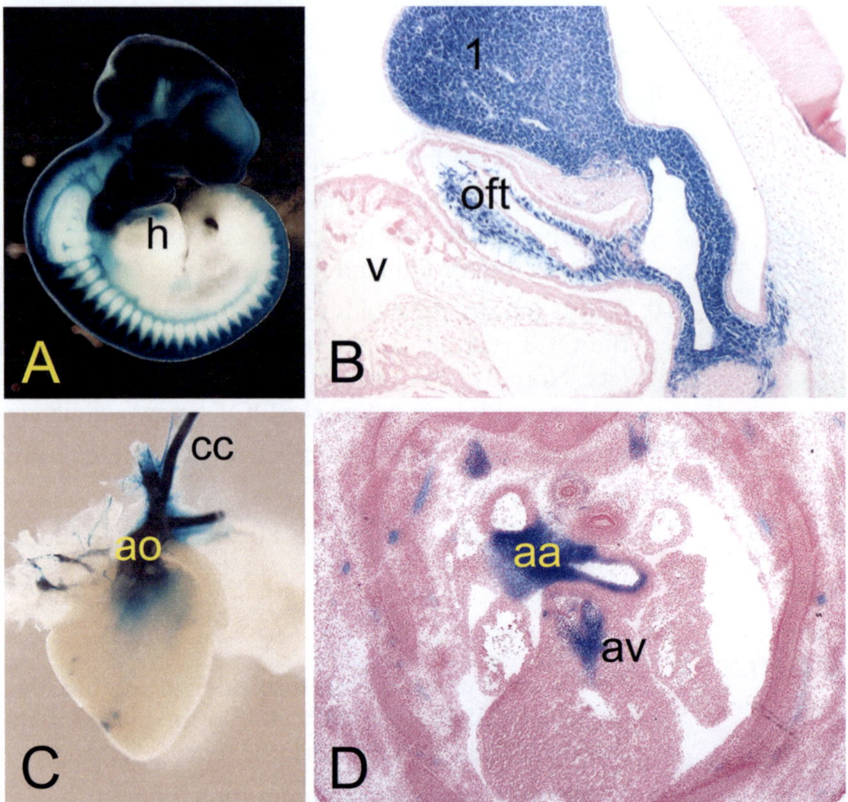

Fig. 1. Visualization of neural crest cells in *lacZ*/β-gal-stained embryos. (**a**) Whole mount-stained E10.5 *Wnt1-Cre;R26R* embryo. Neural crest cells are stained in dark blue following the cleavage of X-gal by β-gal. (**b**) Section through the outflow tract (oft) of a whole mount-stained E10.5 embryo. The section is counterstained with eosin. (**c**) Whole mount-stained heart and great vessels from an E18.5 embryo. (**d**) Section through the cardiac region of an E13.5 embryo counterstained with Nuclear Fast Red. Neural crest cells are observed in the aortic arch (aa) and in the cells of the developing aortic valve (av). *1* first pharyngeal arch; *ao* aorta; *h* heart; *v* ventricle.

6. Rinse slides three times for 10 min each in *lacZ*/β-gal rinse solution.
7. Incubate the slides in *lacZ*/β-gal staining buffer overnight at 37°C.
8. The next day, rinse the slides in PBS for 5 min, then in distilled water (see Note 5).
9. Proceed for counterstaining with either eosin (go to Subheading 3.5 after completing step 10) or Nuclear Fast Red (see Subheading 3.6; Note 6). If using salmon-gal as a substrate for the β-gal enzyme, we recommend using methyl green to counterstain the sections (see Note 7).
10. Dehydrate sections in 70% ethanol for 30 s with gentle agitation (only if doing the eosin counterstaining).

3.4. Embedding and Sectioning of Whole Mount-Stained Embryos

1. After rinsing in PBS (see Subheading 3.2, step 6), incubate embryos in distilled water for 5 min.
2. Rinse one time each in 25 and 50% ethanol (for amount of time, see Note 8).
3. Rinse twice in each concentration of alcohol (75, 95, and 100%) (see Note 9).
4. Rinse twice in cedar (cedarwood) oil (see Note 10).
5. Rinse twice in paraffin; use a vacuum chamber.
6. Proceed with embedding.
7. Once the blocks are cooled, section the embryos at 8 or 10 μm with a microtome.
8. Collect sections on positively charged slides.
9. Once dry, deparaffinize slides by heating them at 58°C for 45–60 min and then rinsing them twice in xylene for 5 min.
10. Rehydrate the sections by rinsing the slides twice for 10 min each in 100 and 95% ethanol.
11. Rinse for 5 min in 70% ethanol. Slides are now ready for counterstaining with eosin (proceed to Subheading 3.5) or continue to the next step.
12. Rinse for 5 min in 50% ethanol.
13. Rinse in distilled water for 5 min. Slides are now ready for counterstaining with Nuclear Fast Red. Proceed to Subheading 3.6.

3.5. Counterstaining with Eosin

1. After the 70% ethanol step, counterstain the section with working eosin for 1 min, agitating every 10 s with a gentle dipping motion. Let the slides drain briefly without drying.
2. Rinse for ten dips in 95% ethanol for about 1 s each (same length for the other dipping).
3. Rinse in 95% ethanol for five dips.
4. Dehydrate in two different 100% ethanol solutions for five dips each.
5. Transfer the slides to xylene (see Notes 10 and 11).
6. Proceed rapidly with mounting using a coverslip and xylene-soluble mounting solution (i.e., Permount).
7. After drying, sections are ready for microscopic observation and photography (see Fig. 1b).

3.6. Counterstaining with Nuclear Fast Red

1. After rinsing with water, counterstain sections in Nuclear Fast Red for 5 min.
2. Rinse slides in distilled water for 30 s, dipping ten times for 1 s at the beginning.

3. Dehydrate sections in 70% ethanol for 1 min.
4. Rinse in 95% ethanol for ten dips of about 1 s each (same length as for the other dipping).
5. Rinse for five dips in 95% ethanol.
6. Dehydrate in two different 100% alcohol solutions for five dips each.
7. Transfer the slides to xylene (see Notes 10 and 11).
8. Proceed rapidly with mounting using a coverslip and xylene-soluble mounting solution (i.e., Permount).
9. After drying, sections are ready for microscopic observation and photography under brightfield conditions (see Fig. 1d).

3.7. Isolation of Neural Crest Cells by FACS

1. Isolate the E8.5–E11.5 embryos in PBS, as described in Subheading 3.1, using a plate containing a 2% agarose bed (see Note 12).
2. Cut the section of the embryo from where the neural crest cells are wanted and transfer the tissue into a 1.5-mL microcentrifuge tube.
3. Remove the PBS and add 100–200 μL of trypsin.
4. Digest for 3–15 min at 37°C, pipetting up and down with a P1000 or P200 tip every 2–3 min to help dissociate the cells.
5. Once a single cell suspension is obtained, add 800 μL of PBS/10% FBS to the tube.
6. Centrifuge the cells for 8–10 min (500–1,000 × g).
7. Discard the supernatant, resuspend the cells in PBS/10% FBS, and centrifuge again.
8. Resuspend the cells in 1–3 mL of PBS in a tube fitting the flow cytometry apparatus. Keep the cells on ice.
9. Perform an initial analysis of the cells to adjust the settings of the apparatus (i.e., gain) and gate the cells such that the cell debris or negative cells are not collected (see Note 13) (42–44).
10. Proceed with the cell sorting and collect the eYFP-positive cells (see Fig. 2).
11. Rapidly add PBS or PBS/10% FBS to the cells and keep the cells on ice while processing the other samples (for viability).
12. Centrifuge the cells for 8–10 min.
13. Discard the supernatant.
14. Add the RNA or protein extraction solution or wash once more the cells if primary cell culture is desired.

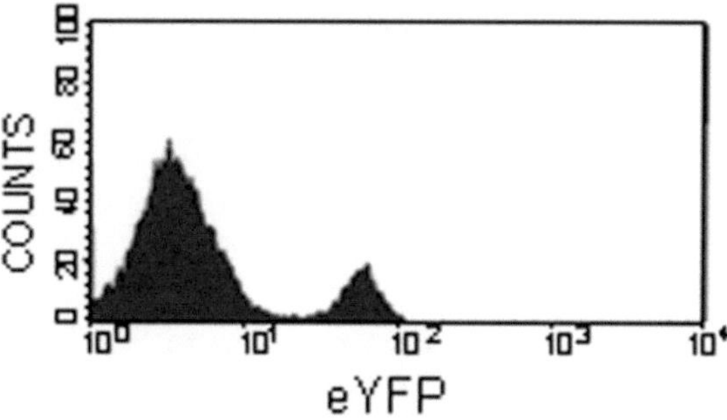

Fig. 2. Neural crest cell sorting using flow cytometry. Neural crest cells were genetically labeled by breeding the *Wnt1-Cre* and *R26R-eYFP* mouse lines together. Yellow-green fluorescent neural crest cells (*right peak*) can be identified and separated from other cells by flow cytometry.

4. Notes

1. Direct embedding in OCT gives satisfactory sections of the cardiac tissues with a strong signal. However, softer tissues such as the lungs and liver will easily break under this condition. To remediate this problem, we recommend prefixing the embryos prior to embedding following the protocol described above.
2. Dry ice pellets work better than larger chunks or blocks. We recommend that the ethanol level not be more than half the height of the molds. Since the ethanol can be reused several times, we suggest recycling it by pouring it into a bottle with a funnel. However, wait a few hours before tightly closing the cap to degasify the liquid and avoid an explosion.
3. This technique can be used to stain whole tissues such as the heart and the attached large blood vessels. In this case, simply dissect the tissue of interest and proceed as indicated in the protocol. We recommend making a small incision at the apex of the heart to allow the penetration of the staining solution inside the ventricles.
4. Incubating the embryos at 37°C increases the signal as well as the background and is recommended for lines with a weaker signal expression. With the *Wnt1-Cre* line, incubation at room temperature gives a satisfactory signal.
5. Avoid using double-distilled deionized water to preserve the integrity of the sections.
6. It is a matter of preference, but based on experience, using Nuclear Fast Red with younger embryos (E11.5 and less) and eosin with older embryos or tissues is recommended. Eosin produces a better

contrast of tissue density and composition, allowing the recognition of sub-anatomical structures [for example, the different nuclei of the brain (45) that would not be visible with Nuclear Fast Red. However, in younger embryos, the tissue density is too low to provide a nice contrast between the blue from the *lacZ*/β-gal staining and the surrounding pink/red tissue with eosin, making nuclear fast red a better choice. As an alternative, staining with eosin and Nuclear Fast Red can be combined, beginning first with the Nuclear Fast Red and staining with eosin after dehydrating the slides with 70% alcohol.

7. For Methyl green staining, prepare the Methyl green 0.5% solution (0.5 g in 100 mL of 0.1 M sodium acetate buffer, pH 4.2) and proceed as when staining sections with Nuclear Fast Red for 5 min. To prepare the buffer, use 1.36 g of sodium acetate trihydrate (MW 136.1) in 80 mL of water and use glacial acetic acid to bring the pH to 4.2; add enough water to make 100 mL. We recommend using ethyl violet-free Methyl green from Sigma (198080).
8. For E8.5 and E9.5 embryos, 10 min per step is sufficient. For E10.5–E12.5 embryos, 30 min for each step should be considered. For E13.5–E15.5 embryos, 60 min per step is recommended, and for older embryos or fatty tissues like the brain, 90 min per step will be necessary.
9. You can use histological reagent alcohol (95 parts ethanol, 5 parts isopropanol) instead of the 100% absolute ethanol.
10. Xylene is not recommended since it bleaches the X-gal staining.
11. We recommend counterstaining a limited number of slides at one time (10–12) to limit the fading of the X-gal staining. The slides can be kept for a longer period in water (before nuclear fast red staining) or in 70% ethanol (before eosin staining) without affecting the results.
12. We recommend making an agarose bed at the bottom of the plate to protect the tip and sharpness of microdissection instruments.
13. The initial gating should be made on the dot plot with the forward scatter (FSC, cell size) on the *X* axis and the side scatter (SSC, cell granularity, or density) of the *Y* axis to avoid collecting cell debris that tend to populate the lower left portion of the graph. Draw a polygon (gate) around the live cells that need to be analyzed. In the fluorescence analysis panel, the gain should be adjusted ("compensated") so that both peaks representing the negative and eYFP-positive cells are well separated, ideally with the 10^1 log scale marker between the peaks (see Fig. 2). Draw a line above the positive (right) peak to set your "collecting" gate or revert into the dot blot mode and draw a polygon around the eYFP-positive cells. For more information, please refer to these publications (42–44).

Acknowledgments

The authors would like to thank Ms. Jeanne Santa Cruz for editing the manuscript and Dr. Chantale Lacelle for helping with the FACS. This work was supported by the NIH/ NIDCR U24 DE16472 (LBR) and T32 DE018380 (YZ) and a Research Development Grant (LBR) from the Office of the Vice President for Research & Graduate Studies/Texas A&M Health Science Center.

References

1. Hoffman, J. I., and Kaplan, S. (2002) The incidence of congenital heart disease, *J Am Coll Cardiol 39*, 1890–1900.
2. Hoffman, J. I., Kaplan, S., and Liberthson, R. R. (2004) Prevalence of congenital heart disease, *Am Heart J 147*, 425–439.
3. Harvey, R. P. (2002) Patterning the vertebrate heart, *Nat Rev Genet* **3**, 544–556.
4. Stennard, F. A., and Harvey, R. P. (2005) T-box transcription factors and their roles in regulatory hierarchies in the developing heart, *Development 132*, 4897–4910.
5. Srivastava, D. (2006) Genetic regulation of cardiogenesis and congenital heart disease, *Annu Rev Pathol 1*, 199–213.
6. Srivastava, D., and Olson, E. N. (2000) A genetic blueprint for cardiac development, *Nature 407*, 221–226.
7. Creazzo, T. L., Godt, R. E., Leatherbury, L., Conway, S. J., and Kirby, M. L. (1998) Role of cardiac neural crest cells in cardiovascular development, *Annu Rev Physiol 60*, 267–286.
8. Kirby, M. L., and Waldo, K. L. (1995) Neural crest and cardiovascular patterning, *Circ Res 77*, 211–215.
9. Hutson, M. R., and Kirby, M. L. (2003) Neural crest and cardiovascular development: a 20-year perspective, *Birth Defects Res C Embryo Today 69*, 2–13.
10. Abu-Issa, R., Waldo, K., and Kirby, M. L. (2004) Heart fields: one, two or more?, *Dev Biol 272*, 281–285.
11. Waldo, K. L., Hutson, M. R., Ward, C. C., Zdanowicz, M., Stadt, H. A., Kumiski, D., Abu-Issa, R., and Kirby, M. L. (2005) Secondary heart field contributes myocardium and smooth muscle to the arterial pole of the developing heart, *Dev Biol 281*, 78–90.
12. Waldo, K. L., Hutson, M. R., Stadt, H. A., Zdanowicz, M., Zdanowicz, J., and Kirby, M. L. (2005) Cardiac neural crest is necessary for normal addition of the myocardium to the arterial pole from the secondary heart field, *Dev Biol 281*, 66–77.
13. Chai, Y., Jiang, X., Ito, Y., Bringas, P., Jr., Han, J., Rowitch, D. H., Soriano, P., McMahon, A. P., and Sucov, H. M. (2000) Fate of the mammalian cranial neural crest during tooth and mandibular morphogenesis, *Development 127*, 1671–1679.
14. Crane, J. F., and Trainor, P. A. (2006) Neural crest stem and progenitor cells, *Annu Rev Cell Dev Biol 22*, 267–286.
15. Trainor, P. A. (2005) Specification of neural crest cell formation and migration in mouse embryos, *Semin Cell Dev Biol 16*, 683–693.
16. Jones, N. C., and Trainor, P. A. (2005) Role of morphogens in neural crest cell determination, *J Neurobiol 64*, 388–404.
17. LaBonne, C., and Bronner-Fraser, M. (1999) Molecular mechanisms of neural crest formation, *Annu Rev Cell Dev Biol 15*, 81–112.
18. LaBonne, C., and Bronner-Fraser, M. (1998) Induction and patterning of the neural crest, a stem cell-like precursor population, *J Neurobiol 36*, 175–189.
19. Kirby, M. L., Gale, T. F., and Stewart, D. E. (1983) Neural crest cells contribute to normal aorticopulmonary septation, *Science 220*, 1059–1061.
20. Stoller, J. Z., and Epstein, J. A. (2005) Cardiac neural crest, *Semin Cell Dev Biol 16*, 704–715.
21. Sieber-Blum, M. (2004) Cardiac neural crest stem cells, *Anat Rec A Discov Mol Cell Evol Biol 276*, 34–42.
22. Jiang, X., Rowitch, D. H., Soriano, P., McMahon, A. P., and Sucov, H. M. (2000) Fate of the mammalian cardiac neural crest, *Development 127*, 1607–1616.
23. Gittenberger-de Groot, A. C., Bartelings, M. M., Deruiter, M. C., and Poelmann, R. E. (2005) Basics of cardiac development for the understanding of congenital heart malformations, *Pediatr Res 57*, 169–176.

24. Ramsdell, A. F. (2005) Left-right asymmetry and congenital cardiac defects: getting to the heart of the matter in vertebrate left-right axis determination, *Dev Biol 288*, 1–20.
25. Waldo, K. L., Kumiski, D. H., Wallis, K. T., Stadt, H. A., Hutson, M. R., Platt, D. H., and Kirby, M. L. (2001) Conotruncal myocardium arises from a secondary heart field, *Development 128*, 3179–3188.
26. Nagy, A. (2000) Cre recombinase: the universal reagent for genome tailoring, *Genesis 26*, 99–109.
27. Soriano, P. (1999) Generalized lacZ expression with the ROSA26 Cre reporter strain, *Nat Genet 21*, 70–71.
28. Moses, K. A., DeMayo, F., Braun, R. M., Reecy, J. L., and Schwartz, R. J. (2001) Embryonic expression of an Nkx2-5/Cre gene using ROSA26 reporter mice, *Genesis 31*, 176–180.
29. Agah, R., Frenkel, P. A., French, B. A., Michael, L. H., Overbeek, P. A., and Schneider, M. D. (1997) Gene recombination in postmitotic cells. Targeted expression of Cre recombinase provokes cardiac-restricted, site-specific rearrangement in adult ventricular muscle in vivo, *J Clin Invest 100*, 169–179.
30. Christoffels, V. M., Grieskamp, T., Norden, J., Mommersteeg, M. T., Rudat, C., and Kispert, A. (2009) Tbx18 and the fate of epicardial progenitors, *Nature 458*, E8-9; discussion E9-10.
31. Kisanuki, Y. Y., Hammer, R. E., Miyazaki, J., Williams, S. C., Richardson, J. A., and Yanagisawa, M. (2001) Tie2-Cre transgenic mice: a new model for endothelial cell-lineage analysis in vivo, *Dev Biol 230*, 230–242.
32. Yang, L., Cai, C. L., Lin, L., Qyang, Y., Chung, C., Monteiro, R. M., Mummery, C. L., Fishman, G. I., Cogen, A., and Evans, S. (2006) Isl1Cre reveals a common Bmp pathway in heart and limb development, *Development 133*, 1575–1585.
33. Macatee, T. L., Hammond, B. P., Arenkiel, B. R., Francis, L., Frank, D. U., and Moon, A. M. (2003) Ablation of specific expression domains reveals discrete functions of ectoderm- and endoderm-derived FGF8 during cardiovascular and pharyngeal development, *Development 130*, 6361–6374.
34. Ruest, L. B., Dager, M., Yanagisawa, H., Charite, J., Hammer, R. E., Olson, E. N., Yanagisawa, M., and Clouthier, D. E. (2003) dHAND-Cre transgenic mice reveal specific potential functions of dHAND during craniofacial development, *Dev Biol 257*, 263–277.
35. Danielian, P. S., Muccino, D., Rowitch, D. H., Michael, S. K., and McMahon, A. P. (1998) Modification of gene activity in mouse embryos in utero by a tamoxifen-inducible form of Cre recombinase, *Curr Biol 8*, 1323–1326.
36. Li, J., Chen, F., and Epstein, J. A. (2000) Neural crest expression of Cre recombinase directed by the proximal Pax3 promoter in transgenic mice, *Genesis 26*, 162–164.
37. Ruest, L. B., Xiang, X., Lim, K. C., Levi, G., and Clouthier, D. E. (2004) Endothelin-A receptor-dependent and -independent signaling pathways in establishing mandibular identity, *Development 131*, 4413–4423.
38. Abe, M., Ruest, L. B., and Clouthier, D. E. (2007) Fate of cranial neural crest cells during craniofacial development in endothelin-A receptor-deficient mice, *Int J Dev Biol 51*, 97–105.
39. Stottmann, R. W., Choi, M., Mishina, Y., Meyers, E. N., and Klingensmith, J. (2004) BMP receptor IA is required in mammalian neural crest cells for development of the cardiac outflow tract and ventricular myocardium, *Development 131*, 2205–2218.
40. Vincentz, J. W., Barnes, R. M., Rodgers, R., Firulli, B. A., Conway, S. J., and Firulli, A. B. (2008) An absence of Twist1 results in aberrant cardiac neural crest morphogenesis, *Dev Biol 320*, 131–139.
41. Luo, Y., High, F. A., Epstein, J. A., and Radice, G. L. (2006) N-cadherin is required for neural crest remodeling of the cardiac outflow tract, *Dev Biol 299*, 517–528.
42. Jaroszeski, M. J., and Radcliff, G. (1999) Fundamentals of flow cytometry, *Mol Biotechnol 11*, 37–53.
43. Cunningham, R. E. Overview of flow cytometry and fluorescent probes for flow cytometry, *Methods Mol Biol 588*, 319–326.
44. Radcliff, G., and Jaroszeski, M. J. (1998) Basics of flow cytometry, *Methods Mol Biol 91*, 1–24.
45. Ruest, L. B., Hammer, R. E., Yanagisawa, M., and Clouthier, D. E. (2003) Dlx5/6-enhancer directed expression of Cre recombinase in the pharyngeal arches and brain, *Genesis 37*, 188–194.

Chapter 13

Indirect Immunostaining on Mouse Embryonic Heart for the Detection of Proliferated Cardiomyocyte

Jieli Li, Marc Antonyak, and Xu Peng

Abstract

The heart is the first organ to form and become functional in a developing embryo and its proper function is critical for most, if not all, subsequent stages of an animal's development. The formation of the heart relies heavily upon the rapid proliferation of cardiomyocytes at a specific stage during early development, and interfering with the ability of these cells to replicate during this time frame results in heart defects that include thin ventricle walls, as well as malformed ventricular septums. Since cardiomyocyte proliferation represents a key step in early cardiac development and identifying the mechanisms that underlie cardiomyocyte proliferation has become an important area of study, techniques to identify and study proliferating cardiomyocytes in vivo are needed. Immunofluorescence and immunohistochemistry staining are powerful tools for studying cardiomyocyte proliferation in the developing animal. The phosphorylation of histone H3 at Ser10 (pH3) only occurs in cells undergoing mitosis, making pH3 a marker for labeling proliferating cells. In this manuscript, we described two immunostaining methods (immunofluorescence and immunohistochemistry) for detecting the pH3-positive cardiomyocytes in formalin-fixed, paraffin-embedded heart tissues.

Key words: Cardiomyocyte, Proliferation, Immunohistochemistry, Immunofluorescence

1. Introduction

The heart is the first formed organ during embryogenesis, and nearly all other subsequent stages of development of the animal depend upon its proper function. During the first two thirds of gestation, the majority of cardiomyocytes are mononucleated and embryonic heart growth relies heavily on the proliferation of cardiomyocytes via mitosis. However, during the final third of gestation cardiomyocytes undergo a maturation or differentiation process and the number of double nucleated cardiomyocyte is increased due to

Xu Peng and Marc Antonyak (eds.), *Cardiovascular Development: Methods and Protocols*, Methods in Molecular Biology, vol. 843, DOI 10.1007/978-1-61779-523-7_13,

a failure of the cells to complete cytokinesis after karyokinesis (1–3). Coinciding with this maturation process, the proliferative capacity of the cardiomyocytes is reduced, with nearly all of the cells exiting the cell cycle at the neonatal stage in mammalian animals (4, 5). Since various forms of genetic intervention have been shown to affect cardiomyocyte DNA synthesis, karyokinesis, and in some cases, cytokinesis, the specific elimination of a gene in cardiomyocytes using cre/loxp technology (6) has become a powerful tool to investigate cardiomyocyte cell cycle regulation, particularly in the developing embryo.

Histone H3 is one of the core components of the nucleosome (7). During mitosis, the phosphorylation of histone H3 at Ser 10 is necessary for the initiation of chromosome condensation in mammalian cells (8). The phosphorylation of histone H3 begins during prophase, reaches its highest levels during metaphase, and decreases to basal levels during telophase (9–11). Since histone H3 is only phosphorylated at Ser 10 in cells undergoing mitosis, the phosphorylation status of histone H3 can serve as a marker for proliferating cells. Phospho-histone H3 staining is a straight-forward and reliable method for quantifying the proliferative capacities of various cell types, including cardiomyocyte (12, 13). The present work describes immunohistochemistry and immunofluorescence staining for phospho-histone H3 (Ser10) procedures, using unconjugated primary polyclonal antibodies, to investigate cardiomyocyte proliferation in mouse embryonic heart.

2. Materials

1. Phosphate-buffered saline (PBS) (1×): dissolve 8 g of NaCl, 0.2 g of KCl, 1.44 g of Na_2HPO_4, and 0.24 g of KH_2PO_4 in 1 L ddH_2O. Adjust the pH of the solution to 7.4, sterilize it, and then store the PBS at room temperature.
2. 4% Paraformaldehyde (PFA): dissolve 4 g of PFA in 100 mL of PBS by heating the mixture at 60°C, with constant stirring, until the solution becomes clear. Allow the solution to cool to room temperature and then adjust the pH to 7.4 using 10 N NaOH (around 0.1 mL will be needed) (see Notes 1 and 2).
3. Ethanol (75, 95, and 100%).
4. PBST (1×): 0.05% (v/v) Tween 20 in PBS (prepare fresh).
5. Antigen retrieval buffer: 3.7 g/L ethylenediaminetetraacetic acid disodium salt dihydrate (EDTA), pH 8.0.
6. Antibodies: Rabbit anti-phospho-Histone H3 (Ser10), Mouse Troponin T, Cardiac Isoform Ab-1 (Clone 13–11), dilute to 1:100 in PBST or serum just prior to use.

7. Avidin and Biotin blocking solution (Dako).
8. Peroxidase blocking reagent: 3% (v/v) H_2O_2.
9. Rabbit ImmunoCruz™ Staining System (Santa Cruz Biotechnology, Inc).
10. 3, 3′-Diaminobenzidine tetrahydrochloride (DAB) solution: Dissolve 1 DAB tablet (Sigma) in 5 mL Tris-buffered saline (pH 7.6) and add 12 μL of 30% hydrogen peroxide (H_2O_2). Filter DAB solution before use.
11. Tris-buffered saline (TBS): 2.4 g/L Tris base, 8 g/L NaCl, Using HCl to adjust pH to 7.6.
12. Permount* Mounting Medium.
13. Humidity box.
14. Antigen retriever (2100 Retriever, Prestige Medical).
15. Hematoxylin.

3. Methods

3.1. Prepare Paraformaldehyde-Fixed, Paraffin-Embedded Tissue Sections

1. Harvest embryonic day (E) 14.5 mouse embryos from time-crossed pregnant female mice. Sacrifice the pregnant female mice using carbon dioxide asphyxiation. Using scissors make a T-shaped cross-section in the abdominoperineal region of the mouse and cut away the skin to expose the gut. With forceps and scissors, remove the uterus and place it into a petri dish containing ice-cold PBS.
2. Isolate the embryos from the uterus and then remove each embryo from their embryonic sac. Transfer the embryos to a second petri dish containing ice-cold PBS by pipet. Gently remove the extraembryonic membranes from the embryos using Dumont #3 forceps.
3. Immerse the embryos in the 4% PFA solution for fixation at 4°C for overnight (see Note 3).
4. Using a surgical knife, make an incision in the embryo transversally between the upper liver level and the lower neck level.
5. Dehydrate and embed the specimen in paraffin using a standard protocol.
6. Section the specimen to a thickness of 4 μm using a microtome.
7. Place the slides on a slide warmer (~37°C) overnight.

3.2. Immunohistochemistry Staining

1. Deparaffinize the sections in xylene, 10 min × 2.
2. Hydrate specimens in 100% EtOH, 5 min × 2; 95% EtOH, 3 min × 2; 75% EtOH, 3 min × 2; and ddH_2O, 5 min × 2.

3. Antigen retrieval: Place the slides in a plastic container and add around 50 mL antigen retrieval buffer. Put the container and slides into the antigen retriever for thermally processing and leave the slides in the machine for overnight. The next day, remove the slides from the antigen retriever (see Note 4).
4. Wash the slides in tap water for 2 min × 2.
5. Carefully wipe the water from the back and edges of each slide using tissue wipers.
6. Place the slides on a flat surface and draw a line around the section of tissue to be stained with a PAP pen. This will help prevent the blocking solution from running off the edges of the slides.
7. Place the slides in the humidity box and incubate the slides with Avidin blocking solution for 10 min at 37°C.
8. Wash the slides with PBST for 10 min × 2 at room temperature (see Note 5).
9. Remove the PBST from the slides with a flick of the wrist and then wipe the back and edges of each slide with tissue wipers. Vacuum aspiration is then used to carefully remove any remaining liquid from the slides (see Notes 6–8).
10. Place the slides in the humidity box and incubate them with biotin blocking solution for 10 min at 37°C (see Note 9).
11. Repeat steps 8 and 9.
12. Incubate the slides with peroxidase blocking buffer for 10 min at 37°C to quench endogenous peroxidase activity.
13. Repeat steps 8 and 9.
14. Place the slides in the humidity box and then block the sections with (donkey) serum (~500 μL) at 37°C for 30 min.
15. Dilute the primary rabbit anti-phospho-Histone H3 (Ser10) antibody 1:100 in a microcentrifuge tube containing either PBS or serum. Centrifuge the microcentrifuge tube briefly to pellet any insoluble particulate and then add the supernatant to the tissue sections (~200 μL), and incubate the slides in a humidity box at 37°C for 60 min (see Note 10).
16. Repeat steps 8 and 9.
17. Incubate the slides with the biotin-labeled secondary antibody (~3 drops) at 37°C for 60 min.
18. Repeat steps 8 and 9.
19. Incubate the slides with horseradish peroxidase (HRP)-labeled streptavidin to bind the biotin-conjugated secondary antibody at 37°C for 30 min (see Note 11).
20. Repeat steps 8 and 9.

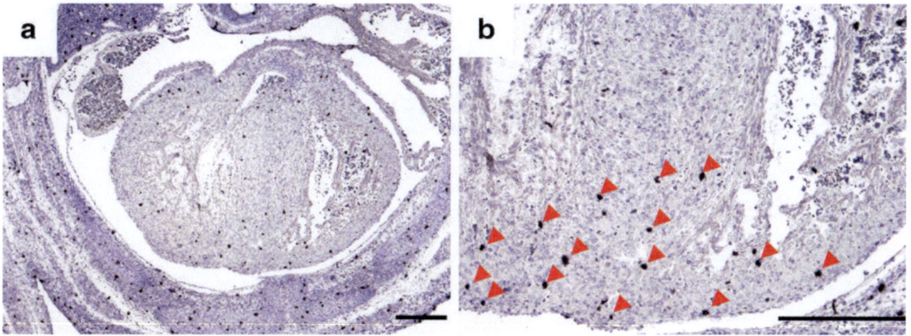

Fig. 1. Immunohistochemistry staining of phosphorylated histone H3 on the E14.5 heart. The majority of phosphorylated histone H3-positive cells distributes in the compact zone of the ventricle (*arrowheads*). *Left panel* is lower magnification (40×) and *right panel* is higher magnification (100×) (bar: 500 μm).

21. Add DAB solution (~3 drops) to each slide and incubate for different lengths of time (from several seconds to 5 min) at room temperature (see Note 12).
22. Wash the slide with room temperature tap water for a few minutes.
23. Counterstain the slides with Hematoxylin in a staining jar for 3 min at room temperature.
24. Wash the slide in tap water for 3 min.
25. Dehydrate the slide successively in 95% ETOH 3 min × 2, 100% ETOH 5 min × 2, and then xylene 10 min × 2.
26. Add Permount* Mounting Medium to the slides and then cover them with a coverslip. Allow the slides to dry at room temperature overnight.
27. Take images of the stained tissues using an upright brightfield microscope (see Fig. 1).

3.3. Immunofluorescence Staining

1. Begin by following steps 1–6 of Subheading 3.2.
2. Place the slides in a humidity box and then block the sections with (donkey) serum (~500 μL) at 37°C for 30 min.
3. Wash the slide with PBST (10 min × 2) at room temperature (see Note 5).
4. Remove excess PBST from the slides with a flick of the wrist. Wipe the back and edges of the slides with tissue wipers, and then carefully vacuum aspirate any residual liquid from the slides (see Notes 6–8).
5. Dilute the primary rabbit anti-phospho-Histone H3 (Ser10) antibody 1:100 in a microcentrifuge tube containing either PBS or serum. Centrifuge the microcentrifuge tube briefly to pellet any insoluble particulate and then add the supernatant

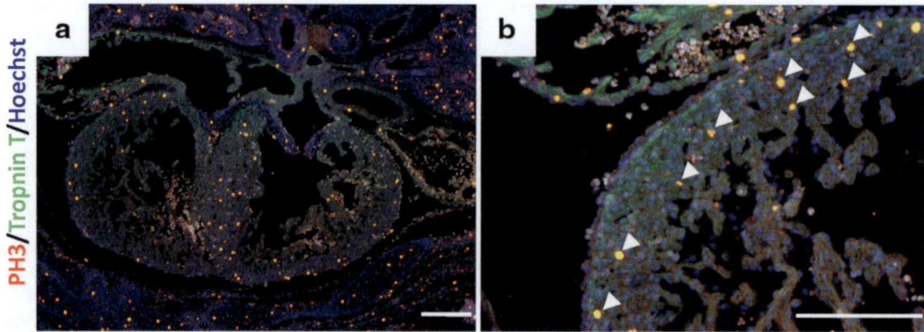

Fig. 2. Immunofluorescence staining of phosphorylated histone H3 on the E14.5 heart. The *arrowheads* show phosphorylated histone H3, and the cardiomyocytes are stained by Troponin T in *green* color. The *blue* ones are Hoechst 33342 staining which shows nucleus of cells.

to the tissue sections (~200 μL) and incubate the slides in a humidity box at 37°C for 60 min.

6. Repeat steps 3 and 4.
7. Dilute the secondary antibodies (Rhodamine Red™-X goat anti-rabbit IgG and Alexa Fluor® 488 goat anti-mouse) in PBST and then add the antibody dilutions to the slides and incubate them in a humidity box at 37°C for 60 min in the dark (see Note 13).
8. Repeat steps 3 and 4.
9. To label nuclei, add Hoechst 33342 diluted in PBST (1:5,000) to the slides and incubate them in the dark for 5 min.
10. Add anti-fade reagent COMPONENT A to the slides and then cover the tissue sections with coverslips.
11. Seal the edges of the coverslips with clear nail polish and allow the slides to dry at room temperature for several minutes in the dark.
12. Take images of the stained tissues under a fluorescence microscope (see Fig. 2).

4. Notes

1. PFA is toxic. Do not inhale the powder and perform all of the steps involving the use of PFA in a fume hood.
2. PFA is the solid form polymerized formaldehyde. The solution should be made fresh before use, but can be kept for up to several weeks at −20°C.

3. The volume of PFA solution used for fixation should be approximately ten times the volume of the embryos. Tissue fixation is one of the most important steps in immunostaining. Incomplete or delayed fixation can lead to autolysis and destroy tissue morphology, whereas prolonged fixation could affect antibody binding and cause false negative results.
4. Heat-induced epitope retrieval is a reliable and convenient method of antigen retrieval. The pH of retrieval buffer is a key factor for obtaining satisfied results. In addition, proteolytic enzyme digestion and microwave can also be used for antigen retrieval.
5. Triton X-100 is the most popular detergent used for improving antibody penetration of frozen and paraffin sections for immunohistochemical analysis.
6. The entire staining process involves many steps of vacuum aspiration. If the supernatant is not carefully aspirated from the slides, tissue samples can be damaged or lost. To reduce tissue damage/loss during vacuum aspiration, a 200-μL pipet tip can be attached to a vacuum tube and touch this tip near the edges of tissues, but not directly on the tissue sections.
7. Do not leave excess buffer rinse on the slide or the antibody, when added to the tissue samples, can become too diluted, resulting in weak staining.
8. Insufficient rinsing at all steps of the protocols outlined can give rise to high background. Mixing new buffers and increasing the washing steps could help alleviate this problem.
9. Endogenous biotin exists in embryos. Pretreatment with biotin blocking reagent is needed.
10. Incubation with primary antibodies can also be done overnight at 4°C.
11. Streptavidin, derived from streptococcus avidin, comes up as substitution of avidin. The streptavidin molecule is uncharged relative to animal tissues, while avidin has an isoelectric point. Therefore, the use of HRP-conjugated streptavidin can significantly reduce background.
12. Incubate with DAB for short periods of time, because the signal will develop quickly (on the order of seconds to minutes depending on the antibody used) and can be a source of high background.
13. During the immunofluorescence staining protocol, the sealed slides should be protected from light. Slides may be stored in the dark at –20°C for a couple of weeks.

Acknowledgments

This work was supported by American Heart Association Scientist Development Grant and Texas A&M Health Science Center Startup Grant to Xu Peng.

References

1. Soonpaa, M. H., Kim, K. K., Pajak, L., Franklin, M., and Field, L. J. (1996) Cardiomyocyte DNA synthesis and binucleation during murine development, *Am J Physiol 271*, H2183–2189.
2. Clubb, F. J., Jr., and Bishop, S. P. (1984) Formation of binucleated myocardial cells in the neonatal rat. An index for growth hypertrophy, *Lab Invest 50*, 571–577.
3. Li, F., Wang, X., Capasso, J. M., and Gerdes, A. M. (1996) Rapid transition of cardiac myocytes from hyperplasia to hypertrophy during postnatal development, *J Mol Cell Cardiol 28*, 1737–1746.
4. Rumyantsev, P. P. (1977) Interrelations of the proliferation and differentiation processes during cardiact myogenesis and regeneration, *Int Rev Cytol 51*, 186–273.
5. Pasumarthi, K. B., and Field, L. J. (2002) Cardiomyocyte cell cycle regulation, *Circ Res 90*, 1044–1054.
6. Minamino, T., Gaussin, V., DeMayo, F. J., and Schneider, M. D. (2001) Inducible gene targeting in postnatal myocardium by cardiac-specific expression of a hormone-activated Cre fusion protein, *Circ Res 88*, 587–592.
7. Workman, J. L., and Kingston, R. E. (1998) Alteration of nucleosome structure as a mechanism of transcriptional regulation, *Annu Rev Biochem 67*, 545–579.
8. Van Hooser, A., Goodrich, D. W., Allis, C. D., Brinkley, B. R., and Mancini, M. A. (1998) Histone H3 phosphorylation is required for the initiation, but not maintenance, of mammalian chromosome condensation, *J Cell Sci 111 (Pt 23)*, 3497–3506.
9. Gurley, L. R., D'Anna, J. A., Barham, S. S., Deaven, L. L., and Tobey, R. A. (1978) Histone phosphorylation and chromatin structure during mitosis in Chinese hamster cells, *Eur J Biochem 84*, 1–15.
10. Jordan, M. A., Wendell, K., Gardiner, S., Derry, W. B., Copp, H., and Wilson, L. (1996) Mitotic block induced in HeLa cells by low concentrations of paclitaxel (Taxol) results in abnormal mitotic exit and apoptotic cell death, *Cancer Res 56*, 816–825.
11. Chadee, D. N., Hendzel, M. J., Tylipski, C. P., Allis, C. D., Bazett-Jones, D. P., Wright, J. A., and Davie, J. R. (1999) Increased Ser-10 phosphorylation of histone H3 in mitogen-stimulated and oncogene-transformed mouse fibroblasts, *J Biol Chem 274*, 24914–24920.
12. Ajiro, K., Nishimoto, T., and Takahashi, T. (1983) Histone H1 and H3 phosphorylation during premature chromosome condensation in a temperature-sensitive mutant (tsBN2) of baby hamster kidney cells, *J Biol Chem 258*, 4534–4538.
13. Peng, X., Wu, X., Druso, J. E., Wei, H., Park, A. Y., Kraus, M. S., Alcaraz, A., Chen, J., Chien, S., Cerione, R. A., and Guan, J. L. (2008) Cardiac developmental defects and eccentric right ventricular hypertrophy in cardiomyocyte focal adhesion kinase (FAK) conditional knockout mice, *Proc Natl Acad Sci U S A 105*, 6638–6643.

Chapter 14

Isolation and Characterization of Vascular Endothelial Cells from Murine Heart and Lung

Yixin Jin, Yang Liu, Marc Antonyak, and Xu Peng

Abstract

The formation of blood vessel networks is a fundamental event in vertebrate embryo development. Angiogenesis and vasculogenesis are the essential processes in vascular formation. Endothelial cells play a key role during angiogenesis and vasculogenesis, and cultured vascular endothelial cells provide an indispensable model for exploring the molecular mechanisms of angiogenesis and vasculogenesis. In this chapter, we described a protocol using PECAM-1-coated Dynabeads for the isolation of vascular endothelial cells from mouse heart and lung. This method will provide up to 10^7 endothelial cells with high purity (>85%). The isolated endothelial cells retain their in vivo characteristics, such as the expression of the cell surface markers PECAM-1 and ICAM-2.

Key words: Cardiovascular development, Angiogenesis, Vasculogenesis, Endothelial cells, In vitro cell culture

1. Introduction

The cardiovascular system transports life-sustaining nutrients and oxygen to all organs and plays an essential role in embryo development. Two different processes are involved in blood vessel formation: Angiogenesis, the budding and branching of new vessels from preexisting vessels; and vasculogenesis, which is the de novo formation of blood vessels by in situ differentiation of endothelial cells from mesoderm (1, 2). In addition to embryogenesis, new blood vessel formation is involved in many physiological and pathological events in the adult, such as wound healing, tissue regeneration and remodeling, coronary heart disease, diabetes, rheumatoid arthritis, and tumor neovascularization (3, 4).

Angiogenesis and vasculogenesis need to coordinate a series of events, including activation of endothelial cells and pericytes,

Xu Peng and Marc Antonyak (eds.), *Cardiovascular Development: Methods and Protocols*,
Methods in Molecular Biology, vol. 843, DOI 10.1007/978-1-61779-523-7_14,

angiogen-stimulated degradation of the basement membrane by proteases, migration and proliferation of endothelial cells, differentiation of endothelial cells back into the quiescent endothelial cell phenotype with reestablishment of cell–cell contact and, ultimately, lumen and tubule formation (5, 6). Vascular endothelial cells are central players in the cascade of events in angiogenesis and vasculogenesis, which includes the generation and release of pro-angiogenic growth factors, endothelial cell activation and proliferation in response to the binding of angiogenic factors to their surface receptors, endothelial cell migration towards the source of angiogenic factors, and the formation of new vessels which are then stabilized by recruiting mural cells (7).

Cultured primary vascular endothelial cells are a powerful model for studying the molecular mechanisms of angiogenesis and vasculogenesis. Endothelial cells isolated from human umbilical veins were first cultured in vitro in 1973 (8, 9) and are used widely for studying the molecular mechanisms of blood vessel formation. However, with the advancement of molecular biology, genetically modified mice became one of the most dominant tools for exploring angiogenesis mechanisms and allowed the isolation of endothelial cells from mice directly. In this protocol, we describe a method in which to isolate mouse heart and lung endothelial cells by endothelial cell-specific antibody (PECAM-1)-coated magnetic beads. In brief, heart and lungs are harvested from mice, minced and digested by collagenase, and then vascular endothelial cells are enriched by incubation with PECAM-1- or ICAM-2-coated Dynabeads. The endothelial cells produced from this method, especially the endothelial cells isolated from knockout and transgenic mice, can then be used for many molecular and cell biological experiments involving cell migration, cell signaling, and drag selection assays.

2. Materials

2.1. Cell Culture Media

1. Basic medium: 500 mL high glucose Dulbecco's modified eagle medium (DMEM) supplemented with 5 mL Penicillin/streptomycin (100×).
2. Isolation and wash medium: 400 mL basic medium with 100 mL fetal bovine serum (FBS).
3. Growth medium: 500 mL EBM-2 medium kit (Lonza) with 5 mL Penicillin/streptomycin (100×).
4. HBSS (Hank's Buffered Salt Solution): dissolve 200 mg of KCl, 30 mg of KH_2PO_4, 175 mg of $NaHCO_3$, 4 g of NaCl, 24 mg of Na_2HPO_4, 500 mg d-Glucose, and 3 g HEPES in

500 mL distilled water. Adjust pH to 7.4 and autoclave. Store in 4°C.

5. PBS (phosphate-buffered saline): add 8 g of NaCl, 0.2 g of KCl, 0.24 g of KH_2PO_4, and 1.44 g of Na_2HPO_4 in 1 L distilled water. Adjust pH to 7.4 and autoclave. Store in 4°C.

2.2. Reagents and Instruments

1. 1-week-old neonatal mice or 4- to 8-week-old young mice are used for endothelial cell isolation (see Note 1).
2. Rat anti-mouse PECAM-1 (CD31) antibody (BD Biosciences) and Rat anti-mouse ICAM-2 (CD102) antibody (BD Biosciences).
3. Collagenase type II (Invitrogen) (see Note 2).
4. 2% Gelatin (Sigma).
5. Dynabeads Sheep anti-Rat IgG and Dynal MPC-S magnetic particle concentrator (Invitrogen).
6. Bovine serum albumin (BSA) (Sigma).
7. Trypsin-EDTA (0.05%) (Invitrogen).
8. Heat-inactivated FBS. Aliquot in 50-mL tubes and stock at −20°C.
9. 5% CO_2 humidified incubator.
10. Tissue culture plates (6-well plates) and Petri dishes.
11. Forceps and scissors.
12. 6-in. 14-G needle.
13. 70-μm cell strainer (BD Falcon Cat. no. 352350) and 0.22-μm syringe filter.
14. Magnetic concentrator (Invitrogen MPC-S).

3. Methods

3.1. Preparation of Magnetic Beads

1. Mix Dynabeads sufficiently by pipetting the beads up and down several times.
2. Resuspend 200 μL Dynabeads in 1 mL PBS with 0.1% BSA (or FBS) in 1.5-mL Eppendorf tube.
3. Place tube on a magnetic concentrator and leave for 1–2 min.
4. Remove supernatant carefully and wash three times with PBS + 0.1% BSA.
5. Resuspend beads in 200 μL PBS + 0.1%BSA.
6. Add 10 μL antibody (PECAM-1 or ICAM-2) into beads.

7. Incubate the antibody and beads at 4°C for overnight or 2 h at room temperature.
8. Place the tube on the magnetic concentrator and wash four times *with* PBS+0.1%BSA.
9. Resuspend beads in 200 μL PBS+0.1%BSA.
10. Store beads at 4°C and use within 1–2 weeks. Can use 0.02% sodium azide to preserve the coated beads, but wash off well before use with PBS+0.1%BSA.

3.2. Gelatin-Coated Plates

1. 6-well plates and Petri dishes are covered with 2% gelatin for 30 min at room temperature.
2. The 2% gelatin solution is aspirated from the plates. The plates are then allowed to dry at room temperature for 4 h in a flow hood.
3. The coated plates can be kept in 4°C for at least 2 weeks. The whole coating process *must be* kept sterile.

3.3. Mouse Dissection

1. Prepare 50 mL 0.2% Collagenase type II with HBSS just before the animal dissection. Prewarm the Collagenase at 37°C, and sterilize using a 0.22 μm syringe filter. Separate into two 50-mL tubes, 25 mL each.
2. Euthanize the mouse by injection of sodium pentobarbital (160 mg/Kg body weight) followed by cervical dislocation and dip in 70% ethanol for 5 min. Usually process 2 mice at one time (see Note 3).
3. Pin mouse supine to a styrofoam board that has two paper towels on the top.
4. Lift up the midabdomen skin with a pair of sterile forceps, incise the skin with sterile scissors and peel the skin to above the chest, then pin the skin down.
5. Incise the thoracic cavity through the ribcage above diaphragm. Cut the sternum and form a T-shaped cross-section.
6. Using another pair of forceps and scissors, gently grasp the heart and lungs, and remove from surrounding connective tissue and mediastinum (see Note 4).
7. Put the heart and lungs in 15 mL HBSS in a 10-cm dish.

3.4. Tissue Dissociation

1. Transfer dish to a laminar flow hood.
2. Remove any remaining tissues around the heart and lungs. Aspirate the HBSS from dish carefully, being careful to avoid the heart and lungs. Add 15 mL new HBSS.
3. Use scissors to cut the heart into two pieces and remove any blood clots in the heart. Transfer the heart to another 10-cm dish.

4. Mince the heart until the pieces are small enough to smoothly go through a 10-mL pipette (see Note 5).
5. Using a 10-mL pipette, take up 7–8 mL of collagenase (total 25 mL) and flush the scissors and dish and aspirate the remaining collagenase. Aspirate gently up and expel down if the tissue sticks to the side of the pipette. Remove all of the tissue from the plate.
6. Cut the lungs into mince. The lung tissue adheres to the side of the pipette more readily than does the heart tissue.
7. Incubate at 37°C with gentle rotation for 45 min. Manually shake the tubes every 10 min to avoid tissue clotting.
8. Using a 30-mL syringe with a cannula, triturate the suspension ten times. Avoid frothing. This breaks up any clumps.
9. Let tissue debris settle. Pipette suspension through a 70-μm disposable cell strainer into a 50-mL centrifuge tube. Wash sieve with 20 mL isolation medium.
10. Spin suspension at 400 × *g*, 8 min at 4°C.

3.5. Cell Sorting

1. Resuspend cells in 1 mL base medium (Normally, 1 mL medium/2 mouse lung or hearts). Add 20 μL/mL anti-mouse PECAM-coated Dynabeads to cell suspension. May modify this volume depending on the mouse and number of cells. Both heart and lung cells are treated identically from this point (see Note 6).
2. Incubate and rotate cells with Dynabeads for 30 min at 4°C.
3. Mount tubes in magnetic separator, and leave for 1–2 min.
4. Remove supernatant and save (for the event of error).
5. Remove tube from magnet and resuspend beads in 1 mL isolation medium by pipetting up and down (not too gently and not too harsh) (see Note 7).
6. Repeat steps 3–5 three to five times until supernatant is clear. For the final wash, use base medium instead of isolation medium.
7. Add 0.5 mL of Trypsin-EDTA (0.05%). Incubate at 37°C for 5 min to remove Dynabeads from cell surface. Stop the trypsinization by adding 0.5 mL isolation medium (see Note 8).
8. Mount tubes in magnetic separator. Transfer supernatant to another tube (the supernatant retains cells).
9. Spin down the cells at 300 × *g* for 10 min and remove supernatant carefully.
10. Resuspend cell pellet in growth medium. Plate in 6-well plate. Normally, one plate accomodates 2 mice: two wells for heart endothelial cells, 4 wells for lung endothelial cells.
11. Incubate at 37°C in 5% CO_2. 2 mL EBM-2 medium per well (see Note 9)
12. The next day, wash the wells with isolation medium and add fresh growth medium.

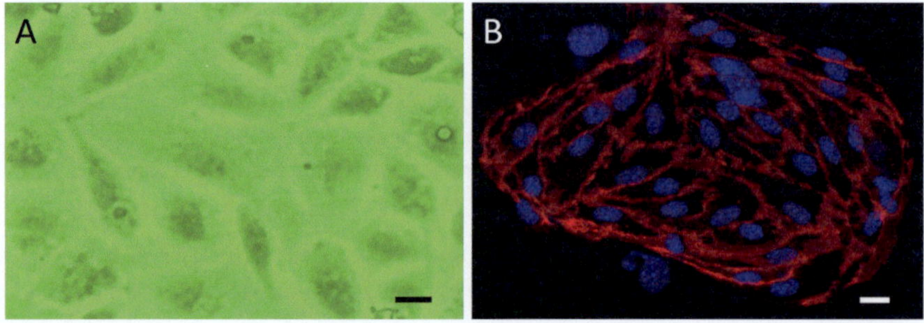

Fig. 1. Isolated and cultured mouse endothelial cells. (**a**) Phasecontrast microscope image of cultured mouse endothelial cells after 7 days culture (×400). (**b**) Immuno-staining by PECAM-1 (*red*) and Hoechst 33342 (*blue*) of isolated ECs after 7 days culture (×400) (bar: 10 μm).

3.6. Second Sorting

Normally, the purity of endothelial cells may reach 80% after the primary sorting. If higher purity is needed, a secondary sorting can be done as follows.

1. Feed with growth medium on Monday, Wednesday, and Friday. Wash each well with 2 mL HBSS, and then add new growth medium.
2. Check cells on Monday. Allow them to grow to confluence 5–9 days after plating. Endothelial cells are satellite cells in packets. Contaminating cells pile up and do not form monolayers.
3. *Trypsinize* cells with warm Trypsin-EDTA (0.05%). First rinse with prewarm HBSS, then add 0.5 mL Trypsin-EDTA and put in the incubator. Leave for 5 min and check to see if all cells are detached from the plate. Avoid prolonged exposure cells to Trypsin-EDTA. Only use Trypsin-EDTA long enough to achieve a suspension of single cells if needed (see Note 10).
4. Add 10 mL of warm isolation medium to inactivate the trypsin. Transfer cells to a 15-mL tube.
5. Spin down cells at 400 ×*g* for 8 min.
6. Remove supernatant and resuspend pellet in 1 mL isolation medium.
7. Add 15 μL ICAM-2-coated Dynabeads and incubate for 10 min, rocking at 4°C.
8. Place in magnet and leave for 1–2 min. Remove supernatant.
9. Wash gently 3× in 3 mL of isolation medium.
10. After final wash, resuspend the cells in growth medium and plate on gelatin-coated plates. Split cells at a ratio of 1:2 to 1:3 (see Fig.1).

3.7. Analysis of Purity of Endothelial Cells by Fluorescence-Activated Cell Scanning (FACS)

1. Remove the medium and rinse the cells with warm HBSS when cell confluence reaches 70–80%.
2. Digest cells with 0.05% EDTA only. Check the cells by microscope until all the cells have detached (see Note 11).

3. Wash the cells with PBS containing 0.1% BSA, then spin down at 300 × *g* for 10 min (see Note 12).
4. Discard the supernatant.
5. Repeat steps 3 and 4.
6. Resuspend cells in 100 μL PBS+0.1% BSA in Eppendorf tube.
7. Add 1 μL Rat anti-mouse PECAM-1 and 1 μL goat anti-mouse VE-cadherin.
8. Incubate cells with antibodies for 30 min on a roller mixer (slow speed setting).
9. Spin down the cells at 3,000 rpm for 5 min.
10. Remove the supernatant carefully. Wash the cell pellet with PBS+0.1% BSA once.
11. Add 1 μL FITC-conjugated anti-goat secondary antibody and 1 μL Alexa 594-conjugated anti-rat secondary antibody.
12. Incubate cells with antibodies for 15 min on a roller mixer (slow speed setting).
13. Add 1 mL PBS+0.1% BSA and centrifuge at 3,000 rpm for 5 min.
14. Wash cells two times with PBS+0.1 BSA.
15. Cells are resuspended in 600 μL PBS+0.1% BSA and ran on the flow cytometer for analysis (see Note 13).

4. Notes

1. The purity and growth ability of endothelial cells isolated from neonatal mice are better than that of endothelial cells from adult mice. If you do not want to do the second sorting, neonatal mice are the best choice.
2. Some protocols for endothelial cell isolation suggest the use of type I collagenase. According to our experience, type II is better than type I collagenase.
3. The mice should not be sacrificed by CO_2 asphyxia, as the CO_2 will damage endothelial cells in the lungs. This prohibits any further endothelial cell culture.
4. After cutting the skin/thoracic cavity, use another set of sterile instruments to remove the organs (to avoid contamination).
5. Mince the heart and lungs into as small pieces as possible, as it will increase cell yield.
6. Anti-ICAM-2-coated Dynabeads can also be used in the primary sorting. However, anti-PECAM-1-coated Dynabeads cannot be used in secondary sorting, because PECAM-1 is a trypsin-sensitive molecule.

7. Pipetting the beads too gently may allow too many contaminating cells, but pipetting too harshly may cause the loss of too many endothelial cells, resulting in a poor yield.
8. Some protocols do not use trypsin when finished with the primary sorting and recommend plating the cells directly into plates or flask together with Dynabeads. We prefer to use trypsin treatment, since the Dynabeads may affect endothelial cell adhesion and decrease yield.
9. Normally, we can get more endothelial cells from lungs than that of heart, but the purity of endothelial cells from heart is better than that of lung.
10. EDTA (0.05%) can only be used for digesting cells from the plate if anti-PECAM-1-coated Dynabeads are to be used for secondary sorting, or PECAM-1 expression will be tested later. The treatment time may be a little longer. Based on our experience, 10 min treatment with EDTA is enough to release endothelial cells from plates.
11. For this FACS analysis, cells were not fixed.
12. BSA may prevent cell loss.
13. Every washing may cause cell loss if care is not taken when removing the supernatant. Do not use a vacuum aspiration system.

Acknowledgments

This work was supported by American Heart Association Scientist Development Grant and Texas A&M Health Science Center Startup Grant to Xu Peng.

References

1. Coultas, L., Chawengsaksophak, K., and Rossant, J. (2005) Endothelial cells and VEGF in vascular development, *Nature 438*, 937–945.
2. Hanahan, D. (1997) Signaling vascular morphogenesis and maintenance, *Science 277*, 48–50.
3. Carmeliet, P. (2005) Angiogenesis in life, disease and medicine, *Nature 438*, 932–936.
4. Costa, C., Soares, R., and Schmitt, F. (2004) Angiogenesis: now and then, *APMIS 112*, 402–412.
5. Folkman, J. (1995) Angiogenesis in cancer, vascular, rheumatoid and other disease, *Nat Med 1*, 27–31.
6. Folkman, J., and Shing, Y. (1992) Angiogenesis, *J Biol Chem 267*, 10931–10934.
7. Eliceiri, B. P., and Cheresh, D. A. (2001) Adhesion events in angiogenesis, *Curr Opin Cell Biol 13*, 563–568.
8. Jaffe, E. A., Hoyer, L. W., and Nachman, R. L. (1973) Synthesis of antihemophilic factor antigen by cultured human endothelial cells, *J Clin Invest 52*, 2757–2764.
9. Nachman, R. L., and Jaffe, E. A. (2004) Endothelial cell culture: beginnings of modern vascular biology, *J Clin Invest 114*, 1037–1040.

Chapter 15

Isolation and Characterization of Embryonic and Adult Epicardium and Epicardium-Derived Cells

Bin Zhou and William T. Pu

Abstract

Epicardium is the outer cell layer of the heart. Its integrity and function are essential for normal heart development. To study the role of epicardium in both fetal and adult hearts, it is desirable to isolate and culture pure populations of these cells. Here we describe methods with Cre-loxP technology to lineage tag epicardial cells (EpiCs) and epicardium-derived cells (EPDCs), dissociate and isolate them by flow-activated cytometry sorting (FACS), and characterize them by quantitative PCR and immunostaining. This platform allows further characterization and manipulation of EpiCs and EPDCs for expression studies and functional assays.

Key words: Epicardium, Epicardium-derived cells, Flow-activated cytometry sorting, Quantitative PCR, Immunostaining

1. Introduction

The epicardium is an epithelial sheet of cells covering the heart. It is gaining recognition as important cells and source of signals that modulate heart development and postnatal heart function (1). Epicardial cells (EpiCs) orginate from the proepicardium (PE), an outgrowth of the embryonic septum transversum. Between E9.5 and ~E11.0, cells from the PE migrate over the surface of the heart to form an epithelial sheet, the epicardium. EpiCs are critical for normal cardiac development, as impaired formation of epicardium leads to midgestation lethality and aberrant heart development, including abnormal thin compact myocardium and deficient

Xu Peng and Marc Antonyak (eds.), *Cardiovascular Development: Methods and Protocols*, Methods in Molecular Biology, vol. 843, DOI 10.1007/978-1-61779-523-7_15,

coronary vessel formation (2–4). Disruption of epicardial genes such as Wilm's tumor (Wt1), retinoid X receptor α (RXRα), β-catenin, erythropoietin (EPO), and integrin α4 likewise cause embryonic lethality and abnormal heart formation (5–9). Epicardium participates in heart development through reciprocal signaling with myocardium, and by undergoing epithelial to mesenchymal transition (EMT) to form epicardium-derived mesenchymal cells (EPDCs). These mesenchymal cells are a major source of coronary vascular smooth muscle and cardiac fibroblasts (4, 10, 11). Recently, we and others found that a subset of epicardial cells differentiated into cardiomyocytes during normal heart development (12, 13).

As a vasculogenic and myogenic signaling center and source of mesenchymal cells and cardiomyocytes in the developing heart, epicardium has great potentials to be reactivated in the mature heart after myocardial infarction (12–14), which yield great interest in the epicardium and its potential roles in regenerative approaches to myocardial injury.

One of the major challenges in characterizing EpiCs and EPDCs in both embryo and adult hearts is to isolate the specific population without contamination of other lineages. We have generated genetic reagents to facilitate studies of EpiCs and their fate. These reagents are based on regulatory elements of Wt1, a transcription factor highly expressed in the developing kidney and in the mesothelial covering of most visceral organs (6, 15). In the fetal heart, Wt1 expression is confined to the PE and epicardium, not within myocardium (6, 10). As EpiCs undergo EMT and migrate into the myocardium, Wt1 is rapidly down-regulated, so that it is not detected in most migrating mesenchymal cells (10, 16). We knocked either GFP or tamoxifen-inducible Cre cDNA into the Wt1 locus, so that Wt1-driven GFP fluorescence marks EpiCs, or Cre-activated reporter gene expression marks EpiCs plus their descendants.

Here we describe the way of using of these genetic reagents to isolate and characterize EpiCs and EPDCs from both embryo and adult hearts. In outline, steps consist of induction of genetic labeling of EpiCs, collagenase-based dissociation of heart cells, FACS isolation of the labeled population, and downstream analysis of the isolated population by quantitative RT-PCR (qRT-PCR), and immunostaining (see Fig. 1a). This system provides a platform to study important biological aspects of EpiCs and EPDCs, such as their differentiation potential, proangiogenic activity, and cardiomyotrophic activity. These methods will allow further genome-wide screening to discover genes and pathways responsible for the beneficial properties of epicardium.

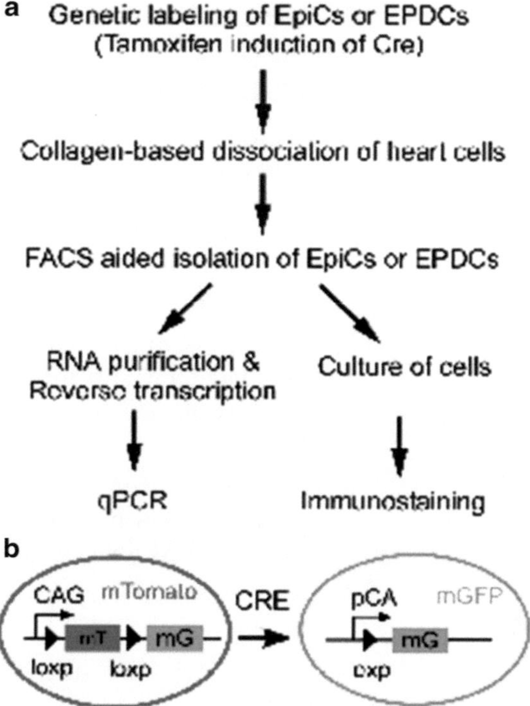

Fig. 1. (**a**) Schematic figure showing the major procedures of isolation and characterization of epicardium cells (EpiCs) and epicardium-derived cells (EPDCs). (**b**) Rosa26$^{mTmG/+}$ reporter shows switching mGFP from mTomato expression after Cre recombination.

2. Materials

2.1. Induction of Labeling

1. Wt1^{GFPCre}, Wt1^{CreERT2}, and Rosa26^{mTmG} mice (Jackson Laboratories, stock numbers 010911, 010912, 007676).
2. Tamoxifen stock solution: Dissolve 25 mg of tamoxifen in 1 mL of 100% ethanol. Store at –20°C.
3. Tamoxifen working solution: Mix tamoxifen stock sol`ution with sesame oil at a 2:1 (v/v). Sonicate for half an hour to mix them at 37°C.
4. Plastic feeding tubes for gavage.

2.2. Dissociation of Heart Cells

1. Digestion stock solution:
   (a) 44.5 mL Hanks' Balanced salt solution.
   (b) 4 mL 1% Collagenase IV. Dissolve collagenase IV in sterile water at 1% (w/v). Stir for half an hour to 1 h at 4°C, filtrate through a 0.45-μm filter, and store at –20°C (see Note 1).
   (c) 1 mL 2.5% trypsin.
   (d) 0.5 mL Chicken serum.

2. Heat inactivated horse serum.
3. Deoxyribonuclease I in PBS buffer at 10 mg/mL. Store at –20°C. Add 1:100 when used in the digestion solution.
4. Surgical tools (Fine scientific tools), ice bucket, 50-mL falcon tubes and shaker in 37°C incubator.

2.3. FACS Analysis and Isolation

1. Collecting medium: mesenchymal stem cell growth medium (MSCGM) with 50% FBS for collection of isolated GFP^+ or GFP^- populations for subsequent cell culture.
2. For immunophenotyping by FACS analysis, we used APC-conjugated rat anti-mouse CD45, CD29, CD90 et al. antibodies (e-Biosciences) together with isotype negative control IgG.
3. FACS buffer is made fresh by adding 0.5 g of BSA (weight/volume 0.5% in final working solution) and 400 μL of 0.5 M EDTA (2 mM final) into 100 mL PBS.
4. 16% Paraformaldehyde solution and 0.5 M EDTA for antibody staining before FACS.
5. Cell strainers (70 μm) for filtrate digested cells to remove clumps.

2.4. qRT-PCR

1. Trizol reagent in 5-mL tube for subsequent RNA isolation.
2. RNase-free or DEPC-treated water for RNA experiments. Dilute 1 mL DEPC in 1 L water and mix overnight at room temperature in the hood. Autoclave it to inactivate DEPC.
3. Superscript III first strand synthesis system.
4. Sybr Green master mix and oligonucleotide primers for qRT-PCR.
5. Some primers that are useful for initial validation of sorting and qRT-PCR are as follows:

   Gapdh, foward acaactttggcattgtgg, reverse gatgcagggatgatgttc.

   Wt1, foward gccttcaccttgcacttctc, reverse gaccgtgctgtatccttggt.

   Raldh2, forward atatgggagccctcatcaag, reverse tctatgccgatgtgagaag.

   Msln, forward tggacaagacctacccacaa, reverse tggtgaggtcacattccact.

2.5. Culture and Immunostaining of EpiC or EPDC

1. 2% Gelatin solution for coating culture dishes to improve cell adhesion.
2. 8-well chamber coated with 2% gelatin.
3. Antibiotic-antimycotic (100×).
4. Mesenchymal stem cell growth medium (MSCGM).
5. 4% fresh PFA for fixation.

6. Triton X-100 for membrane permeabilization.
7. 5% normal donkey serum in PBS for blocking.
8. Antibodies:
   (a) Epicardial markers: WT1 and Epicardin.
   (b) Mesenchymal markers: alpha smooth muscle actin.
   (c) Genetic labeled reporter marker GFP.
   (d) Secondary antibodies. Donkey anti-rabbit or anti-mouse Alexa 555 or 647.
9. VectaShield mounting medium with DAPI to cover slides and stain nucleus. Seal coverslip edges by nail polish.

3. Methods

In heart, Wt1 expression is confined in the epicardium. We used $Wt1^{GFPCre}$ or $Wt1^{CreERT2}$ to enable FACS purification of EpiC or EPDC cells respectively. The $Wt1^{GFPCre}$ allele expresses GFP in $Wt1^{+}$ cells, and therefore GFP^{+} cells represent EpiC. The $Wt1^{CreERT2}$ allele drives CreERT2 expression in the Wt1 expression domain (17). CreERT2 is a fusion protein of Cre recombinase and a portion of the estrogen receptor engineered to be selectively activated by tamoxifen (18). In the absence of tamoxifen, the fusion protein is retained in the cytoplasm (and hence not active as a DNA recombinase). In the presence of tamoxifen, CreERT2 translocates into nucleus, where it catalyzes recombination of loxP sequences. The reporter mouse line we used is $Rosa26^{mTmG/+}$ (19), where a CAG-loxP-mTomato-loxP-mGFP cassette is knocked into the Rosa26 locus (see Fig. 1b). The strong CAG promoter in this permissive locus is widely expressed in most adult tissues including mesothelium. In contrast, other Cre reporters we have tested (e.g., $Rosa26^{fsLz}$ (20) and Z/Red (21)) show less activity in adult mesothelium (BZ and WTP, unpublished). Without Cre recombinase, the cell expresses membrane localized RFP. After excision of the floxed mTomato cassette by Cre, the cell ceases to express mTomato and instead expresses membrane localized GFP, allowing genetic lineage identification. The labeling is irrevocable and heritable, and thus the EpiC and all of its descendants (EPDCs) will express mGFP.

In normal adult mouse epicardium, Wt1 is expressed in a small fraction of cells, making it challenging to isolate enough cells for further characterization. Recently it was reported that after injury, the epicardium reactivates fetal gene organ size-wide (22). Consistent with this observation, we have also found that myocardial injury strongly up-regulated Wt1 expression in large areas of epicardium (Zhou et al., unpublished data). Thus myocardial injury makes it possible to isolate Wt1-expressing cells and their derivatives. Here we surgically ligate the left descending coronary artery to generate an experimental myocardial infarction (MI).

To isolate EpiC or EPDC from embryonic or adult heart, we use collagenase IV and trypsin to dissociate the heart into single cells for subsequent FACS isolation of the GFP^+ population. The purified cells can be directly analyzed by immunostaining or by qRT-PCR, or can be grown in culture medium. When the purified cells need to be cultured for downstream analysis, strict sterile technique should be followed.

3.1. Mouse Breeding and Models

All mice experiments were performed according to protocols approved by the Institutional Animal Care and Use Committee of Children's Hospital Boston. To generate E14.5–E15.5 $Wt1^{CreERT2/+}$;$Rosa26^{mTmG/+}$ embryos for EPDC isolation, we crossed $Wt1^{CreERT2/+}$ male mice with $Rosa26^{mTmG/mTmG}$ female mice. For EpiC isolation, we cross a $Wt^{1GFPCre/+}$ male with wild-type females. Mice were checked each morning for vaginal plugs. Record the age of its embryos as E 0.5 at noon of the day when the vaginal plug is seen. At E10.5, female mice were treated with tamoxifen (0.1 mg/g body weight) via gavage to induce CreERT2 activity (see Note 2). Timed pregnant mice were sacrificed for retrieval of embryos on E14.5 (see Note 3).

For study of adult epicardium, we first inject tamoxifen at 0.2 mg/g body weight twice each week for 3 weeks, and then ligate the left anterior descending artery to generate a model of MI and to induce reactivation of epicardium, thus allowing isolation of enough EpiC or EPDCs for further analysis and culture. The method to make a MI model was described before (23). At 1 week after MI, we sacrificed the mice and obtained the infarcted heart for cell isolation.

3.2. Dissociation of Embryonic EpiCs and EPDCs

1. If cells will be grown in culture medium after sorting, cover the tissue culture dishes with sterile 2% gelatin and incubate at 37°C for 1 h. Remove gelatin and wash with PBS once before adding cells.
2. Prepare 50 mL digestion solution for one-time isolation from a pair of positive and negative samples (see step 3 below). Keep the digestion solution on ice.
3. Remove hearts from embryos or adult mice. Keep the heart intact (i.e., do not mince into pieces as commonly done for cardiomyocyte preparations) as this selectively exposes the epicardial surface for digestion. Wash the isolated hearts in cold HBSS several times to remove excess blood cells. Put hearts with the same genotype (up to four embryo hearts or two adult hearts per pool) into a sterile 5-mL polypropylene tube. For best FACS analysis, it is important to process in parallel equivalent samples known to be GFP^-.

The genotype of adult mice should be known, but for embryos it is useful to identify embryos without the proper genotype (approximately 50% of embryos from the described matings will have the correct genotype). For Wt1$^{GFPCre/+}$ embryos, the green fluorescence of Wt1$^{GFPCre/+}$ hearts is too weak to distinguish from background under a dissecting microscope. However, GFP^{+} kidneys could be observed in Wt1$^{GFPCre/+}$ embryos. Using this way, we pool Wt1$^{GFPCre/+}$ hearts and Wt1$^{+/+}$ littermate control hearts for further isolation (see Fig. 2a). Unlike Wt1$^{GFPCre/+}$ hearts, Wt1$^{CreERT2/+}$;Rosa26$^{mTmG/+}$ hearts are easily identified by their green and red fluorescence (see Fig. 2b, c), while Wt1$^{+/+}$;Rosa$^{mTmG/+}$ littermate controls exhibit only red

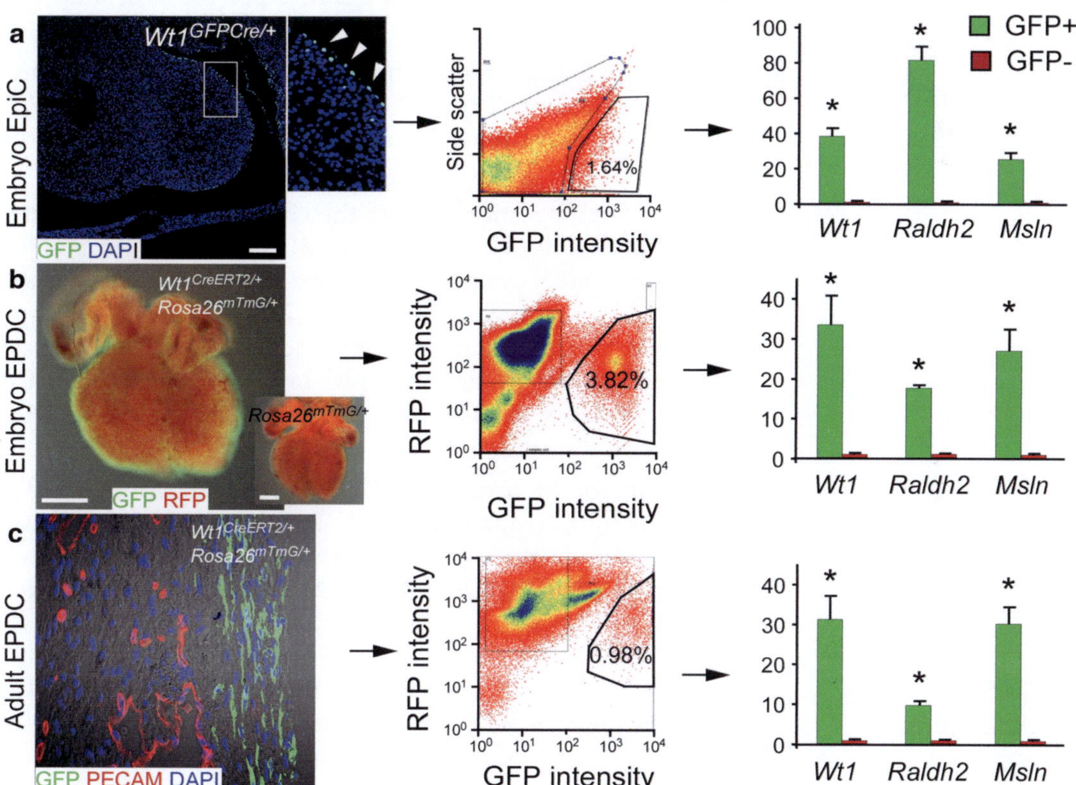

Fig. 2. Isolation of embryonic and adult EpiC and EPDC. (**a**) GFP endogenous expression in E14.5 *Wt1*$^{GFPCre/+}$ heart. Bar = 200 μm. *White arrowheads* indicate the epicardium expression of GFP. GFP^{+} cells were sorted by FACS and analyzed by qPCR. Three epicardium markers *Wt1*, *Raldh2*, and *Msln* were found highly enriched in sorted GFP^{+} cells compared with GFP^{-} cells suggesting the high purity of epicardium cells in GFP^{+} population. (**b**) After tamoxifen injection, E14.5 *Wt1*$^{CreERT2/+}$*;Rosa26*$^{mTmG/+}$ embryo heart shows green fluorescence compared with littermate control *Wt1*$^{+/+}$*;Rosa26*$^{mTmG/+}$. Bar = 500 μm. Quantification of *Wt1*, *Raldh2*, and *Msln* suggests the enrichment of these markers in isolated GFP^{+} population. (**c**) Adult *Wt1*$^{CreERT2/+}$*;Rosa26*$^{mTmG/+}$ mice were treated with tamoxifen and myocardium infarction (MI). The injured heart (7 days post-MI) was stained with GFP and PECAM. GFP^{+} and GFP^{-} cells were isolated by FACS and subsequently analyzed by qPCR. All three epicardium genes were highly up-regulated in GFP^{+} population. $n = 3$, $^{*}P < 0.05$.

fluorescence and no detectable green signal. Pool the double fluorescent hearts (Wt1$^{CreERT2/+}$;Rosa26$^{mTmG/+}$) into one group and red-only embryo hearts (Wt1$^{+/+}$;Rosa$^{mTmG/+}$) as negative control into a second group.

4. Add 4 mL digestion solution to each tube.
5. Rock gently in 37°C shaker (~60 times/min) for 6–7 min. Pipet up and down three times and let the tube stand for 15 s. Remove the supernatant containing dissociated cells to a 50-mL falcon tube and add 0.5 mL horse serum to neutralize the digestion solution. Keep the collecting tube containing dissociated cells on ice throughout all steps.

   If material traps tissues are sticky during digestion, add DNase I (1:100) to cells just after adding digestion solution.
6. Add 4 mL digestion solution again. Pipet the hearts up and down. Repeat step 5.
7. Repeat steps 5 and 6 for seven to eight times (usually the outer layer of the heart will be first digested and come off after 7–8 rounds). To avoid photobleaching, turn off the light in the hood.
8. After the final digestion, filtrate the cells through 70-μm filter and pellet cells by centrifuging at 200 × *g* for 5 min at 4°C. If another marker when co-expressed in EpiC or EPDCs will be analyzed, resuspend the cells in 5 mL FACS buffer and follow the proceed in step 1, Subheading 3.3. If downstream signaling is to be studied on EpiC or EPDCs, resuspend the cells of around 2–5 × 10^6 cells/mL in 0.5 mL HBSS and see step 2 in Subheading 3.3.
9. If the cells will be used for RNA isolation, prepare two FACS collection tubes containing 1 mL Trizol each. If the cells will be used for culture, prepare two FACS collection tubes containing 1 mL 50% FBS-MSCGM for collection of isolated EPDCs.

3.3. FACS Analysis or Isolation of EpiC or EPDCs

For analyzing co-expression of another marker in EpiC or EPDCs, follow Subheading 3.3.1. For isolating purified populations of EpiC or EPDCs for downstream studies, proceed directly to Subheading 3.3.2.

3.3.1. Immunostaining Prior to FACS Analysis

Time estimate: 1 h

1. FACS analysis requires antibody staining for the marker of interest. Since the hearts already have GFP and RFP fluorescence, we use APC or Alexa647 conjugated antibodies to label the cells. Keep antibodies on ice.
2. Wash cell pellets with 5 mL FACS buffer. Spin down cells at 200 × *g* on bench centrifuge for 5 min and then wash again

with 1 mL FACS buffer. Transfer to 1.5-mL Eppendorf tubes. For some intracellular epitopes, a fixation and permeabilization step is necessary. 1% FPA is used for fixation on ice for 10 min and 0.1% Triton X100 to permeabilize the membrane for 5 min.

3. Spin down at 200 × *g* for 5 min, and resuspend the cells with 100 μL FACS buffer containing 1 μL APC-conjugated antibody. Incubate at 4°C for 20 min and mix gently on shaker in dark room or with protection from light in tinfoil paper (see Note 4).
4. Spin down cells at 300 × *g* on bench centrifuge for 3 min and then resuspend the cells with 1 mL FACS buffer. Repeat it for two times.
5. After final centrifugation, suspend the cells with 250 μL 1% PFA fixation on ice.
6. Transfer the samples from Eppendorf tubes to FACS tubes and proceed for FACS analysis. Alternatively, the samples could be stored in the dark at 4°C until analysis.

3.3.2. FACS Isolation

1. Prepare the FACS machine for sterile isolation of cells according to the FACS instrument protocol.
2. Gate on forward and side scatter to focus on single cells, and then gate on GFP and RFP signal intensity to isolate the GFP^+/RFP^- subset (see Fig. 2b, c, middle panels). When using the $Rosa26^{mTmG}$ reporter, two fluorescence colors could be seen: green (GFP^+) and red (RFP^+). Proper control group should be used due to crosstalk between fluorescence channels. The GFP^- control sample is essential to properly set compensation and gating for cells from GFP^+ samples. For APC-conjugated antibodies analysis, a new gate should be set to identify the subset of GFP^+ cells that are also positive for APC.
3. The GFP^+ cells are isolated and put into prepared tubes by FACS. Collection of the GFP^- cells is also necessary. For RNA analysis, collect samples in Trizol at room temperature. For cell culture, collect cells in sterile polypropylene tubes containing culture medium with fetal bovine serum (see Note 5). High speed (around 1,000–2,000 cells/s) is used in the sorted cells to minimize introduction of excess volume into the collection tubes (see Note 6).

3.4. Characterization of EpiC or EPDC by qRTPCR

Prepare everything by using RNase-free or DEPC-treated water. In general, we proceed with Trizol purification immediately, then store RNA until enough samples are collected to proceed to qRT-PCR. It is desirable to have at least three independent samples per group for quantitative comparisons between groups.

1. Purify RNA from cells following the Invitrogen Trizol protocol (see Note 7).

2. At the end of the procedure, dissolve the RNA pellet with 30 μL RNase-free water and incubate for 10 min at room temperature. Measure RNA concentration and quality using a spectrophotometer. Store RNA at –80°C until enough RNA is available to proceed.
3. Reverse transcribe RNA to cDNA. ~0.3–0.5 μg total RNA is needed and the Invitrogen Superscript III protocol using oligo (dT) primers is followed. A control sample lacking RT is highly recommended.
4. Perform qRT-PCR. Sybr Green detection chemistry is used and qRT-PCR is performed with technical triplicates. Expression values are relative to an internal control that is assumed not to vary substantially between conditions. Gapdh is used as an internal control (see Note 8).

3.5. Culture of EpiCs or EPDCs and Characterization by Immunostaining

For immunostaining, it is important not to allow samples to dry between steps. Perform incubations in a humidified slide staining chamber. Examples of immunostained EPDCs are shown in Fig. 3.

1. GFP+ cells were plated onto gelatin-coated wells in MSCGM supplemented with 20% FBS and antibiotic-antimycotic.

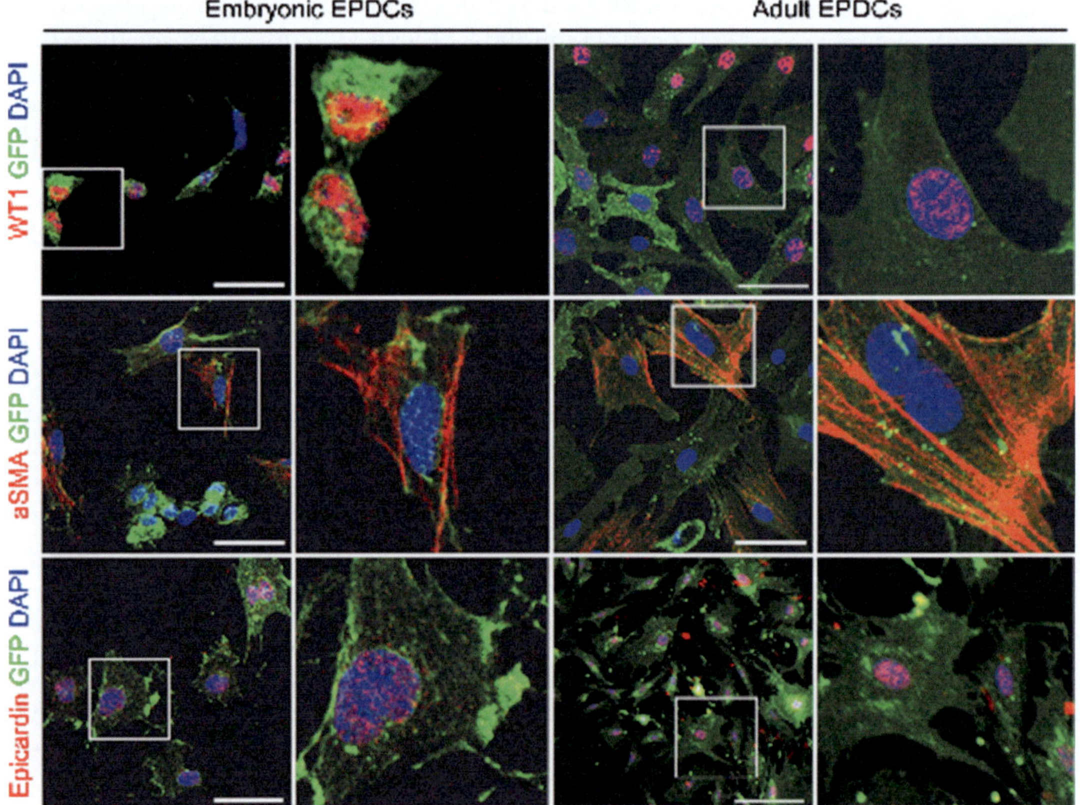

Fig. 3. Representative immunostaining figure of attached primary epicardium-derived cells from embryo or adult hearts. Bar = 20 μm.

Before staining, remove the medium and wash cells twice with PBS. Cells are then fixed in 4% fresh PFA for 10 min, followed by two-time washes in PBS.

2. Antigen block and permeabilization: serum with the same species as the secondary antibody should be used to block nonspecific binding sites. In our case, cells were treated with 5% normal donkey serum and 0.1% Triton X-100 in PBS for 30 min at room temperature. Remove the block solution gently.
3. Primary antibody: incubate the slides overnight at 4°C with primary antibody diluted in block solution. Some antibodies are useful for initial characterization of EpiC and EPDC cultures such as Wt1 1:100, Epicardin 1:100, smooth muscle actin 1:200. After incubation, aspirate primary antibody and wash with PBS three times each for 5 min (see Note 9).
4. Secondary antibody: add donkey anti-mouse or anti-rabbit Alexa 555 or 647 antibodies at 1:1,000. Incubate at room temperature for half an hour in dark room or covered with tinfoil paper (see Note 10).
5. Wash with PBS twice each for 5 min, counter stain with DAPI, and wash with PBS twice again each for 5 min.
6. Add vectashield and mount coverslips. Use nail polish to seal coverslip edges.
7. Acquire images using an epifluorescent or confocal microscope using blue, green, and red or far red channels.

4. Notes

1. Unless stated otherwise, all solutions should be prepared in water that has a resistivity of at least 18.2 MΩ-cm and has been filtered through a 0.22-μm filter. This standard is referred to as "water" in this text.
2. For gavage of tamoxifen, be cautious when inserting the tube, or it will injure the pharynx or esophagus. Make sure the insertion of the tube occurs with the mouse swallowing and align the angle of the tube to that of the esophagus. Insert the tube about 3 cm into the stomach and inject the tamoxifen-sesame oil mixture slowly.
3. Autoclave the surgical tools prior to use and spray the dissecting platform with 70% ethanol. Retrieve embryos under a dissecting microscope in a dissecting hood. It is critical to keep everything sterile during all procedures for culturing the isolated cells. Including 1% antibiotic-antimycotic in culture media helps to avoid contamination by bacteria and fungi.

4. The dilution of each antibody needs to be optimized. For conjugated antibodies we have had good experience starting at a dilution of 1:100.
5. The amount of serum in the collection media influences cell viability. The combination of 50% serum and 50% medium is the best.
6. One E14.5 embryo heart typically yields $\sim 1 \times 10^4$ EpiCs or $2\text{–}3 \times 10^4$ EPDCs. One adult post-MI heart typically yields $\sim 5 \times 10^4$ EPDCs.
7. Usually we obtain 1×10^5 cells or less, making the RNA pellet difficult to visualize. Adding 2 μL glycoblue to 1 mL Trizol reaction at this step enhances recovery and visualization of the pellet.
8. When performing qPCR, primer pairs should be validated in pilot experiments to be highly efficient and to generate a single specific product without significant primer dimers. To avoid issues related to genomic DNA contamination, amplicons should be optimally designed to span an intron.
9. Optimal antibody dilution varies with different antibodies and different lots. The initial testing of dilutions could be 1:100, 1:300, and 1:1,000. The incubation time and temperature also need to be empirically optimized. 2 h at room temperature and overnight at 4°C are both reasonable.
10. The secondary antibody is directed against the species of origin of the primary antibody. If the red channel is available, use Alexa 555. However, if the red channel is occupied, e.g., by the mTomato reporter from $Rosa26^{mTmG}$, then use Alexa 647. $Rosa26^{mTmG}$ expresses either mGFP or mTomato. Therefore, if pilot experiments show that sorting was effective and nearly all cells are GFP^+, then the red channel can be considered unoccupied.

Acknowledgments

The authors would like to thank Elizabeth Boush for aiding FACS isolation. This work was supported by funding from NIH RO1 HL094683 (WTP), an American Heart Association Postdoctoral Fellowship (BZ), and charitable support from James Smith and Gail Federici-Smith (WTP), and the Simeon Burt Wolbach Research Fund (BZ).

References

1. Zhou, B., and Pu W.T. (2008) More than a cover: epicardium as a novel source of cardiac progenitor cells, *Regen Med 3,* 633–635.
2. Manner, J., Perez-Pomares J.M., Macias, D., and Munoz-Chapuli, R. (2001) The origin, formation and developmental significance of the epicardium: a review. *Cells Tissues, Organs 169,* 89–103.
3. Perez-Pomares, J.M., Carmona, R., Gonzalez-Iriarte, M., Atencia, G., Wessels, A., and Munoz-Chapuli, R. (2002) Origin of coronary endothelial cells from epicardial mesothelium in avian embryos, *Int J Dev Biol 46,* 1005–1013.
4. Gittenberger-de Groot, A. C., Vrancken Peeters, M. P., Mentink, M. M., Gourdie, R. G., and Poelmann, R. E. (1998) Epicardium-derived cells contribute a novel population to the myocardial wall and the atrioventricular cushions, *Circ Res 82,* 1043–1052.
5. Yang, J.T., Rayburn, H., and Hynes, R.O. (1995) Cell adhesion events mediated by alpha 4 integrins are essential in placental and cardiac development, *Development 121,* 549–560.
6. Moore, A. W., McInnes, L., Kreidberg, J., Hastie, N. D., and Schedl, A. (1999) YAC complementation shows a requirement for Wt1 in the development of epicardium, adrenal gland and throughout nephrogenesis, *Development 126,* 1845–1857.
7. Zamora, M., Manner, J., and Ruiz-Lozano, P. (2007) Epicardium-derived progenitor cells require beta-catenin for coronary artery formation, *Proc Natl Acad Sci U S A 104,* 18109–18114.
8. Wu, H., Lee, S.H., Gao, J., Liu, X., and Iruela-Arispe, M.L. (1999) Inactivation of erythropoietin leads to defects in cardiac morphogenesis, *Development 126,* 3597–3605.
9. Merki, E., Zamora, M., Raya, A., Kawakami, Y., Wang, J., Zhang, X., Burch, J., Kubalak, S.W., Kaliman, P., Belmonte, J.C., Chien, K.R., and Ruiz-Lozano, P. (2005) Epicardial retinoid X receptor alpha is required for myocardial growth and coronary artery formation, *Proc Natl Acad Sci U S A 102,* 18455–18460.
10. Wilm, B., Ipenberg, A., Hastie, N.D., Burch, J.B., and Bader, D.M. (2005) The serosal mesothelium is a major source of smooth muscle cells of the gut vasculature, *Development 132,* 5317–5328.
11. Dettman, R.W., Denetclaw, W. Jr., Ordahl, C.P., and Bristow, J. (1998) Common epicardial origin of coronary vascular smooth muscle, perivascular fibroblasts, and intermyocardial fibroblasts in the avian heart, *Dev Biol 193,* 169–181.
12. Cai, C.L., Martin, J.C., Sun, Y., Cui, L., Wang, L., Ouyang, K., Yang, L., Bu, L., Liang, X., Zhang, X., Stallcup, W.B., Denton, C.P., McCulloch, A., Chen, J., and Evans, S.M. (2008) A myocardial lineage derives from Tbx18 epicardial cells, *Nature 454,* 104–108.
13. Zhou, B., Ma, Q., Rajagopal, S., Wu, S. M., Domian, I., Rivera-Feliciano, J., Jiang, D., von Gise, A., Ikeda, S., Chien, K. R., and Pu, W. T. (2008) Epicardial progenitors contribute to the cardiomyocyte lineage in the developing heart, *Nature 454,* 109–113.
14. Limana, F., Zacheo, A., Mocini, D., Mangoni, A., Borsellino, G., Diamantini, A., De Mori, R., Battistini, L., Vigna, E., Santini, M., Loiaconi, V., Pompilio, G., Germani, A., and Capogrossi, M. C. (2007) Identification of myocardial and vascular precursor cells in human and mouse epicardium, *Circ Res 101,* 1255–1265.
15. Kreidberg, J. A., Sariola, H., Loring, J. M., Maeda, M., Pelletier, J., Housman, D., and Jaenisch, R. (1993) WT-1 is required for early kidney development, Cell 74, 679–691.
16. Perez-Pomares, J. M., Phelps, A., Sedmerova, M., Carmona, R., Gonzalez-Iriarte, M., Munoz-Chapuli, R., and Wessels, A. (2002) Experimental studies on the spatiotemporal expression of WT1 and RALDH2 in the embryonic avian heart: a model for the regulation of myocardial and valvuloseptal development by epicardially derived cells (EPDCs), Dev Biol 247, 307–326.
17. Zhou, B, A von Gise, Q Ma, YW Hu, and WT Pu. (2010). Genetic fate mapping demonstrates contribution of epicardium-derived cells to the annulus fibrosis of the mammalian heart. Dev Biol 338, 251–261.
18. Feil, R., Wagner, J., Metzger, D., and Chambon, P. (1997) Regulation of Cre recombinase activity by mutated estrogen receptor ligand-binding domains, *Biochem Biophys Res Commun 237,* 752–757.
19. Muzumdar, M. D., Tasic, B., Miyamichi, K., Li, L., and Luo, L. (2007) A global double-fluorescent Cre reporter mouse, *Genesis 45,* 593–605.
20. Mao, X., Fujiwara, Y., and Orkin, S. H. (1999) Improved reporter strain for monitoring Cre recombinase-mediated DNA excisions in mice, *Proc Natl Acad Sci U S A 96,* 5037–5042.

21. Vintersten, K., Monetti, C., Gertsenstein, M., Zhang, P., Laszlo, L., Biechele, S., and Nagy, A. (2004) Mouse in red: red fluorescent protein expression in mouse ES cells, embryos, and adult animals, *Genesis 40,* 241–246.

22. Lepilina, A., Coon, A. N., Kikuchi, K., Holdway, J. E., Roberts, R. W., Burns, C. G., and Poss, K. D. (2006) A dynamic epicardial injury response supports progenitor cell activity during zebrafish heart regeneration, *Cell 127,* 607–619.

23. Tarnavski, O., McMullen, J. R., Schinke, M., Nie, Q., Kong, S., and Izumo, S. (2004) Mouse cardiac surgery: comprehensive techniques for the generation of mouse models of human diseases and their application for genomic studies, *Physiol Genomics 16,* 349–360.

Chapter 16

Vascular Smooth Muscle Cells: Isolation, Culture, and Characterization

Richard P. Metz, Jan L. Patterson, and Emily Wilson

Abstract

Vascular smooth muscle cells (VSMCs) are the cellular components of the normal blood vessel wall that provides structural integrity and regulates the diameter by contracting and relaxing dynamically in response to vasoactive stimuli. The differentiated state of the VSMC is characterized by specific contractile proteins, ion channels, and cell surface receptors that regulate the contractile process and are thus termed contractile cells. In addition to these normal functions, in response to injury or during development, VSMCs are responsible for the synthesis of extracellular matrix proteins, become migratory and proliferate. This phenotype has been termed synthetic cells. To better understand the mechanisms regulating these and other processes, scientists have depended on cultured cells that can be manipulated in vitro. In this chapter, we will discuss in detail the explant method for isolation of VSMC and will compare it to the enzymatic digestion method. We will also briefly describe methods for characterizing the resulting cells.

Key words: Smooth muscle, Isolation, Culture, Explant

1. Introduction

In the adult animal, the vascular smooth muscle cells (VSMCs) are the cellular components of blood vessels that contribute to the structural integrity of the blood vessels and whose primary function is to regulate the diameter of the blood vessels in response to physiological stimuli. To fulfill these functions, normal adult VSMCs are characterized by the expression of a profile of specific contractile proteins, ion channels, calcium handling proteins, and cell surface receptors that serve to regulate contraction of the cell (1, 2). Early attempts to isolate and culture VSMCs provided the evidence of the dynamic nature of VSMC phenotype and the heterogeneity of phenotype in vivo (3–5).

Xu Peng and Marc Antonyak (eds.), *Cardiovascular Development: Methods and Protocols*, Methods in Molecular Biology, vol. 843, DOI 10.1007/978-1-61779-523-7_16,

VSMCs express a wide range of phenotypes in vivo and in vitro cultures. The extremes of the spectrum of VSMC phenotypes have been termed "contractile" and "synthetic" by early investigators based on their primary functions of contraction and synthesis of extracellular matrix proteins. Contractile smooth muscle cells are characterized by 80–90% of the cell volume being occupied by the contractile apparatus (6). Synthetic organelles such as Golgi apparatus, rough endoplasmic reticulum are sparse and located in the perinuclear region in the contractile phenotype. Synthetic smooth muscle cells function almost exclusively to synthesize extracellular matrix. These cells are characterized by large amounts of Golgi apparatus, rough endoplasmic reticulum and contain fewer organized contractile filaments (5). The contractile state is what is considered to be the primary state of VSMC in the normal adult aorta, while the synthetic phenotypes are seen in vivo during development and in response to injury followed by tissue repair. The contractile and synthetic phenotype are considered the extremes of the spectrum of phenotypes that are encountered in vivo and in cultured cells and the precise phenotype is determined by type and location of the blood vessel, the local environment including extracellular matrix, growth and differentiation factors, local mechanical forces, and exposure to vasoactive compounds (7, 8). Additionally, pathologies such as atherosclerosis, hypertension, and diabetes dramatically affect the phenotype of the VSMC and the alteration of VSMC phenotype contributes to these disease states (9).

1.1. Characterization of Vascular Smooth Muscle Cells in Culture

Early attempts to maintain VSMC in culture revealed the propensity of these cells to undergo phenotypic changes from the contractile phenotype to the synthetic/proliferative phenotype. Cells isolated from arteries of adult animals by enzymatic digestion (discussed more fully later in this chapter) are elongated in shape (e.g., fusiform or ribbon-like) and phase dense under the microscope and closely resemble the cells in the intact tissue during the first few days in culture. These cells show a similar ultrastructure to smooth muscle cells in vivo in that they are characterized by a high density of myofilaments and expression of contractile proteins and mRNA for contractile proteins as determined by immunohistochemistry, western blot analysis, and Northern blot or real-time PCR analysis. After several days in culture, the density of myofilaments decreases, the amount of smooth muscle alpha actin (and other contractile proteins) protein and mRNA decreases, and the cells begin to resemble the "synthetic" cells seen during vascular development or that appear upon vascular regeneration. Generally, VSMC cells in culture do not begin to proliferate until after this switch in phenotype has begun after which the cells proliferate logarithmically in the presence of serum (1). Depending on the species, VSMC may undergo a senescent transformation in which they have exhausted their replicative capacity (10).

Factors that ultimately affect the phenotypic status of VSMC in culture include the confluence of the culture, passage number, extracellular matrix, type of medium and growth factors, and vasoactive compounds. The effects of the stimuli on smooth muscle differentiation have been studied extensively in vitro and have led to the development of specific protocols either to help maintain the contractile phenotype in culture or to study factors that induce the phenotypic change to the proliferative/synthetic phenotypes (11, 12). The ability to genetically manipulate and engineer the mouse has led to its use as a model for basic cardiovascular research and for addressing the role of specific gene products in vivo and in vitro. Thus, we will focus on methods of smooth muscle isolation from mouse aorta in this chapter. Two approaches have commonly been used to isolate vascular smooth muscle. The first method that has been used is to explant the vascular tissue and allow the cells to migrate from the vascular tissue and begin to proliferate. The second method involves enzymatic digestion of the vascular tissue followed by plating of the dispersed cells for culture. Both methods have been used extensively in other species and have thus, been adapted for use with mouse tissues.

2. Materials

2.1. Explant Isolation of Vascular Smooth Muscle Cells

1. Small surgical scissors to open mouse chest cavity.
2. Dumont #5 and #7 forceps for dissection of aorta.
3. Spring scissors (6 mm blades) for open aorta.
4. 70% Ethanol.
5. Sodium Pentobarbitol (nembutol) 1 mg/mL.
6. Dissecting Microscope.
7. Phosphate-Buffered Saline (Invitrogen).
8. Antibioltic/Antimycotic Solution (Invitrogen).
9. Lonza Smooth Muscle Basal Media with bullet kit (Lonza).
10. Collagen-coated tissue culture dish (35 mm).
11. Trypsin (0.05%)-with EDTA-4 Na (Invitrogen).
12. Cell culture incubator (37°C 95% air and 5% CO_2).

2.2. Materials for Enzymatic Digestion (in Addition to the Materials Listed Above the Following Reagents Are Needed for This Method)

1. Filter-sterilized Collagenase (1.4 mg/mL basal culture medium, Worthington Biochemical Co. Type II collagenase) (see Note 1).
2. 15-mL Microfuge tube.
3. 15-mL conical centrifuge tubes.
4. Low-speed table top centrifuge.

3. Methods

The basic protocol for isolation of smooth muscle cells by explant culture was developed by Ross (13) using prepubertal guinea pigs. Briefly, sections from abdominal and thoracic aorta were obtained from animals under anesthesia and the aorta was cleaned of all connective tissue and cut into small pieces. The pieces were attached to a bottom of a culture tube and the smooth muscle cells were allowed to migrate out of the tissue pieces. The resulting cultures were initially used after numerous passages. Through the years, others have modified this protocol for specific needs. In the current study we have modified this basic protocol for use with mouse aortic smooth muscle cells.

3.1. Modification of Explant Method for Isolation of Mouse Aortic Vascular Smooth Muscle Cells

1. Mouse is secured and euthanized with intraperitoneal injection Sodium Pentobarbitol (0.25 mL 1 mg/mL) or other approved anesthetic.
2. The thorax is wiped with 70% ethanol and then opened using small surgical scissors.
3. The aorta is dissected from its origin at the left ventricle to the iliac bifurcation using the forceps and spring scissors (see Note 2).
4. The aorta is transferred to a petri dish and irrigated with 1× PBS with 1× antibiotic/antimycotic solution.
5. The connective tissue and adventitia are removed using fine-tipped forceps and small spring scissors.
6. Once the outer surface is clean, the aorta is transferred to a new petri dish containing fresh PBS/antibiotic/antimycotic and the aorta is cut open longitudinally using the small spring scissors and spread open so that the intima is face up.
7. A sterile cotton swabbed is used to gently remove the endothelial layer of cells from the aorta.
8. The de-endothelialized aorta is transferred to an empty collagen-coated culture dish (35 mm) and pressed with the luminal side down on the plate.
9. The aorta is then spread out over as large an area as possible, and allowed to sit 15–30 min until complete adhesion to the plate is achieved.
10. Fresh medium containing 2× antimycotic/antibiotic solution is then slowly added to the periphery of the plate until it just covers the aorta. If the aorta comes off the plate, repeat the procedure as VSMC migration occurs only when the aorta is in direct contact with the plate.
11. The dish is then placed in a 37°C, 5% CO_2 incubator and left undisturbed for 5 days (see Notes 3 and 4).

12. Fresh medium is added, and cells are subcultured as needed thereafter for experiments (see Note 5).

3.2. Isolation of Vascular Smooth Muscle Cells by Enzymatic Digestion

The other primary method used to isolate, culture, and characterize VSMC is the use of enzymatic digestion with the release of smooth muscle cells from their native environment. Critical factors in successful culture of VSMC using enzymatic digestion include the specific enzymatic preparation used and the time of digestion. These factors may vary depending on the source of vascular tissue and the specific vascular bed that is being used because the specific type and amount of connective tissue varies. We have successfully used the methods described by Ray et al. (14) with slight modifications or adjustments. The use of this method is advantageous because it allows for the rapid, reproducible isolation of VSMC from mouse lines where large amounts of tissue might not be readily available.

1. Steps 1–7 are as described for the explant method above.
2. The aorta is then cut into 1–2 mm pieces and transferred to a small culture tube.
3. All remaining manipulations are performed in a laminar flow culture hood.
4. A volume of sterile basal media containing collagenase (1.4 mg/mL culture medium) sufficient to cover the aortic pieces is added to the tube.
5. The aortic pieces are then incubated with the enzyme solution for 4–6 h in a 37°C incubator with 95% air and 5% CO_2 (see Note 6).
6. At the end of the incubation period, the aortic pieces are agitated to release smooth muscle cells into the media and the cell suspension is transferred to a 15-mL sterile conical tube and diluted to a total volume of 3 mL.
7. The cells are concentrated by centrifugation at 300 × *g* for 5 min in a table top centrifuge.
8. The medium is removed and the pellet is washed by resuspension of the pellet in 3 mL medium and repeating the centrifugation.
9. The resulting pellet is resuspened in 0.75 mL of complete smooth muscle culture medium and transferred to a small cell culture dish (35 mm).
10. The resulting culture is placed in a 37°C incubator with 95% air and 5% CO_2 and is left undisturbed for 5 days at which time it may be trypsinized, and transferred to a larger culture dish to expand the cell for experiments (14).
11. The purity of cultured VSMCs can be identified by microscopy observation (see Note 7) and western blotting (see Notes 8–11).

4. Notes

1. It is very important to keep track of the exact source and specific types of enzymes that are used including lot number because enzymes may vary substantially from preparation to preparation.
2. We do not combine tissues from the thoracic and abdominal aorta, but rather separate these tissues because the developmental origin of cells from these regions is different and the responses of the cells to various stimuli is likely to be different.
3. The explant method has the advantage of requiring relatively little hands on time.
4. There are some disadvantages to the explant procedure including the time required for cells to migrate out of the tissue, which can take several days or weeks and the fact that you may be selecting for highly migratory SMCs.
5. McMurray and coworkers reported a standardized method of culturing aortic explants for study of factors affecting phenotypic modulation of cells in culture. These authors suggest that explant cultures provide a system in which VSMC cell growth can be investigated in a seminative environment without fully digesting the tissue and avoid the variability problems associated with enzymatic digestion. These studies were performed making measurements under different conditions and exposure to different growth factors and modulators on migration and proliferation directly from the explant, and subsequent quantification of the rate and number of cells that migrate from the tissue explant (15). Thus, variations on a common approach have been used by many to quantify in vivo changes and to maintain cells in culture.
6. It is our experience that the incubation times with the collagenase may vary somewhat. To optimize the incubation time, samples should be taken at 1 h intervals to determine the number of cells that have been released.
7. Initial characterization of the resulting cells is done on the basis of morphology using light microscopy. Upon initial isolation, VSMC may exhibit an elongated morphology as one would expect from their in viro organization, However, with further time in culture, isolated VSMC show a "hill and valley" organization.
8. Expression of α–smooth muscle actin has been used to verify the smooth muscle phenotype. However, as a better understanding of the expression profile of this protein became clear it is now recommended that multiple differentiation markers should be used to characterize the specific phenotype of cultured VSMC. Among the differentiation markers for the contractile

phenotype that are used in addition to α smooth muscle actin are smooth muscle myosin heavy chain, SM22α, calponin, caldesmon, and smoothelin (16).

9. The synthetic phenotype is characterized by increased expression of extracellular matrix proteins such as Collagen I and III and increased expression of various nonmuscle myosin heavy chain isoforms (17, 18).
10. Quantification of expression of these proteins may be done by Western blot analysis or immunofluorescence microscopy.
11. The culture of vascular smooth muscle has led to a better understanding of the molecular basis of many vascular diseases and to the molecular mechanisms regulating the phenotype of the cells. The varied conditions and sources of the cells have contributed to some controversies as to how the cells respond to different stimuli. Also, because of the variability in phenotype from the native adult cells the use of cultured cells can sometimes be questioned as to their physiological relevance. However, despite these problems the continued use of cultured VSMCs will aid in our understanding of many molecular processes that cannot be understood through the use of isolated vessels or whole animal studies. Additionally, this chapter has focused on the use of mouse arteries as a source of smooth muscle cells. The availability of many genetic models of vascular disease in the mouse make cells isolated from these animals a unique model for studying the involvement of specific genes in the normal function and in pathologies. The development of more standardized culture models will also aid understanding of where specific controversies arise.

References

1. Campbell, G., and Campbell, J. (1995) Development of the Vessel Wall: Overview, in *The Smooth Muscle Cell Molecular and Biolgoical Responses to the Extracellular Matrix* (Schwartz, S., and Mecham, R., Eds.), pp 1–10, Academic Press, San Diego, CA.
2. Owens, G. K. (1995) Regulation of differentiation of vascular smooth muscle cells, *Physiol Rev 75*, 487–517.
3. Campbell, G., and Campbell, J. (1987) Phenotypic modulation of smooth muscle cells in primary culture, in *Vascular Smooth Muscle Cells in Culture* (Campbell, G., and Campbell, J., Eds.), pp 39–56, CRC Press, Boca Raton, FL.
4. Chamley-Campbell, J., Campbell, G. R., and Ross, R. (1979) The smooth muscle cell in culture, *Physiol Rev 59*, 1–61.
5. Chamley-Campbell, J. H., Campbell, G. R., and Ross, R. (1981) Phenotype-dependent response of cultured aortic smooth muscle to serum mitogens, *J Cell Biol 89*, 379–383.
6. Gabella, G. (1984) Structural apparatus for force transmission in smooth muscles, *Physiol Rev 64*, 455–477.
7. Wamhoff, B. R., Bowles, D. K., and Owens, G. K. (2006) Excitation-transcription coupling in arterial smooth muscle, *Circ Res 98*, 868–878.
8. Yoshida, T., and Owens, G. K. (2005) Molecular determinants of vascular smooth muscle cell diversity, *Circ Res 96*, 280–291.
9. Owens, G. K., Kumar, M. S., and Wamhoff, B. R. (2004) Molecular regulation of vascular smooth muscle cell differentiation in development and disease, *Physiol Rev 84*, 767–801.
10. Gorenne, I., Kavurma, M., Scott, S., and Bennett, M. (2006) Vascular smooth muscle cell senescence in atherosclerosis, *Cardiovasc Res 72*, 9–17.

11. Thyberg, J. (1996) Differentiated properties and proliferation of arterial smooth muscle cells in culture, *Int Rev Cytol 169*, 183–265.
12. Pauly, R. R., Passaniti, A., Crow, M., Kinsella, J. L., Papadopoulos, N., Monticone, R., Lakatta, E. G., and Martin, G. R. (1992) Experimental models that mimic the differentiation and dedifferentiation of vascular cells, *Circulation 86*, III68–73.
13. Ross, R. (1971) The smooth muscle cell. II. Growth of smooth muscle in culture and formation of elastic fibers, *J Cell Biol 50*, 172–186.
14. Ray, J., Leach, R., Herbert, J., and Benson, M. (2001) Isolation of vascular smooth msucle cells from a single murine aorta, *Methods Cell Sci 23*, 185–188.
15. Mcmurray, H., Parrott, D., and Bowyer, D. (1991) A standardised method of culturing aortic explants, suitable for the study of factors affecting the phenotypic modulation, migration, and proliferation of aortic smooth muscle cells, *Atherosclerosis 86*, 227–237.
16. Owens, G. K., and Wise, G. (1997) Regulation of differentiation/maturation in vascular smooth muscle cells by hormones and growth factors, *Agents Actions Suppl 48*, 3–24.
17. Majesky, M. W., Giachelli, C. M., Reidy, M. A., and Schwartz, S. M. (1992) Rat carotid neointimal smooth muscle cells reexpress a developmentally regulated mRNA phenotype during repair of arterial injury, *Circ Res 71*, 759–768.
18. Zanellato, A., Borrione, A., Tonello, M., Scannapieco, G., Pauletto, P., and Santore, S. (1990) Myosin isoform expression and smooth msucle cell heterogeneity in normal and atherosclerotic rabbit aorta, *Arteriosclerosis 10*, 996–1009.

Chapter 17

C-kit Expression Identifies Cardiac Precursor Cells in Neonatal Mice

Michael Craven, Michael I. Kotlikoff, and Alyson S. Nadworny

Abstract

Through directed differentiation of embryonic stem cells, it has been demonstrated that mesodermal lineages in the mammalian heart (smooth muscle, endothelial, and cardiac) develop from a common, multipotent cardiovascular precursor (Dev Biol 265:262–275, 2004; Cell 127:1137–1150, 2006; Dev Cell 11:723–732, 2006). Identification of cardiovascular precursor cells at various stages of lineage commitment has been determined by expression of multiple markers, including the stem cell factor receptor c-kit. Utilizing a bacterial artificial chromosome (BAC) transgenic mouse model in which EGFP expression is placed under control of the *c-kit* promoter (c-kit^{BAC}-EGFP), work from our laboratory indicates that c-kit expression identifies a multipotent cardiovascular precursor cell population within the early postnatal heart that can be isolated, expanded, and differentiated in vitro into all three cell lineages that specify the heart (Proc Natl Acad Sci U S A 106:1808–1813, 2009).

Key words: Heart, Cardiomyocyte, Cardiac precursor, C-kit, Fluorescence-activated cell sorting

1. Introduction

C-kit is a type III receptor tyrosine kinase that upon binding stem cell factor (SCF) homodimerizes and triggers an intracellular signaling cascade through tyrosine phosphorylation. This cascade has many downstream effectors including PI3K, the RAS-MAPK pathway, and the Src family kinases, all of which have been implicated in the early migration, self-renewal, and differentiation of various cell types (5, 6).

While c-kit is used widely as a marker of adult hematopoietic stem cells, the SCF receptor is also expressed at various stages during development in germ, mast, stellate, epithelial, endothelial, and smooth muscle cells (5, 7, 8). More recently, c-kit has been identified as a marker of multipotent cardiovascular precursor cells

Xu Peng and Marc Antonyak (eds.), *Cardiovascular Development: Methods and Protocols*,
Methods in Molecular Biology, vol. 843, DOI 10.1007/978-1-61779-523-7_17,

in the developing heart (2, 4), which are capable of generating smooth muscle, endothelial, and cardiac cells (1–4, 9).

Here, we describe the process by which cardiac c-kit⁺ cells can be isolated and purified from the early postnatal heart using enzymatic dissociation and fluorescence activated cell sorting (FACS), to provide a pure population of cells that can be further studied. Investigation into the unique genes involved in specifying cardiovascular precursor status and the mechanisms underlying fate determination in these multipotent cells may advance current gene and cell-based strategies for cardiac repair.

2. Materials

2.1. Breeding and Genotyping

1. C-kit^{BAC}-EGFP homozygote or heterozygote mice generated in Dr. Michael Kotlikoff's laboratory at Cornell University in Ithaca, NY (see Note 1).
2. KL2500 LCD cold light source (Schott Fostec) with safety glasses covered with Wratten filter number 12 (Kodak) (see Note 2).
3. C57Bl/6 wildtype mice (Harlan or Jackson Laboratory).

2.2. Cardiomyocyte Isolation Part I

1. Ethanol: Prepare 70% solution with deionized water.
2. Hank's Balanced Salt Solution, 1× without calcium and magnesium, store at 4°C (HBSS, Mediatech Cellgro).
3. Trypsin vials, NCIS, store at 4°C (Neonatal Cardiomyocyte Isolation System, Worthington).
4. 100×20 mm sterile polystyrene Petri dishes.
5. Surgical tools (see Note 3):
   - (a) Iris Scissors-ToughCut straight 11.5 cm length (FST, Fine Science Tools).
   - (b) Dumont tweezers #2 straight 12 cm length (WPI, World Precision Instruments).
   - (c) Scalpel handle #3 (WPI).
   - (d) Scalpel blade #10 (WPI).

2.3. Cardiomyocyte Isolation Part II

1. Hank's Balanced Salt Solution, 1× without calcium and magnesium, store at 4°C (HBSS, Mediatech Cellgro).
2. L-15 Media Powder (Neonatal Cardiomyocyte Isolation System, Worthington): Reconstitute to 1 L with Millipore water (or other cell culture grade water), filter (0.2 µm filter), and store in 50-mL aliquots at 4°C.

3. Trypsin inhibitor vials, NCIS, store at 4°C (Neonatal Cardiomyocyte Isolation System, Worthington).
4. Collagenase vials, NCIS, store at 4°C (Neonatal Cardiomyocyte Isolation System, Worthington).
5. Cell strainers, 70 μm (BD Falcon).

2.4. Preparation for Cell Sorting

1. Stasis™ Stem Cell Qualified U.S. Origin Fetal Bovine Serum (Gemini Bio-Products): Aliquot into 10 50-mL sterile conicals and store at −20°C. Store working conical at 4°C.
2. Dulbecco's Modified Eagle Medium (DMEM), 1×, no phenol red, store at 4°C (Gibco): Prepare a working solution with 2% Stem Cell Qualified FBS and store at 4°C.
3. Cell strainers, 70 μm (BD Falcon).
4. 12×75 mm Polystyrene round bottom tubes with blue snap cap cell strainer.
5. 12×75 mm Polystyrene round bottom tubes with clear snap cap.
6. F12K Nutrient Mixture, Kaighn's Modification, 1×, store at 4°C (Gibco).
7. Penicillin-Streptomycin, liquid, store at 4°C.
8. bFGF (Invitrogen): Reconstitute in 100 μL of 10 mM Tris–HCL pH 7.6 with 0.1% BSA to yield a 0.1 mg/mL solution. Store in single use aliquots (2.5 μL/tube) at −20°C.
9. ESGRO® (LIF), store at 4°C (Chemicon International).

2.5. Cell Sorting by FACS

1. Becton Dickinson Biosciences FACS Aria with 488 nm excitation laser, 530/30 fluorescein isothiocyanate (FITC) band pass filter, and 585/42 phycoerythrin (PE) band pass filter.
2. Personal computer running Becton Dickinson FACSDiVa software.
3. Ethanol: Prepare 70% solution with deionized water.
4. Bleach: Prepare 10% solution with deionized water.
5. Sample tubes: Polystyrene round bottom tubes with blue snap cap containing cell suspension.
6. Collection tubes: Polystyrene round bottom tubes with clear snap cap containing 500 μL of culture media (see Note 4).

2.6. Culturing C-kit$^+$ Cells Post-FACS

1. Lab-Tek™ II 4-well chamber slides (Nunc) (see Note 5).
2. see Subheading 2.4 for culture media components and see Note 4 for culture media making protocol.

3. Methods

C-kit marks a developmentally heterogeneous population of cardiac precursor cells concentrated within the atrioventricular region, walls of the atria and ventricles, and the epicardial border of the postnatal heart (see Fig. 1) (4). Expression of c-kit peaks around postnatal (PN) days 3–4 and declines rapidly thereafter, with little expression remaining in the adult heart (10). In order to maximize cell yield, it is therefore beneficial to sacrifice pups as close to birth (postnatal day 0) as possible.

C-kit^{BAC}-EGFP neonates can be easily genotyped based on EGFP immunofluorescence in c-kit-expressing melanocytes (8). For control purposes, hearts from genotypically negative littermates (i.e., wildtype littermates) should be included during the dispersal procedure to help quantify the level of background autofluorescence by FACS, thus allowing effective gating and purification of c-kit^{+} cells. To successfully isolate viable cells that can be maintained in culture, it is important to work efficiently and aseptically, adhering closely to sterile techniques, enzyme incubation times, and FACS parameters.

3.1. Breeding and Genotyping

1. Wildtype mice are bred to adult c-kit^{BAC}-EGFP heterozygote and/or homozygote mice to obtain c-kit^{BAC}-EGFP heterozygote pups and their wildtype littermates.

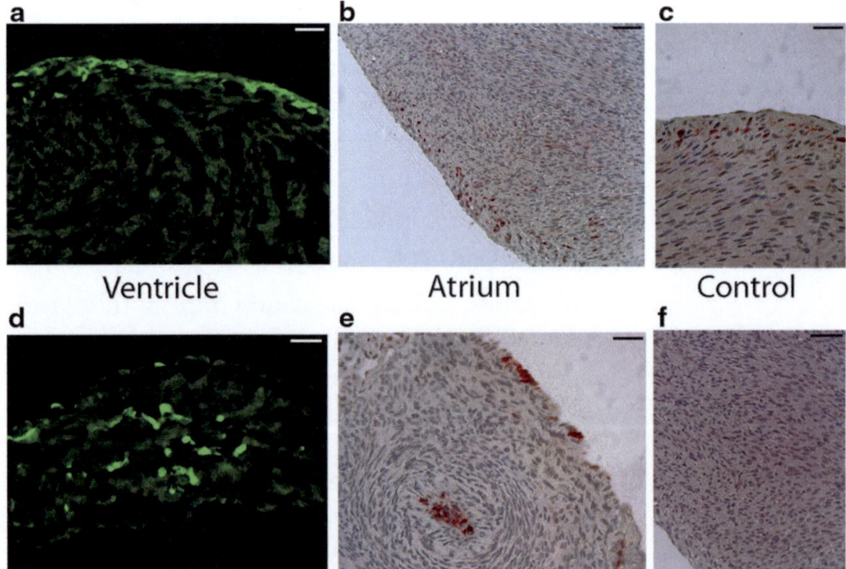

Fig. 1. EGFP expression in c-kit^{BAC}-EGFP mouse hearts. EGFP expression in the ventricular epicardium (fluorescence, **a**) and ventricular (immuno, **b** and **c**) and atrial walls (fluorescence, **d**; immuno, **e**). Control (**f**), no 1° antibody. Fluorescence images from PN1 hearts, immuno images from PN3 hearts (*scale bars*: **a**, **b**, and **f**, 40 μm; **c**–**e**, 20 μm).

2. One day prior to the scheduled sort, preferably in the morning, pups ages PN0–4 are pooled together into one cage with a warmer set underneath to help maintain body temperature (see Note 6).
3. Pups are genotyped by the investigator using a KL2500 LCD cold light source with safety glasses covered with Wratten filter number 12. Pups with the bacterial artificial chromosome (BAC) transgene will appear green while wildtype pups will appear black (see Note 7).

3.2. Cardiomyocyte Isolation Part I (see Note 8)

1. A square ice-bucket is prepared and sprayed with 70% ethanol before being placed inside the tissue culture hood (see Note 9).
2. HBSS is removed from storage at 4°C and placed on ice in the square ice-bucket.
3. Trypsin vials are resuspended in 2 mL cold HBSS (1 trypsin vial per 12–14 hearts) and placed on ice.
4. Sterile 50 mL conicals (one conical per six to seven hearts) are labeled either "wildtype" or "c-kit^{BAC}-EGFP" and set on ice. One wildtype conical typically provides enough cells to establish background autofluorescence.
5. 25 mL of cold HBSS is transferred into each of the labeled 50 mL conicals.
6. Genotyped pups (separated by genotype into small containers), surgical tools, and a small red biohazard bag are placed inside the tissue culture hood.
7. Hearts are removed from wildtype pups by first decapitating with ToughCut Iris Scissors, cutting down the left side of the sternum, and applying pressure to both sides of the incision site until the beating heart is visible. The beating heart is then removed using Dumont tweezers and placed into the HBSS containing wildtype conical. Remaining tissue is placed in the red biohazard bag. This is repeated until the wildtype conical contains 6–7 hearts.
8. Step 7 is repeated for the c-kit^{BAC}-EGFP transgenic pups.
9. Tissue containing conicals are then swirled to wash the hearts and the HBSS is removed by aspiration.
10. Hearts are washed once with 10 mL cold HBSS and swirled.
11. Beginning with the wildtype conical, HBSS is aspirated and the heart tissue is transferred to a labeled Petri dish set over ice. The heart tissue is minced using Dumont tweezers to hold the tissue and a scalpel handle with a #10 surgical blade to cut the tissue.
12. 9 mL of Cold HBSS and 1 mL of reconstituted trypsin are transferred to the Petri dish.

13. Contents of the Petri dish are mixed by swirling and the Petri dish is placed at 4°C overnight.
14. Steps 11–13 are repeated for each remaining c-kit[BAC]-EGFP conical.

3.3. Cardiomyocyte Isolation Part II

1. HBSS and L-15 media are placed inside the tissue culture hood (see Note 10).
2. One trypsin inhibitor vial and one collagenase vial per Petri dish are placed inside the tissue culture hood.
3. Each trypsin inhibitor vial is resuspended in 1 mL HBSS and each collagenase vial is resuspended in 5 mL L-15 media.
4. Petri dishes containing minced heart tissue are removed from the 4°C storage and the contents of each are transferred to a pre-labeled sterile 50 mL conical using a 25-mL serological pipette.
5. The contents of one trypsin inhibitor vial are transferred to each respective conical. Conicals are mixed by swirling.
6. Caps are screwed onto each 50 mL conical and the contents are warmed in a 37°C incubator rotator for 15 min.
7. Warmed conicals are then removed from the incubator and placed inside the tissue culture hood where the contents of one collagenase vial are transferred into each conical. Conicals are mixed by swirling.
8. Caps are screwed onto each 50 mL conical and the contents are warmed in a 37°C incubator rotator for 45 min (see Note 11).
9. Warmed conicals are then removed from the incubator and placed inside the tissue culture hood.
10. Fresh sterile 50 mL conicals corresponding to each warmed conical are prepared with prewetted (1 mL L-15 media) cell strainers.
11. The contents of the wildtype conical are triturated approximately ten times using a 10 mL serological pipette to break up any remaining tissue clumps. Following trituration, the contents of the wildtype conical are filtered through a cell strainer into the corresponding fresh 50 mL conical. The strainer is then rinsed with 2 mL L-15 media.
12. Step 11 is repeated for the c-kit[BAC]-EGFP conicals.
13. After discarding cell strainers, caps are screwed onto each 50 mL conical and the contents are warmed in a 37°C incubator rotator for 20 min (up to 1 h).
14. Warmed conicals are then removed from the incubator and the contents are spun down at room temperature for 12–15 min at a speed of 1,200 rpm.

3.4. Preparation for Cell Sorting

1. Polystyrene round bottom tubes with blue snap cap are pre-coated by adding 2–3 mL Stem Cell Qualified FBS (filter top should be removed before adding FBS). One round bottom tube is prepared for each cell-containing conical. FBS should sit for at least 30 min to 1 h.
2. L-15-media is aspirated from each of the warmed conicals, leaving the cell pellet undisturbed.
3. Cell pellets are resuspended in 2.5 mL of DMEM + 2% FBS by gently pipetting up and down eight to ten times using a 1,000-μL pipette (see Note 12).
4. Fresh sterile 50 mL conicals corresponding to each cell suspension conical are set up with cell strainers (cell strainers should not be prewetted as before).
5. Cell suspensions are pipetted through cell strainers into corresponding fresh conicals using a 1,000-μL pipette.
6. Final cell suspensions are filtered through the blue snap cap filters into corresponding precoated round bottom tubes (FBS should be removed from tube prior to filtering) (see Note 13).
7. One or two polystyrene round bottom tubes with clear snap caps should be filled with 500 μL culture media to serve as collection tubes as detailed in Note 4. Each collection tube can hold approximately 1 million cells.
8. Blue snap cap round bottom tubes containing cell suspensions and clear snap cap round bottom collection tubes are taken to the FACS facility.

3.5. Cell Sorting by FACS (see Note 14)

1. To ensure that there is no contamination of the sample, stringent decontamination procedures are run prior to sorting (see Note 15).
2. All sort surfaces are cleaned thoroughly with 70% ethanol.
3. A 70 μm nozzle is installed on the instrument (see Note 16).
4. The FACS machine is powered on with lasers off, and lasers are then turned on, and allowed 30 min for warm-up.
5. Fluidic levels including sheath, DI water, ethanol, and bleach are checked and filled when required. At this time, waste is emptied if necessary.
6. Fluidics start-up process is initiated and the stream is turned on.
7. Area scaling and laser delay settings are verified (see Note 17).
8. Experimental setup and parameter calibration are executed as follows:
   (a) Create a control experiment folder and label the subfolder, denoted “tube,” as control.

(b) Click on Inspector > Parameters and remove any unnecessary parameters. Only the PE and FITC channels are required to assess background autofluorescence of transgenic-negative control cells and to sort EGFP-positive cells.

(c) Choose Sort > Sort Setup from the menu and select "70 μm" (see Note 18).

(d) To define the Precision mode choose Sort > Sort Precision and select "Purity."

(e) On the "Workspace Toolbar" click on icons to display "Browser," "Instrument," "Inspector," "Worksheet," "Acquisition Controls Frames," and "Sorting."

(f) Before starting, click Instrument > Instrument Configuration and verify current settings.

9. A sample of cardiac cells from transgenic-negative littermate controls is analyzed first in order to establish baseline sorting parameters for c-kit^{BAC}-EGFP cardiac cells.

   (a) Load the control sample tube into the machine and start acquiring data (see Note 19).

   (b) As the data is analyzed, it is presented as acquisition plots in the "Global Worksheet" (see Note 20 for acquisition plot setup).

   (c) Adjust the Forward Scatter (FSC) and Side Scatter (SSC) voltages to display the scatter properties of the control sample.

   (d) Record control events.

   (e) Unload control tube from machine.

10. c-kit^{BAC}-EGFP positive samples are sorted as follows:

   (a) The control template is used as a reference to optimize sorting of the experimental sample.

   (b) Create a new "tube" subfolder within the experimental folder.

   (c) Load the sample tube into the machine.

   (d) Monitor the "Global Worksheet" to gate the sample accordingly, using the same acquisition plots for analysis as stated in Note 20 for control cells. Figure 2 shows an accurate representation of gating parameters for c-kit^{BAC}-EGFP cardiac precursor cells allowing discrimination between the total EGFP (tEGFP) population and the high EGFP-expressing subset (sEGFP) (see Note 21).

   (e) When all events are recorded, print the experimental instrument settings and sort report.

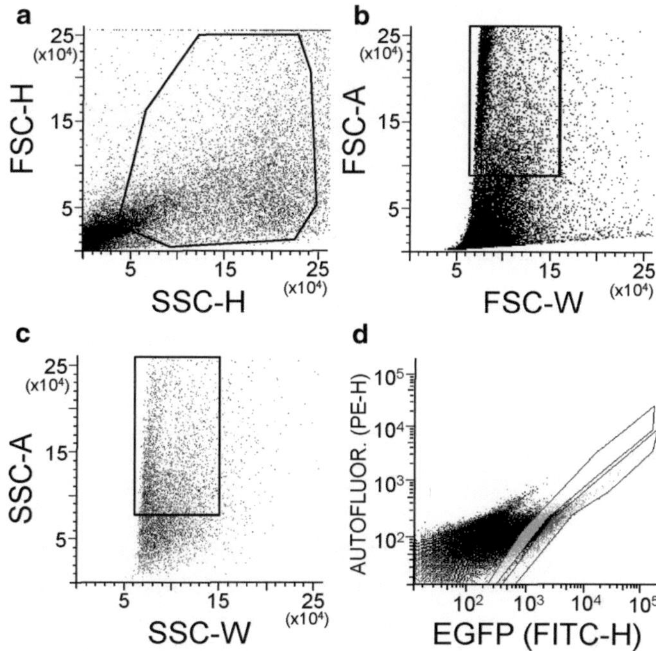

Fig. 2. Acquisition plots demonstrating FACS gating parameters. The total cell population is first gated to exclude debris (**a**) and then to discriminate between singlets and doublets (**b**, **c**). Finally, the c-kit^{BAC}-EGFP sort population is strictly gated to separate a high EGFP-expressing subpopulation equivalent to the brightest 5% of cells (sEGFP, *right window*, **d**), from the overall EGFP-positive population (*left window*, **d**). Note that the gap between the gates is to ensure purity of the sEGFP subpopulation as per our experimental requirements.

(f) Unload the empty sample tube and replace with the next.

(g) If needed, unload the collection tube, cap immediately, and spray with 70% ethanol. Replace with a new collection tube.

(h) When ready, run the next sample and record the data.

(i) Repeat steps 10e–10h until all c-kit^{BAC}-EGFP cells are sorted.

3.6. Culturing C-kit$^+$ Cells Post-FACS

1. Following FACS, cells are diluted to desired concentration using freshly made F12K culture media as described in Note 4 and plated in Lab-Tek™ II 4-well chamber slides. Approximately 50,000 cells are seeded in 600 μL total volume per well (see Note 22).
2. Culture medium is made fresh and changed every 2–3 days. Examples of c-kit^{BAC}-EGFP cell morphologies in culture are presented in Fig. 3.

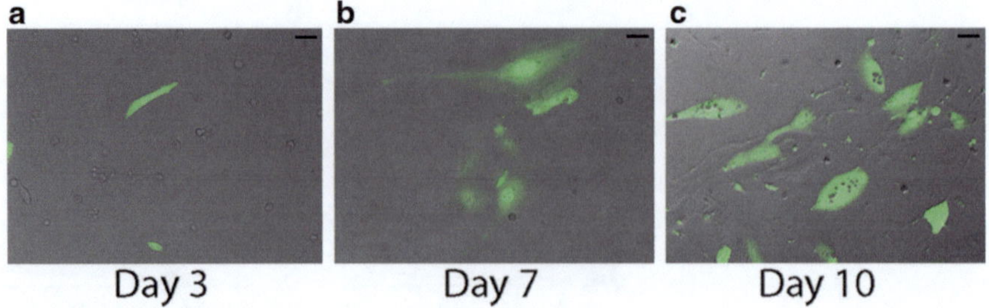

Fig. 3. Combined bright-field and fluorescence images showing differing morphologies of c-kit[BAC]-EGFP cells in culture at 3 days (**a**), 7 days (**b**), and 10 days (**c**) post-FACS (*scale bars*: all 20 μm).

4. Notes

1. Mice are available to the scientific community through a request to the Kotlikoff laboratory. The line is registered with the Mouse Genome Informatics as Tg(RP24-330G11-EGFP)1Mik, Number 3760303 and is on a C57Bl/6 background.
2. c-kit[BAC]-EGFP mice can also be genotyped using the following primers (befarmI: GCAGGTGGAGAAACTGAGCATG; EGFPR1: CCCAGGATGTTGCCGTCCTCCT) (IDT, Integrated DNA Technologies) and cycling parameters (2 min at 94°C; (30 s at 94°C, 30 s at 57°C, 1 min 10 s at 68°C) ×40; 10 min at 68°C; hold at 4°C).
3. Similar surgical tools can be substituted if already available in the laboratory.
4. Culture media should be made fresh according to the following recipe: 50 mL total volume (47 mL F12K culture media, 2.5 mL FBS, and 500 μL Pen-Strep, filter 0.2 μm, after filtration, add 5 μL bFGF and 5 μL LIF).
5. Chamber slides can be substituted with other glass bottom or polystyrene culture vessels as experimentally necessary.
6. PN0 refers to the actual day of birth.
7. Milk spots will autofluorescence and appear green in both the transgenic and non-transgenic pups, be sure not to use this autofluorescence as an indication of genotype.
8. The protocols outlined in Subheadings 3.2 and 3.3 have been adapted from Worthington's Neonatal Cardiomyocyte Isolation System and optimized for use in neonatal mice.
9. All steps for Subheading 3.2 are carried out inside a tissue culture hood. Supplies and reagents must first be sprayed with 70% ethanol before entering the hood to avoid contamination.

10. All steps for Subheading 3.3 unless otherwise noted are carried out inside a tissue culture hood. Supplies and reagents must first be sprayed with 70% ethanol before entering the hood to avoid contamination.

11. In the interest of time, Steps 1 and 7 from Subheading 3.4 can be completed during this 45-min incubation.

12. Clear medium (i.e., no phenol red) or PBS is required for FACS to accurately define background autofluorescence.

13. FBS for coating can be used up to two times if stored in a sterile conical at 4°C.

14. This section details the setup and sorting procedure for c-kit^{BAC}-EGFP cells using a BD FACSAria I controlled by BDFACSDiVa software Version 6.1.1. Other systems and software may vary. It is best to speak to your institution's operator prior to starting any FACS experiment.

15. To ensure no contamination of the sample, select "long clean with bleach" from the Cleaning Modes menu. This requires a 45-min wait time, so it should be carried out in advance. Once finished, the fluidic startup is run twice to remove any residual bleach from within the instrument tubing.

16. Refer to BD FACSAria User's Guide for nozzle installation instructions. Ensure the sort setup is adjusted to 70 μm.

17. Area scaling and laser delay values should be verified each time that the sheath pressure and nozzle are changed. For c-kit^{BAC}-EGFP cardiac cells, a 70-μm nozzle and a sheath pressure of 65 psi are used.

18. On the "70 μm" sort setting, each sample tube should take approximately 20 min to sort. To prevent cells from settling out of suspension during this time, set the sample agitation to a value of 300 rpm.

19. The flow rate is maintained from 3 to 5, depending on the "Threshold Rate" and the "Electronic Abort Rate" (maintained at less than 500 events/s). A flow rate greater than 5 is not used as it affects stream stability and sort output.

20. Default settings in BD FACSDiVa software will produce a plot showing FSC-Area vs. SSC-Area. This should be changed to show FSC-Height (FSC-H) vs. SSC-Height (SSC-H) to ensure all events are incorporated.
    (a) FSC-H vs. SSC-H is an all events plot that allows gating between debris and cell populations.
    (b) FSC-Area vs. FSC-Width and SSC-Area vs. SSC-Width take in cells from the previous gating as the main population and differentiate these events into singlets (single cells) and doublets (clusters).

(c) PE-H vs. FITC-H enables accurate discrimination between EGFP positive cells and autofluorescent cells. Recording control data using this plot will allow effective gating of c-kit^{BAC}-EGFP samples.

(d) It may be helpful to create a histogram showing Cell Count vs. FITC-H in order to visualize the fluorescence distribution of control cells as sorting proceeds. This can then be compared to c-kit^{BAC}-EGFP cells.

21. The tEGFP population is defined as those cells with signal exceeding the Gaussian distribution of heart cells obtained from transgenic-negative littermate controls (4). The sEGFP population is defined as cells having a fluorescence signal greater than fivefold above control cells. On average, the sEGFP population should comprise the brightest 5% of cells gated from the singlet population (4). Autofluorescent cells are identified as cells with a high PE-585/42 to FITC-530/30 signal ratio and excluded.

22. Cells can first be spun down to remove excess DMEM+2% FBS, however, this method results in some cell loss.

Acknowledgments

The authors would like to thank Stanka Semova and Sergei Rudchenko of the Flow Cytometry Facility at the Hospital for Special Surgery in New York, NY and Lavanya Gowri Sayam of the Biomedical Sciences Flow Cytometry Core at Cornell University in Ithaca, NY for their technical input and guidance. The authors would also like to thank their coauthors on the 2009 *PNAS* manuscript (Ref. (4)), without whom this work would not have been possible. This work was supported by R01GM086736 and R01DK065992.

References

1. Martin, C. M., Meeson, A. P., Robertson, S. M., Hawke, T. J., Richardson, J. A., Bates, S., Goetsch, S. C., Gallardo, T. D., and Garry, D. J. (2004) Persistent Expression of the ATP-Binding Cassette Transporter, Abcg2, Identifies Cardiac SP Cells in the Developing and Adult Heart. *Developmental Biology.* ***265***, 262–275.
2. Wu, S. M., Fujiwara, Y., Cibulsky, S. M., Clapham, D. E., Lien, C., Schultheiss, T. M., and Orkin, S. H. (2006) Developmental Origin of a Bipotential Myocardial and Smooth Muscle Cell Precursor in the Mammalian Heart. *Cell.* ***127***, 1137–1150.
3. Kattman, S. J., Huber, T. L., and Keller, G. M. (2006) Multipotent Flk-1+ Cardiovascular Progenitor Cells Give Rise to the Cardiomyocyte, Endothelial, and Vascular Smooth Muscle Lineages. *Dev. Cell.* ***11***, 723–732.
4. Tallini, Y. N., Greene, K. S., Craven, M., Spealman, A., Breitbach, M., Smith, J., Fisher, P. J., Steffey, M., Hesse, M., Doran, R. M., Woods, A., Singh, B., Yen, A., Fleischmann, B. K., and Kotlikoff, M. I. (2009) C-Kit Expression Identifies Cardiovascular Precursors in the Neonatal Heart. *Proc. Natl. Acad. Sci. U. S. A.* ***106***, 1808–1813.

5. Reber, L., Da Silva, C. A., and Frossard, N. (2006) Stem Cell Factor and its Receptor c-Kit as Targets for Inflammatory Diseases. *Eur. J. Pharmacol.* ***533***, 327–340.
6. Naqvi, N., Li, M., Yahiro, E., Graham, R. M., and Husain, A. (2009) Insights into the Characteristics of Mammalian Cardiomyocyte Terminal Differentiation shown through the Study of Mice with a Dysfunctional c-Kit. *Pediatr. Cardiol.* ***30***, 651–658.
7. Yasuda, H., Galli, S. J., and Geissler, E. N. (1993) Cloning and Functional Analysis of the Mouse c-Kit Promoter. *Biochem. Biophys. Res. Commun.* ***191***, 893–901.
8. Alexeev, V., and Yoon, K. (2006) Distinctive Role of the cKit Receptor Tyrosine Kinase Signaling in Mammalian Melanocytes. *J. Invest. Dermatol.* ***126***, 1102–1110.
9. Beltrami, A. P., Barlucchi, L., Torella, D., Baker, M., Limana, F., Chimenti, S., Kasahara, H., Rota, M., Musso, E., Urbanek, K., Leri, A., Kajstura, J., Nadal-Ginard, B., and Anversa, P. (2003) Adult Cardiac Stem Cells are Multipotent and Support Myocardial Regeneration. *Cell.* ***114***, 763–776.
10. Gude, N., Muraski, J., Rubio, M., Kajstura, J., Schaefer, E., Anversa, P., and Sussman, M. A. (2006) Akt Promotes Increased Cardiomyocyte Cycling and Expansion of the Cardiac Progenitor Cell Population. *Circ. Res.* ***99***, 381–388.

Chapter 18

Cardiomyocyte Apoptosis in Heart Development: Methods and Protocols

Dongfei Qi and Mingui Fu

Abstract

Apoptosis is the process of programmed cell death that has been identified in the development of heart. It is likely to be regulated by survival and death signals that are also present in many other tissues. To understand cardiomyocyte apoptosis in normal and abnormal development of heart, the cell death detection techniques were applied to various researches. These methods include morphological, histological, or molecular assays based on recent advances in our understanding of the molecular mechanism of cell death, including: (1) terminal deoxynucleotidyl transferase mediated dUTP nick end-labeling of fragmented nuclei, (2) cardiovascular molecular imaging of apoptosis using Annexin V, and (3) immunohistochemical detection of activated caspases.

Key words: Cardiomyocyte, Apoptosis, TUNEL, Annexin V, Caspase

1. Introduction

The programmed cell death, characterized by a unique phenotype termed apoptosis is now recognized in many life processes, from fertilization to the death of an organism in every animal species (1). During heart development, apoptosis has been identified to contribute to the development of embryonic outflow tract, cardiac valves, conducting system, and the developing coronary vasculature (2). Apoptosis is characterized morphologically by a pattern of nuclear and cytoplasmic condensation, cell shrinkage, long-lasting maintenance of plasma membrane integrity, lack of inflammatory responses in the vicinity of the dying cell, and rapid phagocytosis of apoptotic bodies by adjacent cells (3). Chromatin fragmentation in apoptosis involves the activation or de novo synthesis of endonucleases. The result of the endonuclease activity is the cleavage of

Xu Peng and Marc Antonyak (eds.), *Cardiovascular Development: Methods and Protocols*, Methods in Molecular Biology, vol. 843, DOI 10.1007/978-1-61779-523-7_18,

DNA at linking regions between nucleosomes resulting in the formation of a series of double-stranded fragments that are multiples of 180–200 bp in length (4). During apoptosis, phosphatidylserine (PS) becomes exposed on the surface of apoptotic cells, where it functions as an "eat me" signal for phagocytosis (5). Furthermore, two major biochemical routes dominate apoptotic cell death. They involve the activation of the caspase cascade through either death-receptor-mediated signal transduction or stress-induced release of cytochrome C from mitochondria (6). The intricate scheme of the apoptotic machinery offers several potential targets for molecular imaging. The most widely used method is the terminal deoxynucleotidyl transferase-mediated biotinylated dUTP nick end-labeling (TUNEL) method, annexin V staining, and detection of caspase activity.

1.1. In Situ TUNEL

Extensive DNA degradation is a characteristic event which occurs in the late stages of apoptosis. Cleavage of the genomic DNA during apoptosis may yield double-stranded and single-stranded break. Those DNA strand breaks can be detected by enzymatic labeling of the free 3′-OH termini with modified nucleotides (X-dUTP, X = biotin, DIG or fluorescein). TUNEL is acknowledged as the most suitable choice in the rapid identification and quantification of the apoptotic cells.

1.2. Annexin V Imaging

A change in the plasma membrane is one of the most important morphological features of apoptosis. In normal cells, the appearance of phosphatidylserine (PS) is hidden within the plasma membrane, while it translocated to the surface of the cell during early apoptosis process. Annexin V is a phospholipid binding protein belonging to the Annexin family. In the presence of calcium ions, it exhibits a high affinity for binding selectively to PS. Annexin V is used to stain apoptotic cells by a simple and quick procedure. The stained cells can be measured using flow cytometry. Therefore, annexin V-FITC staining is an established biochemical probe for detecting early apoptosis. When nuclear membranes are disrupted, which is a sign of late apoptosis or necrosis, but not early apoptosis, the propidium iodide (PI) goes into the nuclei and shows positive staining. The partial loss of membrane integrity or functionality is a useful criterion for distinguishing apoptotic from necrotic and living cells.

1.3. Caspase Activity

Caspases are essential in cells for apoptosis, one of the main types of programmed cell death in heart development, and have been termed "executioner" proteins for their roles in the cell. Caspases are enzymes known as proteases, which use a cysteine residue to cleave their substrate proteins at the aspartic acid residue. To date, 14 caspases have been identified. Apoptotic activity can be examined by the measurement of enzymatic caspase activity. Apoptosis was also evaluated by immunostaining for the cleaved form of caspase.

2. Materials

2.1. In Situ TUNEL

1. Terminal deoxynucleotidyl transferase (TdT) Buffer Stock Solution: 125 mM Tris–HCl, 1 M Sodium Cacodylate, 1.25 mg/mL BSA. Adjust pH to 6.6, aliquot, and store at −20°C.
2. Cobalt Chloride Stock Solution: 25 mM Cobalt Chloride in Distilled Water. Aliquot and store at −20°C.
3. TdT Reaction Buffer: 25 mM Tris–HCl, 200 mM Sodium Cacodylate, 0.25 mg/mL BSA, 1 mM Cobalt Chloride. Mix well and store at −20°C.
4. TdT Storage Buffer: 60 mM K-phosphate, pH 7.2, 150 mM KCl, 1 mM 2-Mercaptoethanol, 0.5% Triton X-100, 50% glycerol (see Note 1).
5. Enzyme Reagent: TdT (Roche Diagnostic) is dissolved in TdT Storage Buffer (4%). Mix well and store at −20°C.
6. Label Reagent: Biotin-16-dUTP (Roche Diagnostic) is dissolved in TdT Reaction Buffer (0.4%). Mix well and store at −20°C.
7. TdT Reaction Mixture: Enzyme Reagent and Label Reagent mix just before use at a volume ratio of 1:9.
8. Stop Wash Buffer: 300 mM NaCl, 30 mM Sodium Citrate: Mix to dissolve and store at room temperature.
9. PBS-Tween 20: 8 g/L NaCl, 0.2 g/L KCl, 1.44 g/L Na_2HPO_4, 0.24 g/L KH_2PO_4, and 0.05% Tween 20. Adjust pH to 7.2 and store at RT.
10. DAB, Streptavidin-HRP (DAKO).
11. Proteinase K (Roche Diagnostic).

2.2. Annnexin V-FITC

1. 10× Binding Buffer: 0.1 M HEPES, pH 7.4; 1.4 M NaCl; 25 mM $CaCl_2$. Store at 4°C. Dilute to 1× prior to use.
2. Propidium Iodide (Sigma) (see Note 2).
3. FITC-labeled annexin V (BD Pharmingen).
4. 1× PBS Buffer: 8 g/L NaCl, 0.2 g/L KCl, 1.44 g/L Na_2HPO_4, 0.24 g/L KH_2PO_4. Adjust pH to 7.2, autoclave, and store at RT.

2.3. Caspase Detection

1. Primary antibody: Monoclonal antibody against the cleaved form of caspase 3 (Cell Signaling).
2. 1× PBS Buffer: 8 g/L NaCl, 0.2 g/L KCl, 1.44 g/L Na_2HPO_4, 0.24 g/L KH_2PO_4. Adjust pH to 7.2, autoclave, and store at RT.
3. Blocking buffer: 0.1% Tween 20 in PBS containing 5% horse serum.
4. Second antibody: goat anti-rabbit Cy5 conjugate secondary antibody (Abcam).

3. Methods

3.1. In Situ TUNEL

1. Deparaffinize sections in two changes of xylene for 5 min each, and hydrate with two changes of 100% ethanol for 3 min each, and 95% ethanol for 1 min (see Note 3).
2. Rinse in distilled water.
3. Incubation with proteinase K for 15 min at room temperature.
4. Rinse sections in two changes of PBS-Tween 20 for 2 min each.
5. Incubate sections in 3% H_2O_2 in PBS for 10 min to block endogenous peroxidase activity.
6. Rinse in PBS-Tween 20 for 3 × 2 min.
7. Incubate sections in TdT Reaction Buffer for 10 min.
8. Incubate sections in TdT Reaction Mixture for 1–2 h at 37–40°C in humidified chamber (see Note 4).
9. Wash sections in stop wash buffer for 10 min.
10. Rinse in PBS-Tween 20 for 3 × 2 min.
11. Incubate sections with Streptavidin-HRP in PBS for 20 min at room temperature.
12. Rinse in PBS-Tween 20 for 3 × 2 min.
13. Incubate sections with DAB for 1–2 min.
14. Rinse in tap water.
15. Counterstain with Gill's hematoxylin for 30 s.
16. Wash in running tap water for 5 min.
17. Dehydrate through 95% ethanol for 5 min, 100% ethanol for 2 × 3 min.
18. Clear in xylene for 2 × 5 min.
19. Coverslip with xylene-based mounting medium.

For visualizing by fluorescent, start with step 11 as follows:

11. Incubate sections with streptavidin-FITC (1:50, Vector Labs) in PBS for 30 min.
12. Rinse in PBS for 3 × 5 min.
13. Counterstain with DAPI Working Solution for 10 min at 37°C.
14. Rinse 3 × 5 min in PBS.
15. Coverslip with aqueous mounting medium (FluoroMount) and seal with nail polish.
16. Observation using a fluorescence microscope with appropriate filters. Store slides in the dark at 4°C. An example image of E13.5 mouse heart is shown in Fig. 1.

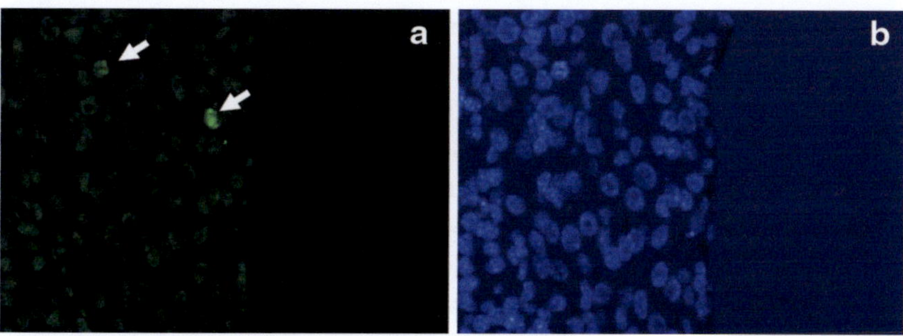

Fig. 1. Apoptosis of myocardium in the mouse heart at E13.5. (**a**) Representative photograph of staining with TUNEL (400×); Arrow pointed at apoptotic cells; (**b**) Nuclei were stained with 4,6-diamidino-2-phenylindole (DAPI; *blue*).

3.2. Annexin V-FITC

1. Cardiomyocyte cells are cultured in 60-mm dishes to 70% confluence. Wash cells twice with cold PBS.
2. Resuspend cells in 1× Binding Buffer at a concentration of 1×10^6 cells/mL (see Note 5).
3. Transfer 100 μL of the solution (~1×10^5 cells) to a 5-mL culture tube.
4. Add 5 μL of Annexin V-FITC and 5 μL of propidium iodide to prepared cell suspension (see Note 6).
5. Gently mix the cell. Keep the tube on ice and incubate for 15 min at RT in the dark (see Note 7).
6. Proceed to A or B below depending on method of analysis.

   A: Quantification by Flow Cytometry, Analyze Annexin V-FITC binding by flow cytometry (Ex=488 nm; Em=530 nm) using FITC signal detector and PI staining by the phycoerythrin emission signal detector (usually FL2).

   B: Detection by Fluorescence Microscopy

   (a) Place the cell suspension from step 6 on a glass slide. Cover the cells with a glass coverslip. Following incubation (6), invert coverslip on a glass slide and visualize cells (see Note 8).

   (b) Observe the cells under a fluorescence microscope using a dual filter set for FITC. Cells that have bound Annexin V-FITC will show green staining in the plasma membrane. Cells that have lost membrane integrity will show red staining (PI) throughout the nucleus and a halo of green staining (FITC) on the cell surface (plasma membrane).

3.3. Caspase Detection

1. Permeabilize the fixed sample slides by incubating in PBS containing 0.1% Triton X-100 for 5 min at room temperature (see Note 9).
2. Wash three times in PBS for 5 min at room temperature.

3. Drain the slides and add 200 μL of blocking buffer (see Note 10).
4. Add 100 μL of the active Caspase 3 antibody diluted 1/200 in blocking buffer (see Note 11).
5. The following day, wash the slides three times, 10 min each in PBS containing 0.1% Tween 20 at room temperature.
6. Drain slides and add 100 μL of goat anti-rabbit Cy5 conjugate diluted 1:500 in PBS. Lay the slides flat in a humidified chamber, protected from light, and incubate for 1–2 h at room temperature.
7. Wash three times in PBS containing 0.1% Tween 20 for 5 min, protected from light.
8. Drain the liquid, mount the slides in a permanent or aqueous mounting medium, and observe with a fluorescence microscope.

4. Notes

1. Stir to dissolve and adjust pH 7.2 using concentrated HCl. Add 50 mL of glycerin (100% glycerol), 0.5 mL of Triton X-100, and 8 μL of 2-Mercaptoethanol (99% Solution. FW 78.13). Store at –20°C.
2. To make a stock solution from the solid form, dissolve in deionized water (dH_2O) at 1 mg/mL (1.5 mM) and store at 4°C, protected from light. When handled properly, solutions are stable for at least 6 months.
3. In this method, slides from cell suspension or preserved tissues can also be utilized. For cell slides: (1) fix air-dried cell samples with a freshly prepared paraformaldeyde solution (4% in PBS, pH 7.4) for 30 min at room temperature; (2) rinse slides with PBS and incubate in permeabilization solution (0.1% Triton X-100, 0.1% sodium citrate) for 2 min in ice and go directly to step 4. For tissue slides: (1) fix tissue sections with 4% paraformaldeyde for 20 min at room temperature; (2) wash 30 min with PBS; (3) incubate slides in permeabilization solution for 2 min in ice and go directly to step 4.
4. To perform each experiment using a blank, a negative control and a positive control sample, is recommended. The blank sample is assessed by substituting equal volume of Label Solution with TdT Reaction mixture to incubate sections. The positive sample, in order to make sure that the method works, is assessed by digesting, after step 6, with DNAse buffer for 10 min at room temperature and wash extensively with PBS-Tween 20 before step 7.

5. Dilute the 10× concentrated binding buffer tenfold with distilled water and place the diluted buffer on ice.
6. For a positive control, incubate the cells with 3% formaldehyde in buffer during 30 min on ice. Wash away the formaldehyde and suspend the cells in cold diluted binding buffer at 10^5–10^6 cells/mL. Proceed with step 5 as described above.
7. The incubation with Annexin V-FITC and propidium iodide should be carried out on ice to arrest further progress of the cells through the stages of life apoptosis secondary necrosis.
8. The cells can also be washed and fixed in 2% formaldehyde before visualization. Cells must be incubated with Annexin V-FITC before fixation since any cell membrane disruption can cause nonspecific binding of Annexin V to PS on the inner surface of the cell membrane.
9. The fixed sample slides from cell suspension or preserved tissues can also be utilized.
10. Use of serum from the host species of the conjugate antibody (or closely related species) is suggested. Lay the slides flat in a humidified chamber and incubate for 1–2 h at room temperature. Rinse once in PBS.
11. You can also prepare a slide with no active Caspase 3 as a negative control. Incubate slides in a humidified chamber overnight at 4°C.

References

1. Poelmann, R.E., and Groot, A.C.G.-d. (2005) Apoptosis as an instrument in cardiovascular development. *Birth Defects Research Part C: Embryo Today: Reviews* 75, 305–313.
2. Fisher, S.A., Langille, B.L., and Srivastava, D. (2000) Apoptosis During Cardiovascular Development. *Circ Res* 87, 856–864.
3. G, M., and I, J. (1995) Apoptosis, oncosis, and necrosis. An overview of cell death. *Am J Pathol* 146(1), 3–15
4. Kunapuli, S., Rosanio, S., and Schwarz, E.R. (2006) "How Do Cardiomyocytes Die?" Apoptosis and Autophagic Cell Death in Cardiac Myocytes. *Journal of Cardiac Failure* 12, 381–391.
5. SJ, Martin., CP, Reutelingsperger., AJ, McGahon., JA, Rader., RC, van Schie., DM, LaFace., and DR, Green. (1995) Early redistribution of plasma membrane phosphatidylserine is a general feature. *J Exp Med* 182(5), 1545–56
6. Scarabelli, T.M., Knight, R., Stephanou, A., Townsend, P., Chen-Scarabelli, C., Lawrence, K., Gottlieb, R., Latchman, D., and Narula, J. (2006). Clinical Implications of Apoptosis in Ischemic Myocardium. *Current Problems in Cardiology* 31, 181–264.

Chapter 19

Adenovirus-Mediated Gene Transfection in the Isolated Lymphatic Vessels

Anatoliy A. Gashev, Jieli Li, Mariappan Muthuchamy, and David C. Zawieja

Abstract

The authors describe technical details of experimental protocol of gene transfection in isolated rat mesenteric lymphatic vessels (MLVs). Authors also refer to the recent publication in *Microcirculation*, which provides wide set of experimental evidences obtained from confocal microscopic imaging and isolated vessels functional tests, which confirmed a successful achievement of the following goals. (1) Optimization of the experimental conditions to maintain the isolated "normal" rat mesenteric vessels in culture for sufficiently long periods of time to permit effective knockdown or overexpression of selected proteins/genes. (2) Development of the effective transfection protocols for lymphatic muscle and/or endothelial cells in intact isolated rat MLVs without nonspecific impairment on lymphatic contractile function due to the transfection protocol per se.

Key words: Lymphatic vessel, Adenoviral transfection

1. Introduction

Modern molecular biology offers a variety of novel experimental techniques to influence genes of interest in different subjects of biological research. In some situations when time, resources, and unique tissue properties allow such, researchers may approach the possibility to target genes in freshly isolated tissue specimens which remains their structural integrity and in situ phenotype. Such experimental approach could widen the ability of investigators to focus on the direct effects of gene modification on isolated tissue specimen, with the characteristic that initial organ morphology and function are still intact or only minimally altered, while the

Xu Peng and Marc Antonyak (eds.), *Cardiovascular Development: Methods and Protocols*, Methods in Molecular Biology, vol. 843, DOI 10.1007/978-1-61779-523-7_19,

experimental conditions are comparatively stable and easy achievable for their permanent control during whole duration of the transfection experiment.

Recently, we developed experimental approaches and protocols to check gene function over the course of up to 2 weeks in lymphatic muscle and/or endothelium from isolated rat lymphatic vessels (1). Technically, rat mesenteric lymphatic vessels (MLV) are particular example of isolated vessels well-suited for gene transfection since the muscle layer is only one to two cells thick, vessel wall only contains one layer of endothelial cells, and the interstitial structures are very thin. Therefore, the experimental protocol presented here is suitable for gene transfection experiments in any isolated blood or lymphatic vessels, which are comparable by size (~100–150 μm in diameter) and wall structure to the vessels of our choice—rat MLV. To develop the techniques of gene transfections in isolated rat MLV, we focused on two major tasks: (1) Optimize the experimental conditions to maintain the isolated "normal" rat MLV in culture for sufficiently long periods of time to permit effective knockdown or overexpression of selected proteins/genes. (2) Develop effective transfection protocols for lymphatic muscle and/or endothelial cells in intact isolated rat MLV without nonspecific impairment on lymphatic contractile function due to the transfection protocol per se. In our recent manuscript in *Microcirculation* (1), we provided wide set of experimental evidences obtained from confocal microscopic imaging and isolated vessels functional tests. These data confirmed that we successfully achieved our goals stated above. In the present manuscript, we describe more technical details of experimental protocol of gene transfection in isolated rat MLV with belief that our experience may serve in future as a good starting point for further development of such molecular tool.

2. Material

1. Dulbecco's phosphate-buffered saline (DPBS) (Invitrogen Corp.).
2. D-MEM/F12 (Invitrogen Corp.) supplemented with antibiotic mixture (Invitrogen) to achieve final concentration of 100 units of Penicillin/100 μg of Streptomycin/mL.
3. Antennapedia leader peptide CT (Anaspec, Inc.) (ALP-CT) stock solution.
4. Standard 0.65-mL plastic tubes (VWR).
5. Fentanyl/Droperidol.
6. Diazepam.
7. Sodium pentobarbital.

8. 1-mL syringes.
9. Petri dishes.
10. Scissors and forceps.

3. Methods

3.1. Dissection of Lymphatic Vessels from Sprague–Dawley Rats

1. Anesthetize the male Sprague–Dawley rats (weighing between 300 and 400 g) according to anesthesia procedure approved for your AUP (in our studies—by intramuscular injection of the combination of Fentanyl/Droperidol (0.3 mL/kg) and Diazepam (2.5 mg/kg)).
2. Using scissors, make a 4-cm long incision in midline abdomen. Separate fascia and muscle layers. Exteriorize a small loop of intestine, 6–7 cm in length.
3. Take out a section of the mesentery containing lymphatic vessels and then put it into a dissection chamber in DPBS under a dissecting microscope. Identify suitable MLVs and clear all surrounding tissues (see Note 1).
4. Carefully dissect sections of 1–1.5 cm MLVs in length. Then euthanize the rat according to euthanasia procedure approved for your AUP (in our studies—by sodium pentobarbital (120 mg/kg body weight IP)) (see Note 2).
5. To eliminate remains of coagulated blood, rinse the exteriorized vessels in standard 35-mm plastic Petri dishes filled with DPBS under a dissecting microscope.
6. Transfer the vessels to another sterile 35-mm Petri dish filled with prewarmed (38°C) D-MEM/F12 with 100 units/mL Penicillin/100 μg/mL Streptomycin for temporary storage (see Note 3).
7. Lightly touch the edges of segments with forceps on the dish bottom to keep the segment submerged under the solution.

3.2. GFP Reporter Gene Transfection in Isolated Rat Mesenteric Lymphatic Vessels

1. Use recombinant adenoviral constructs (in our studies we used a recombinant adenovirus expressing GFP under the control of the cytomegalovirus immediate-early promoter by the AdEasy system (2), as previously described (3)). Purified virus will be used to transfect lymphatic muscle and/or endothelial cells in whole isolated rat MLV.
2. Apply smallest possible volumes as practical for adenovirus transfection. For this purpose, slightly modify the standard 0.65-mL plastic tubes (Fig. 1a).
3. Separate the caps of the plastic tubes (Fig. 1b) and penetrate several holes in tube.

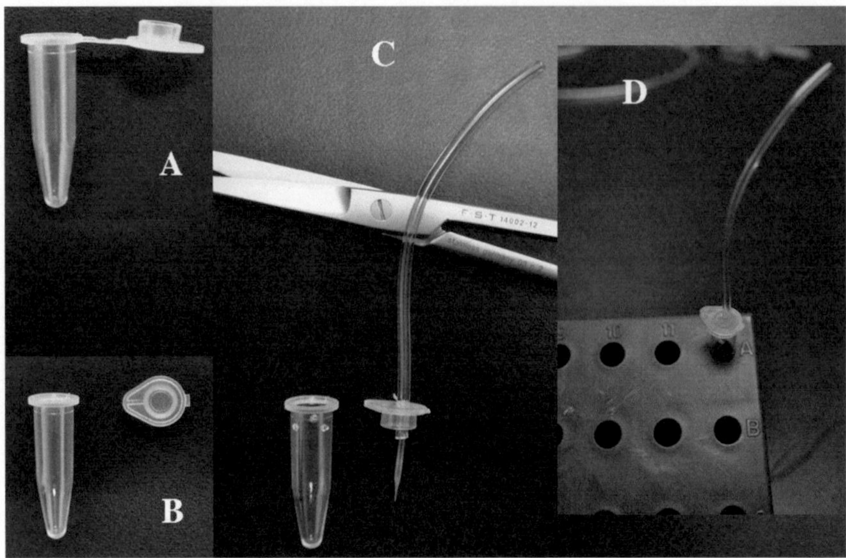

Fig. 1. Preparation of simple 0.65-μL plastic tube-based setup for gene transfection of single vessel. (**a**) Intact plastic 0.65-μL plastic tube. (**b**) Plastic cap and tube separated. (**c**) Holes were penetrated: one hole in plastic cap allowed insertion of a small diameter plastic tubing ~10 cm length. This tubing from the inner cap side was connected with ~1 cm length glass micropipette with a tip diameter of ~100–120 μm. Three holes in separated tube's body helped to relieve pressure inside tube after closure, therefore preventing the prolapse of the lymphatic wall inside the micropipette. Surgical 12-cm scissors presented to reflect dimensions. (**d**) Assembled tube with isolated rat MLV loaded for gene transfection experiment set in tube rack ready for incubation. Other end of tubing (upper) finally opened to atmosphere.

4. Insert a small diameter plastic tube of ~10 cm length to one hole of plastic cap.
5. Connect the tube with a glass micropipette (~1 cm length) with a tip diameter around 100–120 μm. The other end of the plastic tube will be connected with a 1-mL syringe.
6. Keep three holes in separated tube's body to relieve pressure inside tube after closure, therefore preventing the prolapse of the lymphatic wall inside the micropipette (Fig. 1c).
7. Fill the plastic tube and pipette with D-MEM/F12/a/b and put them into a large plastic Petri dish.
8. Cannulate the lymphatic segments at the upstream end onto the micropipette and secure them at the end of the vessel with 6-0 suture, while the output end remains open.
9. Mix equal volumes of ALP-CT stock solution to nondiluted adenoviral construct stock solution (1×10^{13} viral particles/mL) for 30 min at room temperature.
10. Dilute this mixture with D-MEM/F12/a/b to produce a final titer of viral particles ranging between 1.1 and 1.5×10^{10} viral particles/mL.

11. Flush the vessel lumen with ~0.2 mL of D-MEM/F12/a/b using a 1-mL syringe.
12. For endothelial denudation, if desired—disconnect the syringe from the opened input tube and suck ~0.05 mL of air into it. To denude the endothelium, insert air bolus into the vessel lumen. Maintain the vessel for 10–12 s, and then immediately flush it with ~0.2 mL D-MEM/F12/a/b with the syringe to completely replace the air with fluid.
13. Inside the lymphatic vessel, replace the D-MEM/F12/a/b solution with ALP-CT/AdGFP-solution using another 1-mL syringe. Tie the vessel at its output end after it is filled with the virus suspension.
14. Carefully fill the 0.65-μL plastic tube with D-MEM/F12/a/b (with or without virus at 1.1×10^{10} viral particles/mL), and then rapidly transfer the vessel, pipette, and plastic cap from the Petri dish into the plastic tube (see Note 4). Under stereomicroscope, make sure that after this procedure vessel is not damaged or bent.
15. Inject the transfection solution containing 1.1×10^{10} viral particles/mL only into nondenuded vessel to transfect only lymphatic endothelial cells.
16. Inject the solution with 1.5×10^{10} viral particles/mL into endothelium-denuded vessels to transfect only lymphatic muscle cells.
17. To transfect both lymphatic endothelial and muscle cells, put the vessels into the solution containing 1.1×10^{10} viral particles/mL, while injecting with the solution containing 1.5×10^{10} viral particles/mL.
18. Put the plastic tube, containing the cannulated vessel, into a tube rack. Open the end of the plastic tube filled with fluid and place it ~5 cm above the pipette tip to allow the vessel to be pressurized at all times during the subsequent culture (Fig. 1d).
19. Place the tube rack into a cell culture incubator (10% CO_2, 37°C) for the required number of hours for transfection.
20. Check the vessels daily. Discard any vessels with visible signs of contamination.
21. Image the vessels with a Confocal-Multiphoton Microscope System to determine the intensity of the signal in cells of the lymphatic wall. The images were acquired at 0.3-μm intervals via 489 nm of peak excitation wavelength and 508 nm peak emission wavelength. Reconstruct the image in different 3D perspectives using the confocal microscope software.

4. Notes

1. While vessel of interest is still situated in its location in the body, the vessel should be kept at initial natural length and position, so any potential mechanical stress (such as too much distension, wrong direction) during dissection/cleaning procedure will be minimized.
2. Cleaning of vessels selected for incision should be done in situ as much as possible. Clean the vessel carefully to eliminate as much as possible the adipose tissue and other extracellular matrix elements, which later can attract part of transfections constructs, diminishing therefore the power of transfection agent.
3. Procedures must be performed inside biosafety hood to avoid contamination. Everything in contact with the vessel should be single-use sterile (disposable), or alcohol-sterilized (instruments, sutures, vessel chamber, glass pipettes, and glass reservoirs).
4. To eliminate the need to recannulate the vessel when air bubbles formed inside the pipettes, tubing or vessel, or later outside vessel while in incubator, the D-MEM/F12/a/b solution should be continuously heated during all vessel setup procedures to 38°C.

Acknowledgments

This work was supported by National Institutes of Health grants HL-070308, HL-075199, AG-030578, HL-080526, HL-089784, and KO2 HL-086650.

References

1. Gashev, A. A., Davis, M. J., Gasheva, O. Y., Nepiushchikh, Z. V., Wang, W., Dougherty, P., Kelly, K. A., Cai, S., Von Der Weid, P. Y., Muthuchamy, M., Meininger, C. J., and Zawieja, D. C. (2009) Methods for lymphatic vessel culture and gene transfection, *Microcirculation 16*, 615–628.
2. He, T. C., Zhou, S., da Costa, L. T., Yu, J., Kinzler, K. W., and Vogelstein, B. (1998) A simplified system for generating recombinant adenoviruses, *Proc Natl Acad Sci U S A 95*, 2509–2514.
3. Cai, S., Alp, N. J., McDonald, D., Smith, I., Kay, J., Canevari, L., Heales, S., and Channon, K. M. (2002) GTP cyclohydrolase I gene transfer augments intracellular tetrahydrobiopterin in human endothelial cells: effects on nitric oxide synthase activity, protein levels and dimerisation, *Cardiovasc Res 55*, 838–849.

Chapter 20

Isolation of Cardiac Myocytes and Fibroblasts from Neonatal Rat Pups

Honey B. Golden, Deepika Gollapudi, Fnu Gerilechaogetu, Jieli Li, Ricardo J. Cristales, Xu Peng, and David E. Dostal

Abstract

Neonatal rat ventricular myocytes (NRVM) and fibroblasts (FBs) serve as in vitro models for studying fundamental mechanisms underlying cardiac pathologies, as well as identifying potential therapeutic targets. Both cell types are relatively easy to culture as monolayers and can be manipulated using molecular and pharmacological tools. Because NRVM cease to proliferate after birth, and FBs undergo phenotypic changes and senescence after a few passages in tissue culture, primary cultures of both cell types are required for experiments. Below we describe methods that provide good cell yield and viability of primary cultures of NRVM and FBs from 0 to 3-day-old neonatal rat pups.

Key words: Cardiac myocytes, Fibroblasts, Neonatal, Density separation

1. Introduction

Primary cultures of neonatal rat ventricular myocytes (NRVM) and fibroblasts (FBs) are widely accepted as in vitro models in basic cardiac research. These cells readily attach to cell culture surfaces and serve as a means to study a variety of pathophysiologic processes, which lack the influences of hemodynamic factors existing in vivo. In addition, cell culture allows the feasibility to artificially control other concomitant factors using molecular and pharmacologic methods at the cellular level. The use of NRVM and FBs requires that both cell types be isolated as primary cultures. Successful isolation of these cell types from neonatal rat hearts requires that cells be dissociated from the heart tissue and purified. The purification of NRVM from contaminating nonmyocytes is particularly critical for ensuring a constant proportion of myocytes. The procedures

Xu Peng and Marc Antonyak (eds.), *Cardiovascular Development: Methods and Protocols*,
Methods in Molecular Biology, vol. 843, DOI 10.1007/978-1-61779-523-7_20,

described below provide approximately 1×10^6 NRVM from one animal, with 90% viable cells. The complete procedure takes 8 h, which includes digestion periods and 2.5 h purification.

2. Materials

The materials required for isolating primary cultures of NRVM and FBs from neonatal rat hearts are listed below. Although specific sources for the equipment, chemicals, and tissue culture supplies are given, in most cases equivalent products are available from other vendors.

2.1. Equipment

1. Horizontal laminar flow hood.
2. Digital heating circulating water bath, 6 L.
3. Digital stir plate with LED speed display (Corning).
4. Slide warmer (Lab-line, Thermo Scientific).
5. Refrigerated centrifuge (equipped with swinging bucket rotor).
6. Tissue culture microscope.
7. Portable filler/dispenser (Drummond Portable Pipet-Aid, Multispeed XP model).
8. Hemocytometer (Reichert Bright-Line).
9. 200-μm Monofilament open mesh filter material (Sefar America).
10. Jacketed double sidearm cell spinner flask (Wheaton).
11. 1-L Beaker.

2.2. Surgical Instruments

1. Small surgical scissors (Roboz).
2. Small surgical forceps (Roboz).
3. Fine “needle-nose” forceps (Roboz).
4. Fine surgical scissors (Roboz).
5. Gem single-edge razor blades (American Safety razor).

2.3. Tissue Culture Reagents and Enzymes

1. Ampicillin (100×) solution.
2. Arabinosylcytosine (Ara-C, Sigma Chemical Company).
3. α-Chymotrypsin (Sigma Chemical Company).
4. Collagenase type II (Invitrogen-Gibco).
5. Low Glucose Dulbecco’s Modified Eagle’s Medium (DMEM, Invitrogen-Gibco).
6. Fetal bovine serum (Invitrogen-Gibco).
7. Calcium- and magnesium-free Hank’s balanced salt solution (HBSS) (Invitrogen-Gibco).

8. *N*-2-hydroxyethylpiperazine-*N*′-2-ethanesulfonic acid (HEPES) (J.T. Baker).
9. Horse serum (Gibco, Invitrogen-Gibco).
10. L-Glutamine (Sigma).
11. Medium 199 (10×) (Invitrogen-Gibco).
12. Percoll (Amersham Pharmacia).
13. Sodium bicarbonate 99.5% (Fisher Scientific-MP Biomedicals).
14. Trypan blue (Kodak).
15. Bovine Trypsin (3×) (Worthington).

2.4. Tissue Culture Plastic Ware

1. 15-mL Sterile conical centrifuge tubes.
2. 50-mL Sterile conical centrifuge tubes.
3. 100×20-mm Style culture dishes.
4. T75 cell culture flasks.
5. 10-mL Serological transfer pipets.
6. 500-mL (0.45 μm Pore size) polyethersulfone bottle top filters.

2.5. Media and Reagents for Cardiac Cell Dispersion

1. Dispersion media: Combine DMEM and M199 in a 4:1 ratio and supplement with 10% horse serum, 5% fetal bovine serum, and 34 μg/mL ampicillin. pH to 7.4 and filter sterilize.
2. Hanks-HEPES: Add 6 g of HEPES/L HBSS (25 μM final HEPES concentration), pH to 7.4, and filter sterilize.
3. Enzyme solution: Prepare by adding 750 U of bovine trypsin, 825 U of α-chymotrypsin, and 150 U of collagenase type II to 300 mL of Hanks-HEPES. Prepare the enzyme solution just prior to use and filter sterilize (see Notes 1 and 2).
4. Percoll density gradient buffer (12.5×): Combine 8.47 g of NaCl, 5.96 g of HEPES, 0.17 g of NaH_2PO_4, 1.24 g of glucose, 0.5 g of KCl, 0.25 g of $MgSO_4$ in a total volume of 100 mL of deionized water, pH to 7.4 and filter sterilize.

3. Methods

The dispersion and purification methods described below have been optimized for the isolation of NRVM and FBs from 40 Sprague Dawley neonatal rat pups, which are 0–3 days of age.

3.1. Dispersion Preparation

1. Warm the dispersion media, Hanks-HEPES, and enzyme solution to 37°C by placing on the slide warmer, located in the laminar flow hood (see Fig. 1).
2. Connect the cell stir with water bath and ensure the temperature of the running water is 37°C.

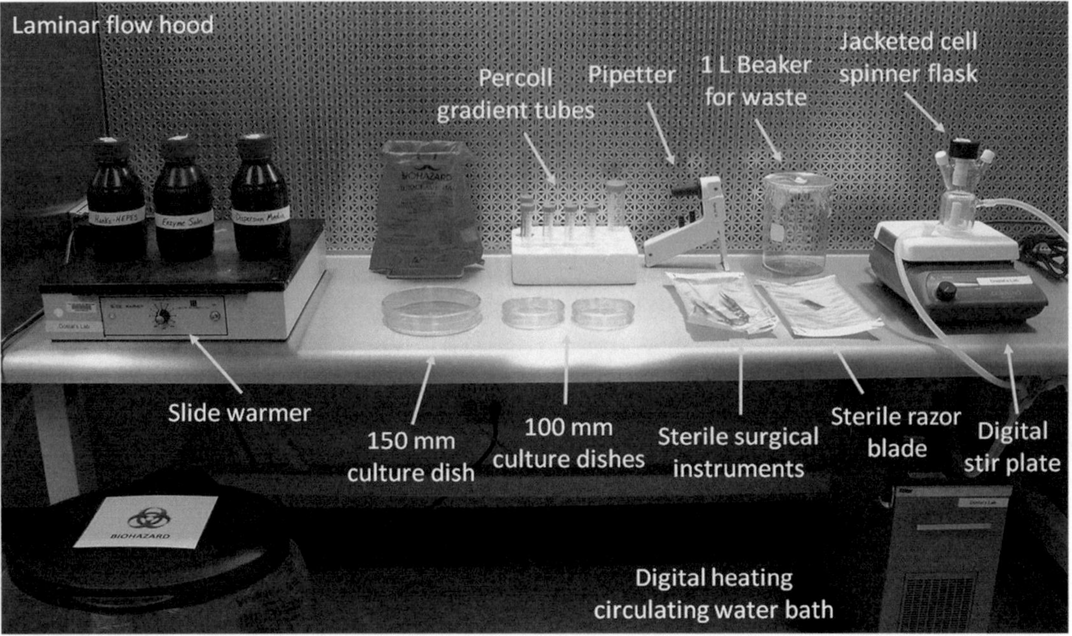

Fig. 1. Preparation for neonatal rat cardiac cell dispersion. Items required for harvesting neonatal rat heart ventricles, dissociation of cardiac tissue, and density gradient separation of cardiac cells are shown.

3. Place a 150-mm sterile culture dish in the hood for euthanizing neonate rat pups.
4. Place sterilized surgical instruments in hood.
5. Ensure HEPES solution is filtered prior to use. Refer to 2.5 media and Reagents for Cardiac Cell Dispersion, step 3.
6. Place two 100-mm culture dishes in the hood, and add 15 mL of warm, sterilized Hanks-HEPES solution to one dish and 5 mL to the other dish (see Note 3).

3.2. Harvesting Neonatal Rat Heart Ventricles

1. Following euthanasia, open the chest of the animal with small scissors and use the small forceps to remove the heart.
2. Transfer the heart to a 100-mm dish containing 15 mL of 25°C Hanks-HEPES which serves to remove blood from the heart.
3. Use the surgical forceps to transfer the heart to a second 100-mm dish containing 5 mL of 25°C Hanks-HEPES, and remove the atria using the small surgical scissors.
4. Slice the heart into 1 mm pieces with the scissors.
5. Once all 40 hearts have been processed as described above, use the razor blade to comb the minced tissue to one side of the culture dish. Use a sterile single-edge razor blade to mince ventricles into ~0.5 mm pieces.

6. Use a 10-mL pipette to gently transfer the mincing buffer (~5 mL) and tissue pieces to a 50-mL water-jacketed tissue stirrer.
7. To ensure the complete transfer of the tissue, use 7 mL Hanks-HEPES solution to wash the 100-mL dish, and transfer the solution and any remaining tissue pieces to the cell stirrer.
8. Repeat the above step with two 6 mL aliquots of 25°C enzyme solution. The total volume of the minced cardiac tissue in the cell stirrer should be 24 mL (see Note 4).

3.3. Enzymatic Dissociation of Cardiac Tissue

An enzymatic approach is required to dissociate NRVM and FBs from the neonate rat hearts. Cells in the myocardium are attached by cell-to-cell and cell-to-matrix interactions. Although these are weak interactions, collectively these effectively retain cells to the ventricular tissue. Bovine trypsin, collagenase II, and α-chymotrypsin will be used to break adhesions among the cells and digest extracellular matrix. Trypsin has been widely used as a dissociating agent for neonatal and adult rat hearts since its initial use in NRVM isolation procedures (1). We employ collagenase II to dissociate the collagen fibers in the myocardium. α-Chymotrypsin is a serine protease that hydrolyses peptide bonds with aromatic or large hydrophobic side chains on the carboxyl end of the bond. This enzyme is routinely used for dissociating a variety of tissues since it cleaves cell surface proteins such as selectins and integrins, which attach cells to one another or extracellular matrix. Although cruder preparations of enzymes are typically more efficient due to the presence of other proteases, purer preparations tend to be less cytotoxic. Below are detailed procedures for enzymatic dissociation of cardiac cells from neonatal rat hearts.

1. Secure the cell stirrer lid and adjust the stirring speed to 300 revolutions per minute (rpm).
2. After 12 min, turn off the stirrer and allow the tissue pieces to settle.
3. Use a sterile 10-mL pipette to gently remove the wash solution, being careful not to disrupt the tissue pieces. This is easily accomplished by placing the pipette tip at the surface of the enzyme solution. The wash solution may be discarded into 1-L beaker.
4. Add 30 mL of fresh enzyme solution to the stirrer and digest the cardiac tissue for 15 min with the stirrer set at 400 rpm.
5. After 15 min, stop the stirrer and gently transfer the enzyme solution into a 50-mL centrifuge tube containing 10 mL of 37°C dispersion medium. Use the pipetting technique described above (step 3), being careful not to transfer tissue pieces or partially dissociated cell clumps.
6. Sediment the collected cardiac cells by centrifugation (1,037 × *g*, 10 min at room temperature).
7. Carefully decant the supernatant and discard into a 1-L beaker.

8. Gently resuspend the cell pellet in 5 mL of dispersion medium and collect in a 50-mL tube.
9. Repeat steps 4–8 for an additional four to six digestions to remove remaining cardiac cells from the tissue fragments. Following the final digestion, only extracellular matrix and DNA from damaged cells should remain. The remaining tissue pieces should be white and the cell solution clear.
10. Gently resuspend any cell clumps among the pooled cells by pipetting, and add enough dispersion medium for a final volume of 35 mL.
11. Pass resuspended cells through 200 μm open mesh Nitex mesh fabric to remove cell debris, and collect the cells in a sterile 50-mL tube.
12. Sediment (1,037 × *g*, 10 min at room temperature) and resuspend collected cells in 8 mL of dispersion medium.

3.4. Density Gradient Separation of NRVM and FBs

In this procedure, a two-step discontinuous Percoll gradient will be used to separate NRVM and nonmyocytes into highly pure populations. The steps for preparing the Percoll solutions used to make the density gradient and separation of cardiac cells for 40 rat hearts are described in Subheading 2.5, step 4. Use Table 1 to prepare these solutions for additional numbers of rat hearts.

1. To each of four 15-mL conical centrifuge tubes, create a two-layer density gradient by carefully layering 3 mL of the 1.060 g/mL Percoll solution on top of 3 mL of the 1.086 g/mL Percoll solution. The tube can be tilted to help minimize mixing of the Percoll layers during layering (see Fig. 2).
2. Use a sterile 5-mL pipette to slowly add 2 mL of cell suspension (obtained in Subheading 3.3) to each of the tubes prepared above.

Table 1
Preparation of discontinuous Percoll gradients

Number of pups	Number of gradient tubes	Volume of resuspended cells (mL)	Layer	12.5× Density buffer (mL)	Sterile water (mL)	Percoll (mL)
40–50	4	8	Low density	1.04	6.64	5.32
			High density	1.04	4.02	7.94
60–70	6	12	Low density	1.56	9.96	7.98
			High density	1.56	6.03	11.91
80–90	8	16	Low density	2.08	13.28	10.64
			High density	2.08	8.04	15.88

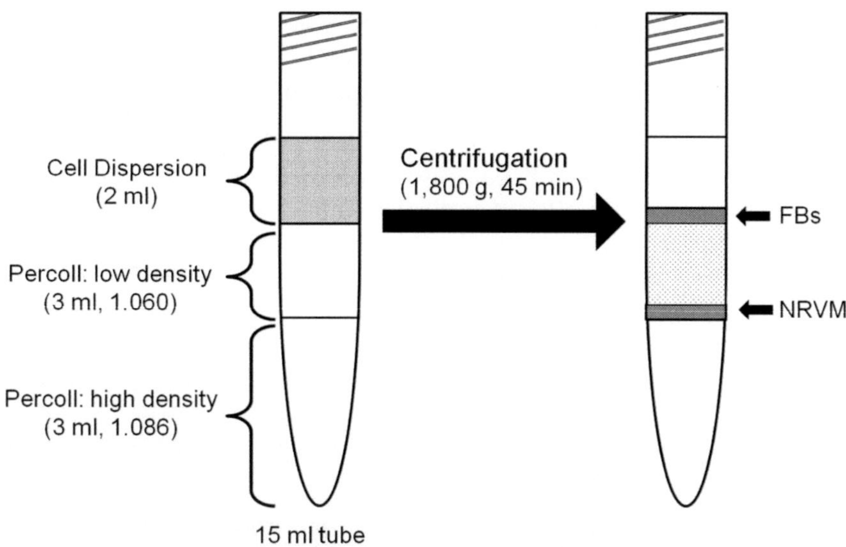

Fig. 2. Percoll gradient tube preparation and isolation of cardiac cells. The low-density Percoll solution (3 mL) is slowly layered over 3 mL of the high-density Percoll solution to form a discontinuous gradient. The cell suspension (2 mL) is then layered on the top of the low-density Percoll solution. After centrifugation, the FB band is located at the top of the low-density Percoll, whereas the neonatal rat ventricular myocytes (NRVM) are located at the interface of the low- and high-density gradients.

3. Centrifuge the tubes at 1,800 × *g* for 45 min, at room temperature.
4. After centrifugation, use sterile 5-mL transfer pipettes to harvest cells in the upper band (primarily FBs) and lower band (NRVM) (see Fig. 2) into separate 50-mL tubes containing 15 mL of dispersion medium. Starting with the first tube, remove and discard the medium above the first band. Next, use the same pipet to harvest the top band of nonmyocytes.
5. Repeat step 4 for the remaining three tubes.
6. Starting with the first tube, remove the volume above the bottom band. This portion of the gradient contains a mixture of stem cells, immature NRVM, coronary smooth muscle cells, and endothelial cells, which can be discarded or harvested in a separate tube as described in step 4.
7. Repeat this procedure with the remaining three tubes.
8. Use a fresh 5-mL transfer pipet to harvest the bottom Percoll band containing NRVM.
9. To each of the 50-mL tubes containing harvested cardiac cells, add dispersion media to make a final volume of 25 mL.
10. Sediment the harvested cells (1,800 × *g*, 10 min, 25°C) and discard the supernatant.
11. Add 5 mL of dispersion media and gently resuspend the cell pellets by pipetting.

12. Use the 5-mL pipet to measure the volume of resuspended FBs. This should be carefully performed to prevent shearing of the cells, in case the pipet tip has sharp edges.
13. Repeat step 12 for the tube containing NRVM.
14. Add sufficient dispersion medium to the tubes containing FBs and NRVM to final volumes of 24 and 15 mL, respectively.

3.5. Determination of NRVM Yield and Viability

Prior to plating, it is important to determine the viability and number of NRVM by counting the number of cells that exclude trypan blue dye. Cells which exclude the blue stain are considered viable and used to calculate an index of viability. The above isolation and purification procedures typically provide ~1×10^6 NRVM per neonate rat heart with 70–90% viability. These determinations are performed as described below:

1. Add 10 μL of the cell suspension to a 1.5-mL microcentrifuge containing 10 μL of trypan blue (0.4%) and allow 1–2 min for dye absorption. Count both the total number of cells and the number of stained (dark) cells by a hemocytometer. Determine the yield and viability of NRVM using the following calculations:

$$\text{Yield} = (\text{total number of cells in four grids}/4)\times(5\times10^4)\times(\text{volume cell suspension})$$

$$\text{Percent viability} = (\text{total cells counted} - \text{stained cells})/\text{total cells counted}\times100$$

2. Once the number of viable cells has been determined, use the equation below to calculate the final dilution volume for the harvested NRVM.

$$\text{Calculated volume} = \text{yield}/(\text{desired cell density per plate})\times(\text{required volume per plate})$$

$$\text{Final dilution volume} = (\text{calculated volume}) - (\text{volume cell suspension})$$

3. Prior to plating, add cytosine arabinoside (0.1 μM final concentration) to prevent cell division of nonmyocytes.

3.6. Differential Plating and Counting of FBs

The upper band of cells generated by the Percoll density gradient (described in Subheading 3.4) primarily contains FBs. However, this layer also contains a small number of endothelial cells and NRVM. Most of these contaminating cells can be removed using differentially plating procedures. This purification procedure takes advantage of the ability of FBs to more readily attach to the culture dish, compared to other cells types. Details of this procedure are follows:

1. Equally divide the 24 mL volume of FBs harvested in Subheading 3.4, step 2 to two T75 flasks and incubate for 90 min at 37°C in the tissue culture incubator.
2. Remove the flasks from the incubator and firmly tap the bottom of the flask on the surface of the laminar flow hood to dislodge nonfibroblasts.
3. Remove the media by aspiration and add 12 mL of warm dispersion medium to each of the flasks and incubate cells for 24–48 h until confluent. At this point, FBs can be passaged into experimental culture dishes.
4. To passage, wash FBs cultures with warm phosphate buffer solution and incubate with 3-mL/T75 flask of warm TrypLE (37°C) for 3–6 min. During this time, most of the cells should detach from the culture dish.
5. Transfer dissociated FBs into 15 mL of dispersion media, count and plate cells as described in Subheading 3.5.

3.7. Cardiac Cell Attachment

Within 1 day after plating, NRVM should be attached and exhibit spontaneous beating. On the second day, the NRVM should start to elongate and a small number will be binucleated (see Fig. 3). On day 3, the NRVM typically form a monolayer in which cells form cell-to-cell contacts with each other by growing pseudopodia (see Fig. 4). FBs, which are mononucleated, are characterized by a flat, irregular shape. In culture, FBs proliferate to form a confluent monolayer with indistinguishable cell–cell adhesion contacts.

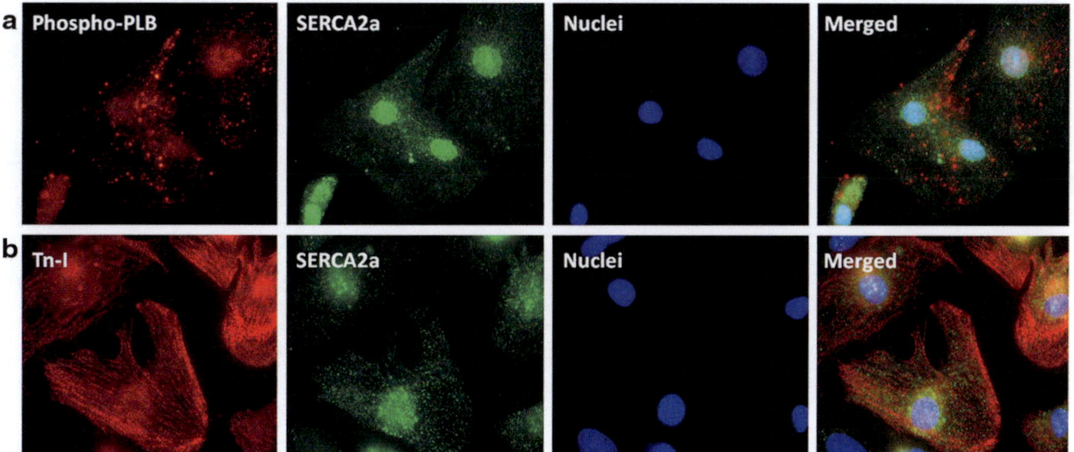

Fig. 3. Myofilament and sarcomeric arrangement in NRVM. Immunostaining of (**a**) phospho-phospholamban (PLB) and SERCA2a reveals sarcomeric structure, while (**b**) troponin-I (Tn-I) defines myofibrillar alignment in NRVM. Nuclei were stained with Hoechst dye. Images were captured by confocal microscopy (60×, oil).

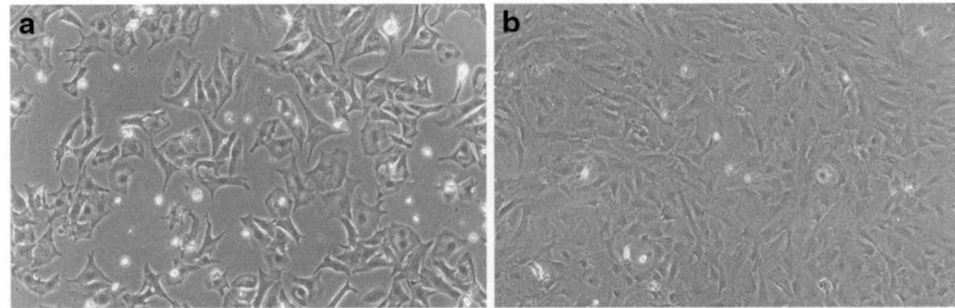

Fig. 4. Morphological features of NRVM and FBs in culture. (**a**) NRVM plated on a collagen I-coated (1 μg/cm^2) 6-well plate, at a density of 0.8×10^6 cells/well, display cell spreading, but also maintain cell–cell contact. (**b**) FBs after 2 days of culture, plated on a collagen I-coated (1 μg/cm^2) 6-well plate at a density of 0.4×10^6 cells/well.

4. Notes

1. Allow enzyme containers to reach room temperature, prior to weighing. This will minimize moisture absorbed from the air.
2. Enzymes can substantially vary in efficiency of dissociation and toxicity among batches. Several lots of enzyme may need to be tested to obtain optimal results. Some vendors, such as Worthington Biochemical Company, provide a sampling program that can be used to choose the optimal batch of enzyme. Worthington Biochemical Company also maintains a web-based database (http://www.worthington-biochem.com/cls/match.php) which can be used to match previous lots of the company's enzyme when reordering.
3. It is important to maintain the proper physiologic pH (7.35–7.4) for the buffers, enzyme solutions, and media used in the dispersion procedure.
4. Hearts must be isolated, minced, and transferred as quickly as possible to the enzyme solution to minimize cell death.

Acknowledgments

This work was supported by the National Institutes of Health (5R01-HL068838-06) and Scott and White Hospital.

Reference

1. Harary, I. and Farley, B. (1963) In vitro studies on single beating rat heart cells. I. Growth and Organization. Experimental Cell Research **29**, 451–465.

Part III

New Techniques

Chapter 21

The Application of Genome-Wide RNAi Screens in Exploring Varieties of Signaling Transduction Pathways

Shenyuan Zhang and Hongying Zheng

Abstract

Cardiovascular development is a precisely coordinated process at multilevels. It involves cross-talking among numerous signaling transduction pathways to ensure proper cell polarity, migration, proliferation, differentiation, and programmed death. Here, genome-wide RNA interference screens in *Drosophila* cells are introduced as novel approaches to discover potential regulators, with special emphases on (1) cell growth and viability, and (2) receptor tyrosine kinase and extracellular-signal-regulated kinase signaling pathway.

Key words: S2 cells, Genome-wide, RNAi, Growth and viability, RTK, ERK

1. Introduction

The phenomenon of RNA interference (RNAi) on gene expression was originally identified in *Caenorhabditis elegans* as a self-defensive mechanism against double-stranded RNAs (dsRNAs) from viruses (1, 2). Nowadays, applications based on this mechanism have been broadly utilized for targeted gene silencing (3). In mammalian systems, mRNAs of individual gene can be triggered for degradation by transfecting cells/tissues with its corresponding small interfering RNA (siRNA). The typical length of siRNAs is around 20–25 nucleotides. However, the inhibitory effect varies, depending on both the transfection efficiency and the structures of individual siRNA species. Plus, siRNA and reagents for siRNA transfection are costly. By contrast, RNAi in cultured *Drosophila* cells is relatively easy and cheap. They can uptake long dsRNA from serum-free medium without transfection and cut-off dsRNA into siRNA by the endogenous Dicer enzyme (4, 5).

Xu Peng and Marc Antonyak (eds.), *Cardiovascular Development: Methods and Protocols*,
Methods in Molecular Biology, vol. 843, DOI 10.1007/978-1-61779-523-7_21,

Initiated in 2003, Dr. Norbert Perrimon and his research group set up the *Drosophila* RNAi Screening Center (DRSC) at Harvard Medical School as an HHMI-supported state-of-the-art facility open to the public (http://www.flyrnai.org) (6, 7). Taking the advantage of cracked details on fly genome (8), a collection of ~20,000 dsRNAs was generated, targeting nearly all identified and predicted *Drosophila* genes, for genome-wide RNAi knockdown. Several automated signal detection systems were established to acquire functional data following RNAi in 384-well cell culture plates, including plate-reader (Analyst GT) based assays, infrared plate-reader (LiCor Aerius) based assays, and high-content imaging assays with a fluorescent confocal system (Perkin Elmer) (9).

Drosophila Schneider 2 (S2) cells with variant sublines are commonly used in the DRSC for RNAi screens. This cell line was derived from a primary culture of late stage (20–24 h old) *Drosophila melanogaster* embryos (10). S2 cells grow at room temperature without CO_2 as a loose, semi-adherent monolayer in tissue culture plates/flasks. There are other available *Drosophila* cell lines or primary cells being adapted for genome-wide RNAi screens in DRSC, but this issue will not be discussed in details here.

2. Materials

2.1. S2 Cell Culture

1. S2 cells (Invitrogen).
2. S2 cell complete culture medium: Mix Schneider's *Drosophila* Medium (Invitrogen) with 10% (v/v) heat-inactivated fetal bovine serum (FBS). Penicillin-Streptomycin can be added to the complete medium as an option. The final concentration should be 50 units penicillin G and 50 μg streptomycin sulfate/mL of medium.
3. S2 cell freezing medium: contains 45% conditioned complete Schneider's *Drosophila* Medium, 45% fresh complete Schneider's *Drosophila* Medium, and 10% DMSO.

2.2. Synthesis of dsRNA

1. cDNA mixture from S2 cells can be generated through two steps: total mRNA isolation through RNeasy Mini Kit (Qiagen) and reverse transcription via SuperScript III First-Strand Synthesis System (Invitrogen). Alternatively, individual cDNA clones may be found and ordered from DGRC (https://dgrc.cgb.indiana.edu).
2. Customized primers can be ordered from Sigma (http://www.sigmaaldrich.com/life-science/custom-oligos/custom-dna.html).
3. Platinum Pfx DNA Polymerase (Invitrogen) or other high-fidelity polymerase chain reaction (PCR) enzymes.

4. QIAquick PCR purification kit (Qiagen) or equivalent products.
5. MEGAscript T7 kit (Ambion).
6. MEGAclear kit (Ambion).

2.3. Drosophila Genome-Wide RNAi Collection

1. The DRSC Genome-wide RNAi Library (DRSC 2.0) is a collection of dsRNAs covering the entire *Drosophila* genome. It is supplied in a set of 63 × 384-well cell culture plates. Based on the detection method that will be used, different types of plates can be chosen to increase the signal/noise ratio.
2. DRSC 2.0 targets ~14,000 genes, with an average of 1–2 dsRNAs/gene.

2.4. Cell Population Measurement

1. White, polystyrene 384-well plates (Corning) equipped with DRSC 2.0.
2. CellTiter-Glo Luminescent Cell Viability Assay (Promega).

2.5. ERK Activation Measurement

1. A stable S2R+ cell line (Rolled-YFP S2) overexpressing Rolled-YFP, *Drosophila* extracellular-signal-regulated kinase (ERK) ortholog tagged with YFP at the C-terminus (11).
2. Bovine insulin (Sigma) for ERK stimulation.
3. Phosphate buffer saline (PBS), formaldehyde, and Triton X-100 (all from Sigma) for cell fixation, permeabilization, and washing.
4. Monoclonal antibodies (Cell Signaling Technologies) targeting dually phosphorylated ERK (dpERK) (12).
5. Alexa Fluor 647 Protein Labeling Kit (Invitrogen) to label primary antibodies.
6. Bovine serum albumin (Sigma) for blocking nonspecific antibody staining.

3. Methods

The base of performing a genome-wide RNAi screen in *Drosophila* S2 cells is to have a clear cellular phenotype which can be monitored in 384-well cell culture plates, for example cell morphology, cell viability, the location of a protein, the expression level of a fluorescent molecule, or signals from a dye. The key for a successful screen is to have robust signal/noise ratio of the phenotype being recorded. Thus, before executing a screen in the DRSC center, it is requested on the application form (http://www.flyrnai.org/DRSC-APP.html) to demonstrate the feasibility of the assay in 384-well format, normally with both positive and negative controls (control dsRNAs or conditions that can mimic the positive and negative phenotypes upon the application).

The other essential issue that should be considered before carrying out a genome-wide screen is how to analyze and follow up the data generated from the screen. It is typical to have numerous interesting candidate genes (hits) popped-up from a screen, few with strong phenotypes and more with weaker phenotypes. A general strategy is to statistically rate all the hits, and then validate the top hits in details at first, with possible extension to their mammalian homologs.

3.1. Culturing S2 Cells

1. Frozen stocks of S2 cells should be quickly thawed at 30°C (see Note 1). Transfer ~1×10^7 (one vial) cells from the vial to 5 mL room temperature complete Schneider's *Drosophila* Medium, and centrifuge at $1,000 \times g$ for 5 min to pellet cells. Remove the supernatant which contains DMSO. Resuspend cells in 5 mL fresh room temperature complete medium and plate in a 25-cm² flask (see Note 2).
2. Cultured S2 cells are generally passed every 2–3 days with the cell density maintained between 1×10^6 and 2×10^7 cells/mL (see Note 3). Once the cell density is below 0.5×10^6 cells/mL, it will significantly influence cell growth.
3. To prepare frozen S2 cell stocks, pellet healthy cells and resuspend in the freezing medium with a density of 1.1×10^7 cells/mL. Aliquot cells into cryovials and freeze slowly to −80°C. For long-term storage, transfer the cryovials to liquid nitrogen.

3.2. Generation of dsRNA Against the Positive Control Gene

dsRNAs can be manually produced with lower cost compared to manufactured siRNAs. Typically, the synthesis procedure is a T7 RNA polymerase based in vitro transcription on a PCR-generated DNA template containing the T7 promoter sequence on both ends.

1. Define the target gene of interest (the positive control, see Note 4).
2. Select a proper region from the cDNA sequence of the target gene as the PCR template. The size of the region should be between 300 bp and 1 kb for an efficient in vitro transcription in the next step. To avoid off-target effects of RNAi, the sequence of the template should not have any 19-mer or longer homology to other predicted genes in *Drosophila* genome (see Note 5).
3. Design a pair of primers corresponding to both ends of the selected cDNA fragment. The melting temperature (T_m) of both primers should be equal to or higher than 55°C for an efficient PCR reaction. Add the T7 promoter sequence (TAATACGACTCACTATAGGG) to the 5′ end of both primers.
4. Set up a 100 μL PCR reaction on ice with the following components: 67 μL autoclaved and distilled H_2O, 20 μL Pfx

Amplification Buffer, 2 μL 50 mM $MgSO_4$, 3 μL 10 mM dNTP mixture, 3 μL 10 μM forward primer, 3 μL 10 μM reverse primer, 1 μL PCR template (20 pg to 400 ng in total, a cDNA clone of the target gene or S2 cell cDNA mixture), 1 μL Platinum Pfx DNA Polymerase. The PCR conditions may vary, depending largely on the sequences of PCR templates and primers (see Note 6). We recommend starting with the following conditions:

Step 1, denaturing temperature (94°C) for 5 min.

Step 2, denaturing temperature (94°C) for 30 s.

Step 3, annealing temperature (may take the lower primer T_m) for 30 s.

Step 4, extension temperature (68°C) for 1 min (30 s/500 bp).

Step 5, Repeat steps 2–4 for 35 times.

Step 6, extension temperature (68°C) for 10 min.

Step 7, the reaction can be maintained at 4–10°C after step 6.

5. PCR products should be examined on an agarose gel to verify the size and specificity (single band) and to determine the concentration (see Note 7). The DNA templates can be purified and enriched, but not necessary, before the transcription reaction.
6. The in vitro transcription can be achieved with the Ambion MEGAscript T7 kit. Following the instruction, the reaction (20 μL in total) is assembled with 8 μL DNA templates, and 8 μL supplied NTP solution, 2 μL 10× reaction buffer, plus 2 μL enzyme mix. The mixture is incubated at 37°C for 4 h to create dsRNA. 1 μL TURBO DNase will then be added to the system to remove the DNA templates by 15-min incubation at 37°C.
7. dsRNA can be purified through Ambion MEGAclear kit and stored at −20°C. The RNA yield can be quantified by measuring the UV light absorbance at 260 nm (A_{260}). dsRNA concentration (μg/mL) = A_{260} × 45 (extinction coefficient) × dilution factor. It is expected to have ~100 μg dsRNA out of one 20 μL transcription reaction.

3.3. Genome-Wide RNAi in S2 Cells

1. RNAi in *Drosophila* S2 cells (4): to examine the positive control, 2×10^6 S2 cells are seeded in a 25-cm^2 flask with 2 mL of S2 complete medium. Cells are allowed to attach and the medium will be removed and replaced with 2 mL of serum-free S2 medium. 10 μg dsRNA (~37 nM) will be added and cells will be incubated at room temperature (~22°C) for 30–45 min with gentle rocking. 4 mL of complete medium will then be added and cells will be incubated for 3–5 days before testing (see Note 8).

Genome-wide RNAi screen

Treat 10^4 S2 cells 3-5 days with dsRNA

Functional assays via:
1) Plate-reader
2) Infrared plate-reader
3) Confocal imaging system
x 384 wells/plate
x 63 plates
x 2 experimental runs for each dsRNA

Analysis

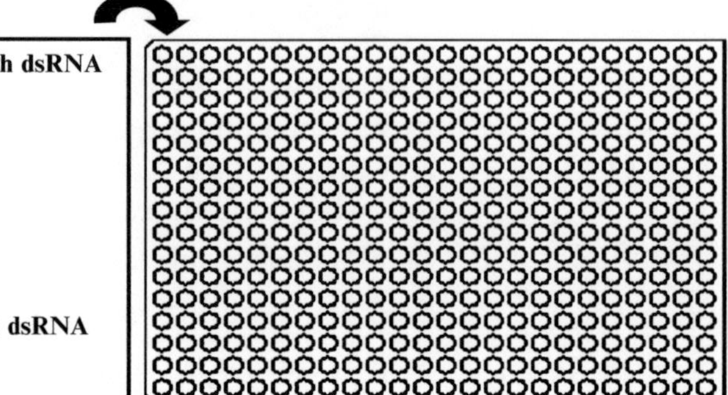

Fig. 1. Genome-wide RNA interference (RNAi) screen in *Drosophila* S2 cells: time lapse of general procedure. The entire *Drosophila* genome is represented in a set of 384-well plates, each well containing a dsRNA (amplicon) targeting a particular gene. S2 cells will be incubated with dsRNA for 3–5 days. Then, functional measurements will be systematically taken in each well. There are 63 plates for each genome set.

2. RNAi in 384-well plate format (see Fig. 1) (13): *Drosophila* S2 cells (~10^4 cells in 10 μL serum-free medium/well at the beginning) are cultured in 384-well plates containing ~0.25 μg dsRNA in 5 μL of 1 mM Tris pH 7 per well. Here, each well of 63 separate 384-well plates contains an individual dsRNA amplicon (see Note 9). Each plate includes an empty well, which will be loaded with customized dsRNA to serve as the positive control. 20 μL of complete medium will be added to each well after 45-min room temperature incubation. After 3–5 days, cells will be screened (see Note 10). Assays are normally carried out in duplicate (two sets of 63 × 384-well plates).

3.4. Screening for Genes Involved in Cell Growth and Viability

1. After 5 days of RNAi treatment, cell numbers are evaluated through an indirect quantitative luciferase-based assay for ATP-levels and read by an Analyst HT 384-well plate reader. In principle, by adding a single reagent (CellTiter-Glo, 30 μL/well) without washing (just wait for 10 min after adding the reagent and mixing), this homogeneous method determines the number of viable cells in culture based on quantitation of the ATP present, an indicator of metabolically active cells (see Fig. 2) (7). The reduction of signal represents less viable cells, as revealed by RNAi of the positive control, D-IAP1, which is known to inhibit apoptosis (14).
2. To evaluate the reproducibility, correlation coefficient can be calculated between duplicated screens (see Note 11).
3. To assess and analyze the screen data, the numerical readouts can be normalized by mean-centering per 384-well plate. The averaged *z*-score for each amplicon from the duplicated screens (calculated separately) will be considered as its statistic index

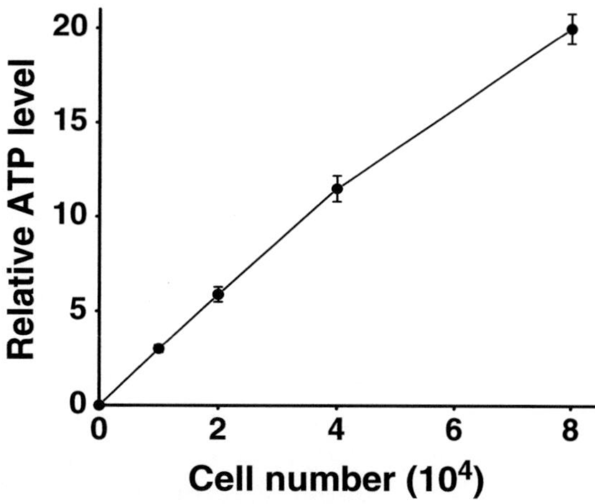

Fig. 2. Cell growth and viability assay. The relative intracellular ATP levels, indicated by quantitative luciferase-based assays, are correlated with numbers of S2 cells in wells from a 384-well plate.

(see Note 12). In general, a threshold of three standard deviations and above can be set to identify hits with 99.9% confidence (see Note 13).

4. To validate top hits from genome-wide RNAi screen, a package of amplicon DNA templates (cherry-picks) can be ordered from DRSC to produce dsRNAs through in vitro transcription (see Note 14).
5. Information of the validated hits can be obtained from http://www.flybase.org. In parallel, search http://www.ncbi.nlm.nih.gov/homologene for their mammalian homologenes.

3.5. Screening for Regulators of ERK Signaling Pathway

There is one single ERK gene, Rolled, in *Drosophila* (15). It was demonstrated to be downstream of multiple receptor tyrosine kinases (RTKs), including the *Drosophila* insulin receptor (InR), *Drosophila* EGFR (DER), and the PDGF/VEGF homologue receptor (PVR) (11, 15). Insulin stimulation on S2 cells, which express InR, can activate the ERK signaling pathway (4). This is evident by the boosted dually phosphorylated active form of Rolled. RNAi treatment against known ERK pathway components had expected regulation on ERK activation. For example, the effect was negative in the case of DSOR1, the *Drosophila* mitogen-activated protein kinase kinase, which phosphorylates Rolled (4).

1. Four days after RNAi treatment to Rolled-YFP S2 cells in 384-well plates, cell media are replaced by either PBS ("baseline") or PBS with 25 μg/mL bovine insulin ("Stimulated"). Duplicated screens (two sets of 63 × 384-well plates) should be performed with each condition. After 10 min incubation at room temperature, total YFP fluorescence from live cells is measured in

individual wells, using an Analyst GT plate reader (Molecular Devices). This set of values will be used to exclude false-negative hits with low cell numbers, which will lead to low signals in the screen.

2. Cells will be fixed in the plates with PBS containing 4% formaldehyde at room temperature (10 min) and then washed with PBS containing 0.1% Triton X-100 (PBST) twice.
3. The monoclonal antibodies targeting dpERK are pre-conjugated with Alexa 647 dye, using Alexa Fluor 647 Protein Labeling Kit. Cells will be labeled with 750 ng/mL antibodies in PBST containing 3% bovine serum albumin at 4°C (overnight). At last, the plates are washed with PBST twice to remove unbound antibodies, therefore reducing the background.
4. Fluorescent signals from YFP and Alexa 647 will be recorded sequentially in each well to represent total Rolled-YFP (excluding endogenous Rolled) and activated Rolled (dually phosphorylated).
5. Both raw signals will be background-subtracted to minimize the influence from autofluorescence of the plastic screening plates. The numerical readouts from activated Rolled will be divided by those from total Rolled-YFP to create a normalized value representing the relative activation level of ERK. *z*-scores of every amplicons are calculated based on the mean of individual plates, and are used to yield a list of hits.

4. Notes

1. S2 cells should be handled with sterile techniques.
2. S2 cells can be cultured in a 25–28°C incubator/container with no requirement of CO_2.
3. S2 cells may start to clump at a density of ~5×10^6 cells/mL. To pass them, use a pipette to gently wash off adherent cells from the bottom surface of the flask with the conditioned medium, and then pipette up and down for several times to break up clumps of cells.
4. A positive control is required before performing a genome-wide RNAi screen in DRSC. Usually, it represents a gene, upon RNAi knock-down, that is known to have a statistically severe phenotype through the designed assay. By contrast, a negative control means a gene, after RNAi treatment, has nondetectable phenotype.
5. "Off-target effects of RNAi" means in addition to expected degradation of the mRNA from the targeted gene, there are other genes being silenced. In dsRNA-mediated RNAi treatment,

off-target effects occur when the applied dsRNA has at least 19-mer homology to other genes. In this case, after Dicer-directed random truncation of the dsRNA fragment, it will create siRNA species recognizing off-target genes.

6. In the step of generating DNA templates for in vitro transcription, the PCR conditions (annealing temperature, extension time, number of PCR cycles, etc.) can be optimized for higher product yield. For high-GC PCR templates, up to 10% DMSO of total reaction volume can be added for better results.
7. A second-round PCR reaction with the T7 primers can be performed to re-amplify from the diluted original PCR products and to increase the yield.
8. RNAi efficiency can be verified by reverse transcription polymerase chain reaction (RT-PCR). Information for optimized RNAi in S2 cells can be found in ref. (4).
9. "Amplicons" are referred to dsRNA species (generated by in vitro transcription and used to direct RNAi against individual genes) in this text.
10. Edge-effect: in some cases, cells in the edges of the 384-well plates (wells numbered A1 to A24, A1 to P1, A24 to P24, and P1 to P24) will grow slower due to changed microenvironment (higher evaporation rate of those wells). This phenomenon of growth retardation may severely affect the phenotypic readouts. To avoid an edge-effect, assay plates may be stored in sealed plastic boxes with bottoms covered by wet paper towels. It is also suggested to analyze wells in edge separately if necessary.
11. Correlation coefficient represents a measure of the strength of linear association between two variables. Its value ranges from −1.0 (negative relationship) to +1.0 (positive relationship). Formula:

$$\text{Correlation}(r) = N\Sigma XY - (\Sigma X)(\Sigma Y) /$$
$$\text{Sqrt}\left\{\left[\text{N}\Sigma X^2 - (\Sigma X)^2\right]\left[N\Sigma Y^2 - (\Sigma Y)^2\right]\right\}$$

where N = Number of values or elements

X = First score

Y = Second score

ΣXY = Sum of the product of first and second scores

ΣX = Sum of first scores

ΣY = Sum of second scores

ΣX^2 = Sum of square first scores

ΣY^2 = Sum of square second scores

12. z-Score indicates how many standard deviations an observation is above or below the mean. Formula:

$$z = (x - \mu) / \sigma$$

where z = z-Score

x = A raw score or an observation to be standardized

μ = Mean of the population

σ = Standard deviation of the population

13. A hit means a candidate gene which may be involved in the signaling pathway screened for. Upon RNAi targeting this hit, it shows statistically significant phenotype by the assay used in the screen.

14. Cherry-picks: DRSC offers a customized collection of up to 250 amplicons (as DNA templates) for hits validation after the primary genome-wide RNAi screen. Amplicons from cherry-picks are independent amplicons. They are different from the corresponding amplicons in the screening set (DRSC 2.0), targeting different regions of candidate genes.

Acknowledgments

The authors would like to thank Professor Norbert Perrimon, and staff of the *Drosophila* RNAi Screening Center at Harvard Medical School.

References

1. Siomi, H., and Siomi, M. C. (2009) On the road to reading the RNA-interference code, *Nature 457*, 396–404.
2. Fire, A., Xu, S., Montgomery, M. K., Kostas, S. A., Driver, S. E., and Mello, C. C. (1998) Potent and specific genetic interference by double-stranded RNA in *Caenorhabditis elegans*, *Nature 391*, 806–811.
3. Castanotto, D., and Rossi, J. J. (2009) The promises and pitfalls of RNA-interference-based therapeutics, *Nature 457*, 426–433.
4. Clemens, J. C., Worby, C. A., Simonson-Leff, N., Muda, M., Maehama, T., Hemmings, B. A., and Dixon, J. E. (2000) Use of double-stranded RNA interference in *Drosophila* cell lines to dissect signal transduction pathways, *Proc Natl Acad Sci U S A 97*, 6499–6503.
5. Jinek, M., and Doudna, J. A. (2009) A three-dimensional view of the molecular machinery of RNA interference, *Nature 457*, 405–412.
6. Friedman, A., and Perrimon, N. (2004) Genome-wide high-throughput screens in functional genomics, *Curr Opin Genet Dev 14*, 470–476.
7. Boutros, M., Kiger, A. A., Armknecht, S., Kerr, K., Hild, M., Koch, B., Haas, S. A., Paro, R., and Perrimon, N. (2004) Genome-wide RNAi analysis of growth and viability in *Drosophila* cells, *Science 303*, 832–835.
8. Rubin, G. M., Yandell, M. D., Wortman, J. R., Gabor Miklos, G. L., Nelson, C. R., Hariharan, I. K., Fortini, M. E., Li, P. W., Apweiler, R., Fleischmann, W., Cherry, J. M., Henikoff, S., Skupski, M. P., Misra, S., Ashburner, M., Birney, E., Boguski, M. S., Brody, T., Brokstein, P., Celniker, S. E., Chervitz, S. A., Coates, D., Cravchik, A., Gabrielian, A., Galle, R. F., Gelbart, W. M., George, R. A., Goldstein, L. S., Gong, F., Guan, P., Harris, N. L., Hay, B. A., Hoskins, R. A., Li, J., Li, Z., Hynes, R. O.,

Jones, S. J., Kuehl, P. M., Lemaitre, B., Littleton, J. T., Morrison, D. K., Mungall, C., O'Farrell, P. H., Pickeral, O. K., Shue, C., Vosshall, L. B., Zhang, J., Zhao, Q., Zheng, X. H., and Lewis, S. (2000) Comparative genomics of the eukaryotes, *Science 287*, 2204–2215.

9. Echeverri, C. J., and Perrimon, N. (2006) High-throughput RNAi screening in cultured cells: a user's guide, *Nat Rev Genet 7*, 373–384.
10. Schneider, I. (1972) Cell lines derived from late embryonic stages of *Drosophila melanogaster*, *J Embryol Exp Morphol 27*, 353–365.
11. Friedman, A., and Perrimon, N. (2006) A functional RNAi screen for regulators of receptor tyrosine kinase and ERK signalling, *Nature 444*, 230–234.
12. Bolshakov, V. Y., Carboni, L., Cobb, M. H., Siegelbaum, S. A., and Belardetti, F. (2000) Dual MAP kinase pathways mediate opposing forms of long-term plasticity at CA3-CA1 synapses, *Nat Neurosci 3*, 1107–1112.
13. Zhang, S. L., Yeromin, A. V., Zhang, X. H., Yu, Y., Safrina, O., Penna, A., Roos, J., Stauderman, K. A., and Cahalan, M. D. (2006) Genome-wide RNAi screen of Ca(2+) influx identifies genes that regulate Ca(2+) release-activated Ca(2+) channel activity, *Proc Natl Acad Sci U S A 103*, 9357–9362.
14. Hay, B. A., Wassarman, D. A., and Rubin, G. M. (1995) *Drosophila* homologs of baculovirus inhibitor of apoptosis proteins function to block cell death, *Cell 83*, 1253–1262.
15. Gabay, L., Seger, R., and Shilo, B. Z. (1997) MAP kinase in situ activation atlas during *Drosophila* embryogenesis, *Development 124*, 3535–3541.

Chapter 22

Application of Atomic Force Microscopy Measurements on Cardiovascular Cells

Xin Wu, Zhe Sun, Gerald A. Meininger, and Mariappan Muthuchamy

Abstract

The atomic force microscope (AFM) is a state-of-the-art tool that can analyze and characterize samples on a scale from angstroms to 100 μm by physical interaction between AFM cantilever tip and sample surface. AFM imaging has been used incrementally over last decade in living cells in cardiovascular research. Beyond its high resolution 3D imaging, AFM allows the quantitative assessments on the structure and function of the underlying cytoskeleton and cell organelles, binding probability, adhesion forces, and micromechanical properties of the cell by "sensing" the cell surface with mechanical sharp cantilever tip. AFM measurements have enhanced our understanding of cell mechanics in normal physiological and pathological states.

Key words: Atomic force microscopy, Mechanotransduction, Cardiomyocytes, Vascular smooth muscle cells, Vascular endothelial cells, Cell culture

1. Introduction

Since the invention of atomic force microscope (AFM) in 1986 (1), the AFM has emerged to be a powerful instrument for studying ligand–receptor and cell–cell interactions, as well as the mechanical properties of living cells in the cardiovascular and other biological research. Unlike magnetic twisting cytometry, magnetic tweezers, and optical stretcher used for the study of cell mechanical properties, AFM with a very sharp cantilever tip passively senses the localized forces between atoms and molecules of the scanning tip and sample surface under unique *x*–*y*–*z* axis movements. AFM imaging can provide (1) high sensitivity up to piconewton; (2) high spatial resolution up to nanometer; (3) three-dimensional (3D) surface topographical imaging; (4) directly measuring co-relationship between local mechanical properties with underlying cytoskeleton and cell

Xu Peng and Marc Antonyak (eds.), *Cardiovascular Development: Methods and Protocols*, Methods in Molecular Biology, vol. 843, DOI 10.1007/978-1-61779-523-7_22,

organelles; (5) directly measuring local mechanical properties in freshly isolated and cultured cells and tissues, in situ and in vitro, and in air and in liquid; (6) information regarding binding probability and adhesion forces between molecules; and (7) elasticity of the cells. Furthermore, a powerful future direction for structural and functional studies in mechanotransduction will be the combination of AFM system with patch-clamp technique for dynamic ion channels study, and with other optical imaging techniques, including fluorescence imaging, total internal reflectance fluorescence, fluorescence resonance energy transfer, and confocal microscopy for probing cellular contact function and cellular signaling (2–9).

The principle of AFM: The AFM is a relatively "simple" instrument that based on laser tracking the deflection of microscopic-sized probe (i.e., cantilever) through its nanometer tip interacting with sample surface (see Fig. 1a). The system consists of the AFM probe with a sharp nanometer size tip mounted on each soft cantilever with specific spring constant (also see Fig. 2a, i), the piezo-control (feedback loop) system that allows for monitoring the interaction forces between the tip and sample surface, and controls the piezo-scanner movements through digital/analog converter, the

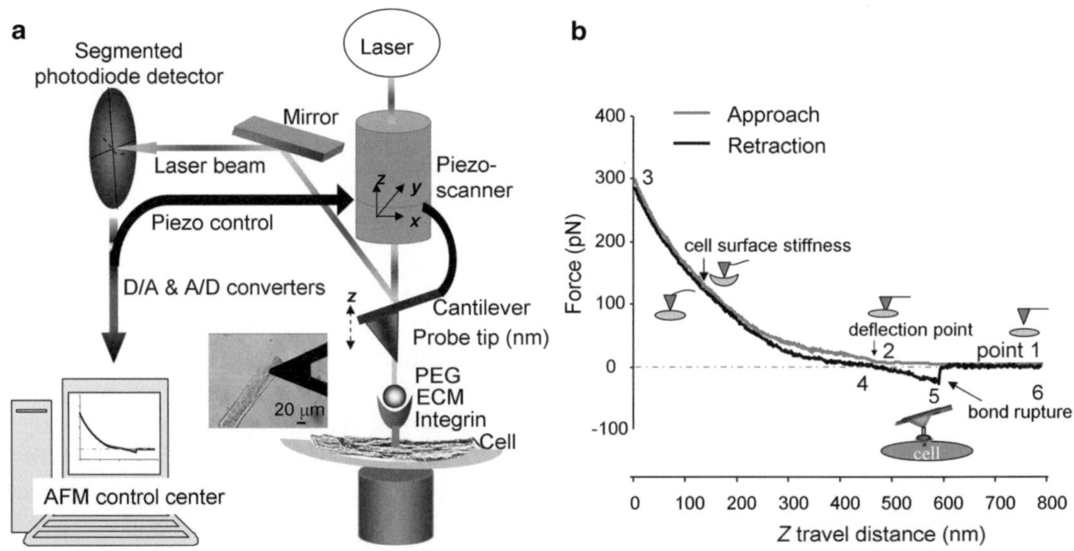

Fig. 1. Schematic representation of the atomic force microscope (AFM) and diagram of a force curve. (**a**) A sharp tip (nanometer in diameter) mounted on a flexible cantilever is rigidly connected to a *xyz* piezoelectric component. A laser beam detects the deflection of the cantilever to segmented photodiode while AFM tip moving at *xyz*-axes. A feedback piezo-control system controlled by NanoScope software senses and controls the deflection and the interaction forces. A labeled AFM probe tip coated with PEG-ECM protein and integrin receptor on the cell surface is also shown. A 3D image or force curve will be recorded by the system. *Inset image* shows the AFM probe approaching a cardiomyocyte. (**b**) Raw force curves generated using FN-coated AFM probe on cardiomyocytes. FN-coated cantilever was controlled to repeatedly (800 nm/s *z*-axis movement at 0.5 Hz frequency) approach (*gray trace*) and retract (*black trace*) from freshly isolated cardiomyocytes while *xy*-axes fixed. The points *1–6* represent stages of approach and retraction (explained in details in the Subheading 3). *PEG* Polyethylene glycol; *ECM* extracellular matrix protein.

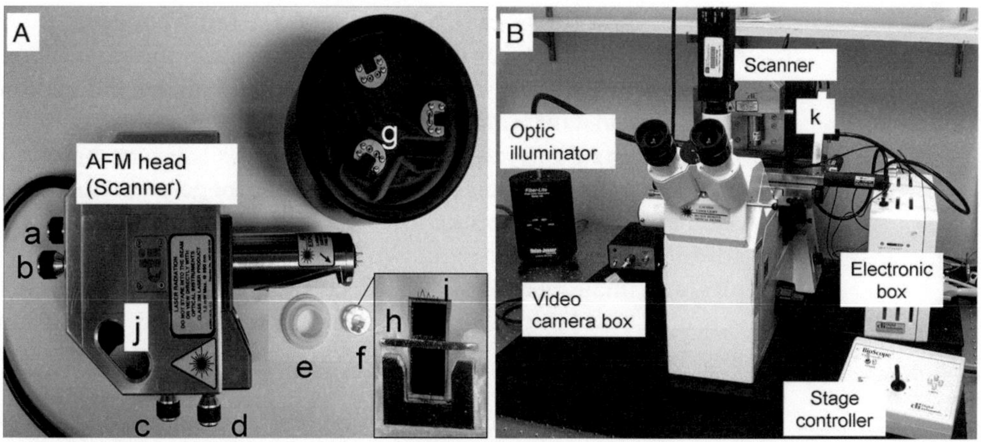

Fig. 2. AFM components. AFM head (or Scanner in **A** and **B**) houses laser, quadrature photodiode detector, and piezoelectric scanner tube. The standard open-loop head (**A**) scans up to 90 μm in *x–y* and up to 6 μm in *z* axis. (**A**) "a and b": Adjustment screws to control position of laser on back of cantilever; "c and d": adjustment screws to control position of laser on the specific position (e.g., center) of the photodiode; "e" : O-ring to seal the fluid holder from the bath solution; "f": AFM probe (fluid) holder; "g": stand for probe holder during inserting and removing the probe; "h": AFM (silicon nitride) probe in the cartridge of the holder ("f"); "i": "V"-shaped cantilevers in the probe, which contains the probe tips (the pyramidal tip of cantilever is shown in Fig. 1); and "j" in AFM head: laser intensity and position indicators. (**B**) "k": *loose* the screw to secure the AFM head and *tighten* the screw to release the AFM head. AFM head in the stand is shown in (**B**).

piezoelectric scanner that moves the tip on the surface of the sample in the *x–y–z* planes, segmented photodiode detector for measuring deflections of cantilever through laser, and analog/digital converter system for recording data. AFM probes consist of a microscopic-sized rectangular or/and "V"-shaped cantilevers, typically constructed from silicon or silicon nitride, with a sharp pyramidal tip (nanometer) or glass/polystyrene beads (micrometer). The property of the soft cantilever determines the sensitivity. The dimension of the tip determines the spatial resolution of the instrument, smaller in tip size and better resolution.

The operation of AFM: The primary AFM imaging can be obtained through contact and tapping (intermittent) mode. *Tapping mode*: the cantilever in AFM probe is oscillated at its resonant frequency under an external electrical excitation, lightly "taps" on the sample surface, and contacting the surface at the bottom (*z*-axis) of each swing at each given *xy*-point. By maintaining constant oscillation amplitude, a constant tip–sample interaction is maintained and an image of the surface is obtained. The advantages of tapping mode are that it allows high resolution scanning of samples that are prone to be easily damaged and could be used for freshly isolated cells that loosely held to a dish bottom. The disadvantages of tapping mode are that it does not offer a good image in liquids and slower scan speeds are needed for tapping mode operation. *The contact mode*: the spring constant of cantilever is much less than sample surface; the cantilever bends when contacted to sample. By maintaining a constant cantilever deflection using the piezo-feedback loop control system, the force between the probe and the sample remains constant and an image of the surface is obtained. The "height" image by contact mode preserves the true height information of the sample. The "deflection" image presents more fine details of the sample but loses the true height information. The advantages of contact mode are fast scanning, good for rough samples, and imaging analysis. The disadvantages are damage or deform action of soft samples by movement on the sample surface and not good for imaging on fresh isolated cells that loosely held to a dish bottom.

Contact mode is easier and more convenient to use than tapping mode, and more conducive to switching between imaging and constant force mode (more details described below in this chapter). Image recorded in imaging mode will be analyzed using AFM Company's software.

In force mode, the AFM tip is brought in contact with the sample surface. The position of the probe was controlled to repeatedly touch and retract (*z*-axis) from the sample surface. The deflection signal from the cantilever tip's indentation is recorded and drawn as *z*-position vs. deflection of the cantilever tip, called as "force curve" (see Fig. 1b). The indentation in the contact point depends on the spring constant of the cantilever, the geometry of the tip on cantilever, and the mechanical properties of the sample.

The application of AFM: The AFM has been used to study a wide variety of samples (i.e., plastic, metals, glasses, and biological samples such as cells and bacteria). The AFM technique has also been successfully applied in cardiovascular research on cardiomyocytes (10, 11), vascular smooth muscle (VSM) cells (12), and endothelial cells (13). In this chapter, we will discuss how to isolate and/or culture cardiomyocytes, VSM, and endothelial cells, and how to operate AFM in contact mode on these cells in physiological state.

The limitation of AFM: AFM has number of limitations: (1) The physical AFM probe used in imaging is not ideally sharp or not correlated with the geometrical feature of the sample. Therefore, an AFM image does not reflect a true topography of the sample, but rather represents the interaction of the probe with the sample surface. Consequently, a contaminated or blunt tip will cause an imaging distortions; (2) Computational methods for analysis stiffness and imaging are critical because the cell membrane has irregular topography and more complex mechanical properties, including heterogeneity, multiphasic material composition, and viscoelasticity; (3) Time consuming that limited number of cells can be recorded and analyzed in a given time; and (4) Possible lateral drag of the cell especially in an un-immobilized sample by the tip during AFM imaging.

2. Materials

2.1. Myocytes Isolation Materials

1. Shaver for shaving animal hair.
2. Stainless scissors ×2: One Scissor (small), iris, 115 mm (4.5 in.), curved for removing small piece tissues from heart; One dissecting Scissors 6 3/4 in. straight (large) for cutting small animal ribs.
3. Stainless steel hemostatic forceps ×2 to help open chest.
4. 10-mL Beakers ×4 with saline solution to transfer heart and for cell isolation.
5. Cooling system for dissecting chamber (4°C).
6. Sylgard 184 Silicone Elastomer for bottom of the chamber.
7. 10-mL Syringe ×1, 1-mL syringe ×3 (one for injecting the heparin, one for anesthesia, and one for dissecting procedure).
8. 10-mL tubes ×2 for cell isolating procedure.
9. Langendorff perfusion system (Radnoti).
10. Lab stand.
11. Falcon tube, 50 mL.
12. Heater/Bath Circulator Pump.
13. Falcon culture dish, 60 × 15 mm.
14. 5-0 Black braided silk.
15. Heparin.
16. 100% O_2.
17. Ethanol, 70%.
18. Forceps.
19. Fine-tip forceps.
20. Dissecting microscope.
21. Thermometer: Cole-Parmer.
22. Timer.
23. Nylon Mesh 250 μm (Small Parts Inc.).
24. Plastic transfer pipette, 2 mm.
25. Pasteur glass fire polished pipette.
26. Vacuum flask.
27. Sodium pentobarbital for anesthesia (Sigma).
28. Collagenases: type 1 and type 2 (Worthington) for adult mouse cardiomyocytes. Weigh out the enzyme(s) in small vials and keep refrigerated (see Note 1).
29. Papain (Sigma), dithioerythritol (Sigma), collagenase (FALGPA U/mL; Sigma), soybean trypsin inhibitor (Sigma), and elastase

(Calbiochem) for VSM cells isolation. Weigh out the enzyme(s) in small vials and keep refrigerated (see Note 1).

30. EZ-Link Sulfo-NHS-LC-Biotin (Pierce).
31. 60-mm Glass bottom dish (WillCo-Dish).
32. Ultrafree-MC filters (Millipore Corp).

2.2. Cannula

The cannula is a very important part of the preparation. It is a 20-gauge needle with the sharp tip cut off (or 20-gauge intramedic luer stub adaptor). It is also useful to make 1-mm notches on the bottom of the cannula (this is important to prevent snagging the aorta when hanging) and to determine how far the cannula is inside the aorta and for holding the silk when tying the aorta:

1. Computer for recording.
2. Inverted microscope.
3. Vibration Cancellation (table) System.
4. AFM system (including software and hardware. Example system: Bioscope Model IIIA, Digital Instruments).

AFM cantilever with (a) silicon nitride, pyramidal-shaped tip (model MLCT-AUHW) diameters was <40 nm and mean spring constant was approximately 14.4 ± 0.6 pN/nm; or (b) 2–5 μm biotin-labeled borosilicate beads as the tip (Novascan).

2.3. Solutions

1. Ca^{2+} free physiological saline solution (PSS) buffer for cardiomyocyte isolation: 133.5 mM NaCl, 4 mM KCl, 1.2 mM NaH_2PO_4, 1.2 mM $MgSO_4$, 10 mM HEPES, and 11 mM glucose, pH 7.4.
2. Arrange 6–50-mL conical centrifuge tubes (marked as buffer #) in the following manner (all solutions bubbled with 100% O_2 for 30 min before experiments):
   (a) #1, 50 mL Ca^{2+} free PSS buffer with 10 mM 2,3-butanedione monoxime (BDM) at 4°C.
   (b) #2, 25 mL Ca^{2+} free PSS buffer containing 1 mg/mL bovine serum albumin (BSA) at 37°C.
   (c) #3, 50 mL 25 μM Ca^{2+} PSS with 62.4 U/mL collagenase type I+73.7 U/mL collagenase type II at 37°C. Weigh out the enzyme(s) in small vials and keep refrigerated. Dissolve it before each experiment in 50 mL Buffer #2 (zero Ca^{2+}).
   (d) #4, 25 mL 100 μM Ca^{2+} PSS at 37°C.
   (e) #5, 25 mL 200 μM Ca^{2+} PSS at 22–24°C.
   (f) #6, 50 mL 1.8 mM Ca^{2+} PSS at 22–24°C.
3. Polyethylene glycol (PEG, Sigma).
4. Dulbecco's Phosphate buffered saline (PBS) with Ca^{2+} and Mg^{2+}.

5. For isolating VSM cells, low Ca^{2+} PSS solution: 144 mM NaCl, 5.6 mM KCl, 0.1 mM $CaCl_2$, 1.0 mM $MgCl_2$, 0.42 mM Na_2HPO_4, 0.44 mM NaH_2PO_4, 10 mM HEPES, 4.17 mM $NaHCO_3$, pH to 7.4 at 37°C.
6. For isolating VSM cells, zero Ca^{2+} PSS solution: 147 mM NaCl, 8.6 mM KCl, 1.17 mM $MgCl_2$, 1.2 mM NaH_2PO_4, 5.0 mM d-glucose, 2.0 mM sodium pyruvate, 0.02 mM EDTA, and 3.0 mM MOPS, pH to 7.4 at 4°C.

2.4. Cell Culture for Cardiomyocyte, VSM Cells, and Vascular Endothelial Cells

1. Fetal bovine Serum (FBS) (Invitrogen).
2. Dulbecco's Modified Eagle Medium (DMEM) (Invitrogen).
3. Laminin (10 μg/mL. Invitrogen) or gelatin (1.5 mg/mL, Invitrogen) for coating culture dish.
4. 35- and 60-mm Culture dishes.
5. 100 U/mL Penicillin.
6. 100 μg/mL Streptomycin.
7. Incubator: 37°C, 5% CO_2, 100% humidification.
8. Trypsin-EDTA (1×, Invitrogen).

3. Methods

3.1. Cardiomyocytes Isolation from Adult Mouse [11]

1. Fill the perfusion system with 50 mL buffer #2 with BSA. Mouse cardiomyocytes require 100% O_2 perfusion throughout the entire procedure (see Notes 2 and 3).
2. Set up the thermometer, light, and timer.
3. Cut several small pieces of 5-0 surgical silk (5–10 cm), knot loosely, and place on the adjustable stage (this will be used to secure the aorta to the cannula).
4. Weigh the mouse (around 30 g for age 12–20 weeks).
5. Anesthetize the mouse with sodium pentobarbital (60 mg/kg, intraperitoneal injection). When the mouse is anesthetized, it will lose consciousness and roll over on its side. Check with a toe pinch to ensure that the mouse is fully anesthetized.
6. Shave the chest, cut the ribs with large scissor, and open the chest with hemostatic forceps. Cut the aorta at about 2 mm from its entry into the heart and quickly remove the heart with small forceps and scissor (see Note 4); immediately place the heart in a 10-mL beaker containing 10 mL cold buffer #1 with BDM (4°C) and view with a dissecting microscope. While in the cold buffer, trim off any excess debris or tissue. Do not cut any part of the heart. A one-way luer valve should be connected to the end of the cannula to protect against trapping air bubbles.

7. Hang the heart by cannulating the aorta. It is helpful to use two fine point tweezers (using microdissecting curved-tip forceps) and to place one of the forceps within the aorta. Using 5-0 surgical silk, tie the aorta onto the cannula filled with the buffer #1 (check the 1-mm notch on the cannula to ensure proper cannulation).
8. Mount the heart in a Langendorff perfusion system fitted with heating coils at 37°C (see Note 5). Dead space in the perfusion apparatus should be minimized to 2 mL. The heart has to perfuse at a pressure of 60 cm H_2O for <5 min with 40 mL buffer #2 (zero Ca^{2+}) and perfuse with buffer #2 for 5 min. The heart should start to beat rhythmically. Maintain the temperature of the heart at 37°C.
9. Subsequently perfuse for 15–20 min with buffer #3 containing 25 μM Ca^{2+} together with specially selected collagenases type 1 (62.4 U/mL) and type 2 (73.7 U/mL). During the perfusion with collagenase solution, the flow will be initially decreased and after a few minutes gradually increased. The length of time for collagenase perfusion should be determined by the palpation method (see Note 6). The perfusion should be stopped when the heart looks like digested (heart will become swollen, turn slightly pale, and feel spongy) or coronary flow increased dramatically.
10. At the end of the perfusion period, remove the heart and transfer to a 30-mL beaker containing 10 mL buffer #4 with 100 μM Ca^{2+}. Trim off any atria or other large vessels present. Cut the ventricles into small pieces, and place the beaker in a 37°C water bath for 5 min during which the pieces should be gently triturated (ten times, see Note 7) with fire polished Pasteur pipette.
11. After the trituration (usually 5 min), filter the cell suspension through a 250-μm nylon mesh (purpose is to separate cells from un-digested small tissue pieces) and collect the cell suspension into a centrifuge tube (10 mL).
12. After permitting the cells to settle under gravity for 5 min (do not centrifuge), remove the supernatant fraction and resuspend the cells in 1 mL fresh PSS containing 200 μM Ca^{2+} (buffer #5). Repeat the above procedure once (i.e., wait for 5 min, remove supernatant, and add 1 mL PSS containing 200 μM Ca^{2+}), and then store the cells at room temperature (22–23°C) until used, normally within 3–5 h. (A good preparation should contain more than 60% rod-shaped myocytes).

3.2. Isolation of Vascular Smooth Muscle Cells (14)

1. Harvest cremaster muscle (left and right) from rat anesthetized with intraperitoneal injection of pentobarbital sodium (120 mg/kg, intraperitoneal injection), and place the tissue in 4°C zero Ca^{2+} PSS for VSM cells containing 1 mg/mL BSA.

2. Isolate the arterioles from the cremaster muscle tissue under dissecting microscope, and then transfer the arterioles into a test tube with 2 mL low Ca^{2+} PSS for VSM cells (see Note 8).
3. Allowing the vessel to settle to the tube bottom, aspirate the majority of the solution and replace with pre-warmed 1 mL of low Ca^{2+} PSS containing: 26 U/mL papain, 1 mg/mL dithioerythritol.
4. Incubate the test tube at 37°C for 30 min, with one agitation after first 5 min of incubation.
5. Gently aspirate the majority of the solution, and replace with pre-warmed 1 mL low Ca^{2+} PSS containing: 0.95 FALGPA U/mL collagenase, 40 U/mL elastase, and 1 mg/mL soybean trypsin inhibitor.
6. Incubate the test tube at 37°C for 15 min.
7. Gently aspirate the majority of the solution, and replace with pre-warmed 1 mL low Ca^{2+} PSS containing 1 mg/mL BSA, allow the vessels to settle to the tube bottom, and let the test tube stand in room temperature for 10 min.
8. Gently aspirate about 1.0 mL of the solution and gently triturate (up to five times) the digested vessels using a fire-polished Pasteur pipette to release the single VSM cells.
9. Transfer the mixture from the tube into a cell culture dish and put it in the 37°C incubator. Let the cell settle down for 2 h; from the side of the dish, gently add in 1 mL of VSM cells culture medium with 10% FBS and 1% PS.
10. Leave the dish undisturbed for 2 days in the incubator. The cell usually will attach and develop processes on substrate after 2–3 days.

3.3. Isolation of Endothelial Cell from Porcine Aorta

1. Obtain porcine aorta from the slaughter house.
2. Wash the aorta with PBS.
3. Remove the non-aortic tissue and trim the adventitia using sterile scissors and forceps. Wash the aorta with PBS to remove the loosened tissues.
4. Gently pipetting PBS through the lumen of aorta to wash off the blood cells retained in the lumen.
5. Clamp a section of the aorta so that there are no branching points on the section, cut away the parts on each end of the clamps.
6. Inject a pre-warmed 140 U/mL collagenase type 2 solution to fill the lumen using a sterile needled syringe, and incubate it for 10 min at 37°C.
7. After incubation, open one clamp and decant the collagenase solution; using a Pasteur pipette gently wash the lumen surface

several times with DMEM medium and collect the wash medium into a cell culture dish; supplement with equal volume of complete endothelial cell culture medium.

8. Incubate the cells for 2–3 days without disturbing.

3.4. Passaging of Cardiomyocytes, VSM, or Endothelial Cells (12, 13)

1. Cardiomyocytes, VSM, and endothelial cells were cultured in a complete cell culture medium (DMEM supplemented with 10% FBS (20% FBS for aortic endothelial cells) and 1% Penicillin + Streptomycin, and used in the experiments at passages 3–10.
2. Aspirate the cell culture medium from a 60-mm culture dish (skip steps 3–7 for cardiomyocyte culture).
3. Wash twice with pre-warmed PBS (5 mL each wash) and aspirate the PBS.
4. Add in warm 0.5–1 mL Trypsin-EDTA (1×, Invitrogen), and incubate at 37°C for 2–3 min.
5. Observe the dish under an inverted microscope with phase contrast; gently shake the dish to dislodge cells from the substrate.
6. Add 2.5 mL pre-warmed complete cell culture medium into the dish, and gently suspend the cells by repeated pipetting.
7. Add 0.5–1 mL of the suspension into new cell culture dishes.
8. Supplemented with 4 mL of warm, fresh complete cell culture medium.
9. Incubate the cell culture dish in the incubator (37°C).
10. Change the medium every 3–4 days.
11. Change the medium to serum-free cell culture medium before AFM experiments as needed.

3.5. AFM Operation Based on Nanoscope IIIa Controller and Nanoscope III Software (Version 5.12)

1. Put a glass bottom dish (<2 mL bath solution in 60-mm culture dish) with one drop of the freshly isolated cells (e.g., cardiomyocytes) in 1.8 mM Ca^{2+} PSS (buffer #6) for at least 30 min or a dish with cultured cells to the inverted microscope stage.
2. Turn on AFM computer (see Note 9).
3. Run Nanoscope software.
4. In the "NanoScope control" window, click on the microscope icon in the upper right corner.
5. Turn on the front button of the AFM system Conditioner, the red light in front of the big controller should be on.
6. The two yellow, one green, and four red lights in front panel of the electronic box (see Fig. 2b) should be on too.
7. Turn on the optic illuminator (see Fig. 2b) and the video camera box controller.

8. Install the probe (see Fig. 2a, h) to the AFM probe holder (see Fig. 2a, f) using a forceps on the black holder stand (see Fig. 2a, g).
9. Prepare the cantilevers (coating with ligands as needed; here using of extracellular matrix protein fibronectin (FN) is given below) on the AFM probe.
10. Labeling of AFM probes with FN (9, 10, 13, 14): For AFM probe with silicon nitride tip, use PEG (Sigma) to cross-link proteins onto silicon nitride tip at room temperature. Incubate the probe first with 10 mg/mL PEG for 5 min, wash with PBS four times, and then incubate with reagents (i.e., FN, 1 mg/mL) for 1 min. Wash the tip again with PBS for four times. For AFM probe with biotin-labeled borosilicate beads, use biotinylation procedure. Prepare biotinylated FN by incubating the 10 mL NHS-LC-Biotin (10 mM, Pierce Chemical Co., Rockford, IL) with 200 mL FN (1 mg/mL) for 30 min at room temperature or for 2 h on ice. To remove unreacted biotin, use ultrafree-MC filters (Millipore Corp., Bedford, MA). Dissolve the filtered biotinylated FN in PBS to a concentration of 0.5 mg/mL. Incubate the AFM probes with biotin-labeled borosilicate beads with avidin (1 mg/mL, Sigma-Aldrich) for 5 min. Wash the probes five times with PBS, incubate with biotinylated FN for 6 min, wash again with PBS for five times.
11. After labeling, install the holder onto the AFM head (Scanner in Fig. 2a), and put on the O-ring seal (see Fig. 2a, e; see Notes 10 and 11).
12. Install the AFM head to the stand in AFM stage (see Note 12). Tighten the releasing screw (see Fig. 2b, k) to lower the AFM head, and then loose the screw to secure the AFM head position.
13. Carefully adjust the two screws (see Fig. 2a, a and b) on the top of AFM head to bring laser onto cantilever (see Fig. 2a, i). Bright red laser light indicator is shown in the window (see Fig. 2a, j) of the AFM head. In addition, a red round cursor presented as laser spot will also be moved into the "photodiode detector," and a white cursor will show the strength of laser light signaling (normally >3) in the "sum" in "NanoScope image" window of the program.
14. Select microscope on the menu in "NanoScope control" window of the program, and then select reset. The four red lights on electronic box (see Fig. 2b) should be off now, and the green light starts flickering.
15. Adjust the focus to see the cell, and then raise the focal plane well above the cells.
16. Using the engage command (the green arrow button in "NanoScope control") to lower the cantilever down into the buffer: click engage button, select manual and pressing on approach, and lower it into the focal plane. Using the three black

knobs (in the stage of microscopy) to bring the tip of cantilever to the blue crosshair in the center of video monitoring ("vision system") window in the program.

17. Adjust the two screws on the left of the AFM head (see Fig. 2a, c and d) to bring the laser spot to the center of the photodiode diagram.
18. Adjust the focus till the cells are clearly visible using the joy stick (see Fig. 2b, stage controller) and bring a desired cell into the crosshair region on the "vision system."
19. Adjust parameters on the AFM "NanoScope control" window of the program. Scan control panel: Scan size (e.g., set as 0), Scan rate (e.g., 0.5 Hz); Feedback Control Panel: Setpoint (e.g., 0.2–0.3 V above vertical deflection), integral gain (e.g., 0.28), proportional gain (e.g., 0.29). Channel 1: Data Scale; Realtime planefit (select line); Offline planefit (select full). Channel 2: Data Scale; Realtime planefit (select line); Offline planefit (select full).
20. Click engage ("Down" arrow) button from "NanoScope control" window, select manual and pressing on approach to bring the cantilever down close to the cell, but the image of the cantilever still looks fuzzy.
21. Click on OK, the step motor will automatically bring the tip down to the cell. AFM will automatically start scanning the cells in Contact mode. For generating topographic image of the cell surface, set the instrument to apply a constant force on the cell. In each horizontal line scan, record both height data (z axis) and the position of the probe (deflection data) in the "NanoScope image" window. The scanned image size will be up to 90×90 μm with a scan speed of 40 μm/s.
22. Click on the "Scale" button in "NanoScope control" window to start the force curve mode operation. The real-time force curves will show in "NanoScope image" window.
23. Click on Setpoint 0 to bring force curve into the middle of y-scale, by moving Scan start back and forth to adjust the force curve position on x-scale. Adjust the Scan rate (e.g., 0.5 Hz), ramp size (e.g., 800 nm) for z-axis movement.
24. Click on menu of "Capture" and then select "continue" to continuously record force curves. Select "capture" again and select abort to stop recording.
25. Force curves are normally recorded by repeated cycles (normally >50 cycles) of AFM probe approach and retraction at a given scan frequency (e.g., 0.5 Hz) and a given z-axis movement (e.g., 800 nm). A typical force curve is shown in Fig. 1b. When the AFM probe with/without coating (e.g., coated with FN) moves to approach the cardiomyocyte cell surface (point 1–2),

force remains at zero level. The cantilever will bend, encounter a resistance, and change the deflection signal after contact with the surface (gray "approach" line, point 2–3). Point 2 represents as "reflection point or contact point." Data in the region of point 2–3 are used to fit using different Models (e.g., the Hertz model) to calculate the cell cortical stiffness. The stiffer the cell, the less the indentation and the steeper the upslope of the force curve. As the probe retraction starts (black "retraction" line), the resistance force will decrease (point 3–4). The snap-off that represents bond rupture (i.e., termed adhesion force) between AFM tip and the cardiomyocyte is shown in retraction line (black-line point 5). As seen in Fig. 1b, the example trace shows one adhesion events (bond rupture) that occurred when the FN coated-probe retracted. When all adhesions between the FN-coated probe and cardiomyocyte have been broken, the retraction curve again overlies the initial approach curve level (point 6) because net forces acting on the cantilever are zero (i.e., equivalent to force acting on the probe during the approach).

26. Click on the "Eye" icon on the upper right corner of "NanoScope control" window to bring back AFM into contact mode imaging. It will take a longer time for a set of imaging depends on the scan size and scan rate.
27. Click on withdrawing button (red "up" arrow button) to withdraw the AFM head from the cell.
28. Click withdraw button several times to raise the AFM probe out of buffer. Tighten the screw (see Fig. 2b, k) on stand to unlock AFM head and lift the head from stand, remove the O-ring and the fluid holder from AFM head. After removing the holder, put the AFM head back onto the stand, and hold with left hand and then release the locking screw (see Fig. 2b, k) to secure the AFM head in the upper position.
29. Turn off the electrical conditioner on the floor to shut off controllers and electronic box. Turn off the camera and the illuminator stand. Remove the cantilever from the holder using a forceps on the black holder stand; clean the holder and O-ring by washing with soap and water.
30. You may blow dry the holder with air duster. Holes in the holder need to be dried with paper tips. Leave the tip dry on the holder stand for next time use.
31. Turn off the Nanoscope software and turn off the computer.
32. The collected data will be analyzed using built-in software programs or customized software programs. To measure cell cortical stiffness (i.e., elastic modulus or cell resistance to shape deformation, see Fig. 1b), use the approach force curves for analysis (gray line in Fig. 1b). Fit the approach force curves

with the Hertz Model between points 2 and 3 (see Fig. 1b) using MATLAB software (Mathwork, Inc.) and use NForceR software (copyright, 2004) to calculate the cortical stiffness based on tip displacement and membrane indentation (12). Use the retraction curve (black line in see Fig. 1b) to analyze the specific adhesion forces related to bonding between AFM tip and cell surface. During retraction, if a specific adhesion event occurs, it will be detected as small sharp shift (bond rupture, see Fig. 1b, point 5) in the deflection curve obtained during probe retraction from the cell surface. No adhesions will be apparent as a smooth retraction curve similar in appearance to the approach curve. These deflection shifts referred to as "snap-offs" will be recorded in the force curve and represent the force required to cause bond failure between the AFM probe and a cell surface molecules (i.e., integrin receptor) (10, 12). With the application of the spring constant of the AFM probe cantilevers, all deflection shifts (snap-offs) in a retraction curve will be detected, quantified, and used to compute the rupture force. Adhesion force between FN and integrins on myocyte plotted as a function of the frequency (events) of occurrence. Single-rupture forces will be determined using Hooke's Law: $F = kd$, where d is the height of the step change in the retraction curve representing bond rupture (in Fig. 1b, point 5) and k is the spring constant of the cantilever. Imaging data in contact mode can be analyzed by using built-in software.

4. Notes

1. Different lot of the same enzymes might yield inconsistent results. Test the enzymes before use for each new lot of enzymes purchased.
2. Mouse myocytes are extremely sensitive to any air bubbles within the tubing of the perfusion system. Make sure that there are absolutely no bubbles anywhere within the tubing. Pipetting up and down is helpful to remove any bubbles found. Therefore, it is imperative to set the Langendorff perfusion buffer tubes in series so that the buffers can be switched quickly.
3. Mouse myocytes require 100% O_2 perfusion throughout the entire procedure.
4. While removing the heart tissue from the anesthetized mouse, remove some of the lung with it in order to have a large aorta to work with.
5. Make sure that the perfusion lines are filled and the temperature is calibrated to remain at 37°C. It may be necessary to set the

water bath at slightly a higher temperature (at 39°C) to maintain this perfusion temperature at 37°C.

6. During enzymatic procedure, the heart will become swollen and turn slightly pale, feels spongy. Perfusion with collagenase for a longer time reduces the cell viability and yield.
7. Do not triturate too much that will damage the freshly isolated cells.
8. Carefully isolate arterioles and arteries and do not stretch the tissues a lot.
9. Always turn on computer first in AFM system.
10. No bath solution over O-ring fluid cantilever holder (Fig. 2a, e) to avoid burning the AFM head.
11. Do not allow the poles on AFM head touch any liquid. If the poles touch the liquid, clean and remove the liquid immediately. No liquid is allowed to touch the electronics above the poles to avoid the AFM head burn.
12. Do not bring the AFM tip all the way down to the cell; you may damage the probe and the cell.

References

1. Binnig, G., Quate, C. F., and Gerber, C. (1986) Atomic force microscope, *Phys Rev Lett 56*, 930–933.
2. Zhang, P. C., Keleshian, A. M., and Sachs, F. (2001) Voltage-induced membrane movement, *Nature 413*, 428–432.
3. Besch, S., Snyder, K. V., Zhang, P. C., and Sachs, F. (2003) Adapting the Quesant Nomad atomic force microscope for biology and patch-clamp atomic force microscopy, *Cell Biochem Biophys 39*, 195–210.
4. Sun, Z., Juriani, A., Meininger, G. A., and Meissner, K. E. (2009) Probing cell surface interactions using atomic force microscope cantilevers functionalized for quantum dot-enabled Forster resonance energy transfer, *J Biomed Opt 14*, 040502.
5. Trache, A., and Meininger, G. A. (2005) Atomic force-multi-optical imaging integrated microscope for monitoring molecular dynamics in live cells, *J Biomed Opt 10*, 064023.
6. Charras, G. T., and Horton, M. A. (2002) Single cell mechanotransduction and its modulation analyzed by atomic force microscope indentation, *Biophys J 82*, 2970–2981.
7. Kassies, R., van der Werf, K. O., Lenferink, A., Hunter, C. N., Olsen, J. D., Subramaniam, V., and Otto, C. (2005) Combined AFM and confocal fluorescence microscope for applications in bionanotechnology, *J Microsc 217*, 109–116.
8. Kellermayer, M. S., and Grama, L. (2002) Stretching and visualizing titin molecules: combining structure, dynamics and mechanics, *J Muscle Res Cell Motil 23*, 499–511.
9. Formigli, L., Meacci, E., Sassoli, C., Chellini, F., Giannini, R., Quercioli, F., Tiribilli, B., Squecco, R., Bruni, P., Francini, F., and Zecchi-Orlandini, S. (2005) Sphingosine 1-phosphate induces cytoskeletal reorganization in C2C12 myoblasts: physiological relevance for stress fibres in the modulation of ion current through stretch-activated channels, *J Cell Sci 118*, 1161–1171.
10. Shroff, S. G., Saner, D. R., and Lal, R. (1995) Dynamic micromechanical properties of cultured rat atrial myocytes measured by atomic force microscopy, *Am J Physiol 269*, C286–292.
11. Wu, X., Sun, Z., Foskett, A., Trzeciakowski, J. P., Meininger, G. A., and Muthuchamy, M. (2010) Cardiomyocyte contractile status is associated with differences in fibronectin and integrin interactions, *Am J Physiol Heart Circ Physiol 298*, H2071–2081.

12. Sun, Z., Martinez-Lemus, L. A., Trache, A., Trzeciakowski, J. P., Davis, G. E., Pohl, U., and Meininger, G. A. (2005) Mechanical properties of the interaction between fibronectin and alpha5beta1-integrin on vascular smooth muscle cells studied using atomic force microscopy, *Am J Physiol Heart Circ Physiol 289*, H2526–2535.
13. Trache, A., Trzeciakowski, J. P., Gardiner, L., Sun, Z., Muthuchamy, M., Guo, M., Yuan, S. Y., and Meininger, G. A. (2005) Histamine effects on endothelial cell fibronectin interaction studied by atomic force microscopy., *Biophys J 89*, 2888–2898.
14. Wu, X., Mogford, J. E., Platts, S. H., Davis, G. E., Meininger, G. A., and Davis, M. J. (1998) Modulation of calcium current in arteriolar smooth muscle by alphav beta3 and alpha5 beta1 integrin ligands., *J Cell Biol 143*, 241–252.

Chapter 23

In Utero Assessment of Cardiovascular Function in the Embryonic Mouse Heart Using High-Resolution Ultrasound Biomicroscopy

Honey B. Golden, Suraj Sunder, Yang Liu, Xu Peng, and David E. Dostal

Abstract

Murine models are currently the preferred approach for studying the molecular mechanisms of cardiac dysfunction resulting from changes in gene expression. Transgenic and gene-targeting methods can be used to generate mice with altered cardiac size and function, and as a result, in vivo techniques are indispensible in evaluating cardiac phenotype. Traditionally, the pathologic assessment of sacrificed hearts was used to study cardiac pathophysiology in small animals. Below we describe the use of ultrasound biomicroscopy-Doppler analysis to temporally assess cardiac function in mouse embryos. Methods are described for obtaining 2D, pulsed-wave Doppler, and M-mode imaging using standard clinical cardiac ultrasound imaging planes.

Key words: Biomicroscopy, Cardiac development, Color Doppler, Echocardiography, Fetal hearts, Mouse embryos, Pulse Doppler

Abbreviations

A	Peak atrial diastolic velocity
AET	Aortic ejection time
CO	Cardiac output
CSA	Valve orifice cross-sectional area
dP/dt	Left ventricular developed pressure
DT	Deceleration time
E	Peak early diastolic velocity
ECG	Electrocardiogram
EF	Ejection fraction
fps	Frames/s
FS	Fractional shortening
HR	Heart rate
ICRT	Isovolumic contraction time

Xu Peng and Marc Antonyak (eds.), *Cardiovascular Development: Methods and Protocols*, Methods in Molecular Biology, vol. 843, DOI 10.1007/978-1-61779-523-7_23,

IVRT	Isovolumic relaxation time
IVS	Interventricular septum
LV	Left ventricle
LVOT	Left ventricular outflow tract
MV	Mitral valve
PA	Pulmonary artery
PRF	Pulse-rate frequency
PSAX	Parasternal short-axis
PSLAX	Parasternal long-axis
PV	Pulmonary vein
RV	Right ventricle
RVOT	Right ventricular outflow tract
SV	Stroke volume
TDI	Tissue Doppler imaging
VTI	Velocity time interval of the Doppler flow profile

1. Introduction

Cardiovascular disease is the leading cause of human mortality globally and ranks as the number one killer in the United States. Mice have proven to be an excellent model system for studying a variety of congenital human heart diseases. Many of the major congenital heart anomalies seen clinically can be reproduced using transgenic mouse models. However, mice with the more serious congenital heart defects frequently die before term. Thus, assessment of fetal mouse cardiac structure and function has become increasingly important for investigating the etiology of human congenital heart disease. Of critical importance in such studies is the availability of tools for fetal mouse cardiovascular phenotyping. Studies have traditionally been based on histological observation after necropsy or surgery. Although an immense body of knowledge has been obtained using this technique, its highly invasive nature makes it inappropriate for sequential dynamic studies on the same animal. Ideally, high-resolution anatomical imaging tools for this type of analysis should be rapid, inexpensive, and noninvasive. Unlike other noninvasive emerging imaging modalities, such as magnetic resonance imaging, microcomputed tomography, or positron emission tomography, echocardiography has an advantage in real-time evaluation of cardiac function including hemodynamic evaluation. Ultrasound methods are commonly used to monitor in utero progress during human pregnancy. However, the maximum frequencies reached by conventional clinical probes are 10–15 MHz. This provides spatial resolution in the order of millimeters, adequate for a macroscopic study of the embryo, but insufficient for visualizing microscopic details in the heart (less than 2 mm at birth) and other tissues (1). While conventional echocardiography, with a 15-MHz frequency transducer, was originally used for the assessment of murine cardiac function, it is not ideal for adequately visualizing small heart size with rapid heart rate.

Advances in imaging technology led to the development of ultrasound biomicroscopy (UBM) instruments which use an ultra-high frequency (30–55 MHz) pulse-echo method. The high frequencies generate images with a resolution of 30–50 μm, close to conventional histology. Improved 2D spatial resolution provided by UBM has allowed very early mouse embryos to be imaged (2, 3). However, relatively slow frame rates (maximum of 8 images/s) or the lack of image-guided Doppler interrogation (2, 3) limit the use of these systems. Given a heart rate of 120–200 bpm, this gives only 2–4 frames for each cardiac cycle. Thus, UBM is most widely used for static, often ex vivo observations rather than for sequential dynamic studies. In this study, we used a recently available digital UBM, which has a frame rate of 740 frames/s (4×4 mm field) to define chamber development and function in mouse embryos.

2. Materials

1. VisualSonics Vevo Color 2100 ultrasound system, equipped with a 40 MHz transducer (MS550D), pulsed-wave (PW) Doppler, color Doppler, and cardiovascular analysis tools software package (VisualSonics, Inc., Canada).
2. Vevo integrated rail system including physiological monitoring unit (VisualSonics, Inc., Canada).
3. Mouse warming platform (VisualSonics, Inc., Canada).
4. Compact gas inhalation system for anesthesia (VisualSonics, Inc., Canada).
5. Heating lamp (Grandrich 20-W halogen lamp or equivalent).
6. Chemical epilator for fur removal (Nair, Church & Dwight Co., Inc.).
7. Aquasonic CLEAR® ultrasound gel (Parker Laboratories, Inc.).
8. Thermosonic® Gel Warmer (Parker Laboratories, Inc.).
9. Isoflurane (Vedco, Inc.).
10. Aquagel® lubricating gel 142 (Parker Laboratories, Inc.).
11. Signagel® electrode gel (Parker Laboratories, Inc.).
12. Sterile lubricant eye ointment (Artificial Tears, Vedco, Inc.).
13. Cotton-Tipped Applicators (Q-Tips™, Kendall Healthcare).
14. Disinfectant (Vimoba, Quip Labs).
15. First aid cloth tape (Johnson & Johnson).

16. Deionized water.
17. 2×2 Gauze pads (12 ply Curity Gauze Sponge, Kendall Healthcare).

3. Methods

Several ultrasound imaging platforms are used to study animal models. This study used the novel Vevo 2100 system with color Doppler capability and the linear phased array MS400 transducer (18–38 MHz). The Vevo 2100 presents images at an axial resolution of 30 μm and a lateral resolution of 62 μm. Presently, the transducer has a 2D acquisition rate of 30 frames/s (fps), a depth of view of 10 mm and the first focal length of approximately 6 mm. B-mode imaging for anatomical visualization and quantification was obtained with enhanced temporal resolution with frame rates up to 740 fps (in two-dimensions for a 4×4 mm field of view) and M-mode at 1,000 fps.

Echocardiography of fetal mice can be used to detect fetal embryos in the mice uterine horns as early as E8.5. Changes in cardiac geometry and function (systolic and diastolic) were obtained serially in C57BL/6 mouse embryos every day from E9.5–18.5 using in utero ultrasound. Mice used for this study were obtained from an established breeding colony and echocardiography was conducted in accordance with an animal protocol approved by the Texas A&M Health Science Center IACUC. (See the "Abbreviations" commonly used in echocardiography.)

3.1. Preparing the Ultrasound Machine and Imaging Platform

1. Prior to anesthetizing the mouse, verify that Vevo 2100 software presets are optimized for embryo hearts.
2. Attach the cable of the 40 MHz transducer to the active port on the Vevo 2100.
3. Secure the transducer probe onto the holder (see Fig. 1a) of the integrated rail system of the Vevo imaging system.
4. Spray the echo platform and anesthesia chamber with disinfectant (e.g., 0.02% chlorine dioxide), which does not contain alcohol or ammonia. Remove the disinfectant solution with a paper towel. Line the bottom of the anesthesia chamber with a paper towel to absorb urine excreted by the animal.
5. Sterile the nose cone with a cotton-tipped applicator moistened with disinfectant.
6. Verify that the echo platform has been adjusted to 37°C.

3.2. Preparing the Pregnant Mouse for Imaging

1. Place the pregnant mouse in the induction chamber and adjust the anesthetic (2–4% isoflurane mixed with 0.8 L/min 100% O_2). Waste gas from the induction chamber should be scavenged using a charcoal filter to provide safety for the operator.

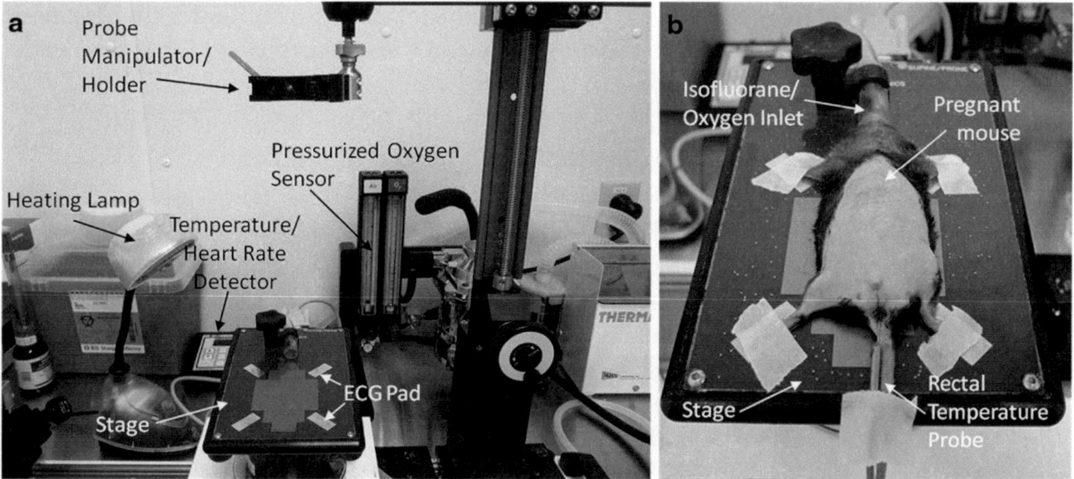

Fig. 1. The Vevo 2100 ultrahigh-resolution ultrasound biomicroscopy (UBM) imaging system for echocardiography and Doppler imaging. (**a**) The VisualSonics integrated rail system with physiological monitoring unit, electrocardiogram (ECG) board, and 40 MHz scan head. (**b**) The mouse is positioned and restrained on the heating board with the four limbs of the mouse taped to the integrated gold ECG electrodes and rectal probe inserted.

2. Remove the anesthetized mouse from the induction chamber and use a cotton-tipped applicator to apply artificial tears eye ointment onto the eyes to prevent drying of the sclera (avoid contacting the cornea with the applicator).
3. Place the anesthetized mouse in a supine position on the heated echo platform and insert its snout into the nose cone used to deliver anesthetic (see Fig. 1b). Maintain a steady-state sedation level throughout the procedure (1.0–1.5% isoflurane mixed with 0.8 L/min 100% O_2). If necessary, adjust the level of anesthesia to maintain a target heart rate of 500 ± 50 bpm.
4. Apply electrode gel to the electrocardiogram (ECG) contacts on the heating pad and secure the four paws and tail to the pad using 1-cm strips of tape.
5. Gently insert the rectal thermometer (after application of a water-based lubricant) to continuously monitor and adjust body temperature via the heating pad (see Note 1).
6. Place a heating lamp approximately 8–10 in. away from the animal to minimize radiant heat loss.
7. Maintain the body temperature and heart rate by adjusting the level of anesthesia and manipulating the heating lamp and/or room temperature. Ambient room temperature should be maintained at 27.5°C (see Notes 2 and 3).
8. Remove fur from the abdomen by applying uniform layer of chemical epilator. This is required to minimize attenuation of the ultrasound.

9. After 1–2 min, use surgical gauze saturated with deionized water to thoroughly remove residual epilator. Repeat as needed (see Note 4).
10. Once dry, apply a generous amount of warmed ultrasound gel onto the hairless surface of the abdomen.

3.3. Locating Embryos

1. Adjust your transducer's orientation on the maternal abdomen laterally across the urethral opening in B-mode (2D imaging).
2. Scan cranially until the urinary bladder becomes visible (see Fig. 2a). Uterine horns containing embryos are located on either side of the bladder. Due to the imaging depths of 20–30 mm and frame width of 10 mm for the 40 MHz probe, a single 2D image can locate multiple fetuses in the uterine horns at the earlier stages (E8.5–12.5) of development.
3. The embryos can be identified by several distinguishing features (see Note 5). At earlier gestational age, the amniotic sac is readily identifiable as a hypoechoic (i.e., low echogenicity or echo reflection) mass containing the fetal mouse. During development, the embryos increase in size and a number of structures become visible, including the presence of vertebra and ribs by E13.5. Color Doppler can be used to identify the descending aorta, which lies on the left side of the spine. Closer to term (>E15.5), the eyes are also discernable from the rest of the structures as large hypoechoic masses located cranially to the heart. Fetal mice can be detected in the uterine horns as early as E8.5, when the linear heart tube begins to beat. However, this method has its limitation since it is more difficult to identify an aborted embryo whose cardiac contractions are not visible.

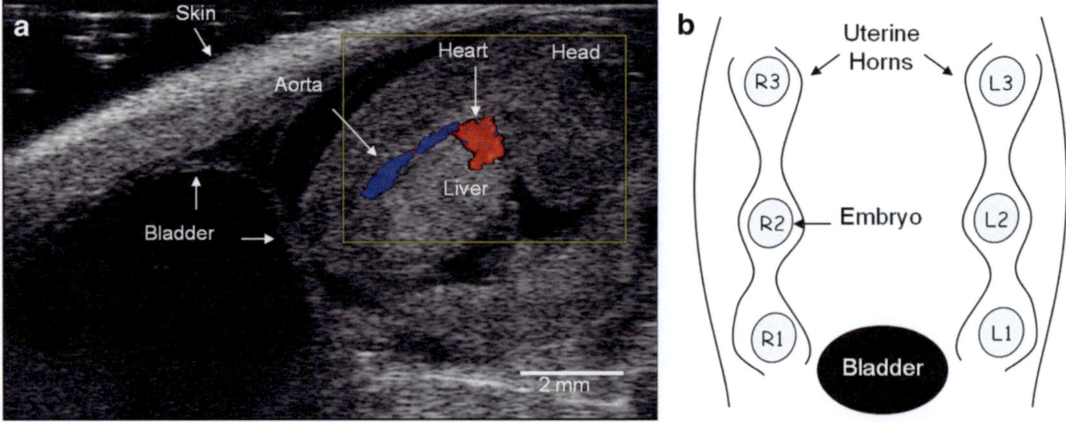

Fig. 2. Locating embryos using echocardiography. (**a**) Murine fetal organs, including the heart and liver, can be viewed by ultrahigh-resolution sonography. Because echocardiography has a limited depth of field, however, this procedure is most easily performed at earlier stages of development, preferably at E10.5 or earlier. (**b**) Location of embryos in the right *(R1, R2, R3)* and left *(L1, L2, L3)* uterine horns is noted.

4. For serial cardiac measurements, the position of the fetus in the uterus can be recorded as shown in Fig. 2b.

3.4. B-Mode Imaging of Fetal Hearts

It is preferable to start the echo protocol in B-mode image. B-mode images allow analysis of the physical parameters of the heart without overlying color images using color Doppler, which can obscure cardiac structures. In the adult mouse and human, the parasternal (along the sternum) long-axis (PSLAX), the parasternal short-axis (PSAX), and the 4-chamber apical axis are the three major cardiac views to assess cardiac dimensions and function. The PSLAX gives a view of the heart in the long axis, the PSAX gives the short-axis of the heart, whereas the apical 4-chamber view allows visualization of the atria, ventricles, and the left ventricular outflow tract (LVOT). However, in the fetus, echocardiographic scanning is performed in the sagittal, frontal, and transverse planes (see Fig. 3). The sagittal and frontal planes in the embryo correspond to the PSLAX and PSAX, respectively, in the adult heart. The transverse plane through the fetal thorax corresponds to the 4-chamber apical view in the adult. Below are some key aspects of scanning using these views in fetal heart echocardiography.

1. Sagittal plane (see Fig. 3a): The entire fetus is readily visible at earlier stages (E8.5–12.5). At later embryonic ages (>E14.5), one of the fetal eyes can be identified in the long-axis view. Unlike the short-axis view, the outline of the fetal head is usually visible along with the outline of one set of ribs. The sagittal view can be used to identify the atrioventricular (AV) valves and the LVOT as well as the vertical portions of the aorta. The two ventricles are readily visible and have synchronous contractions (see Notes 6 and 7).
2. Frontal plane (see Fig. 3b): In this longitudinal view, the head, two fetal arms, ribs, and liver are visible at the level of the

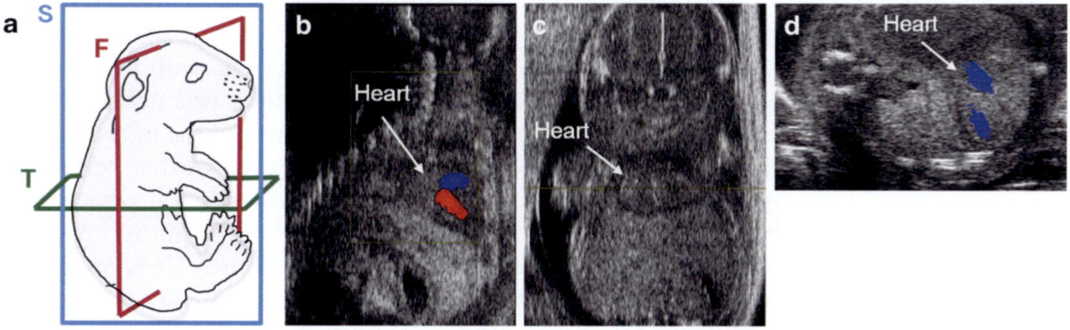

Fig. 3. Ultrasound imaging planes guided by the vertebral column and body axes of the fetal mouse. (**a**) Fetus and the three orthogonal imaging planes (sagittal, S; frontal, F; transverse, T) used for ultrasound scanning of the heart. (**b**–**d**) 2D Images obtained in utero show an embryonic day 16.5 (E16.5) fetus in the sagittal, frontal, and transverse planes. Color Doppler was used to locate the cardiac plane in the sagittal and transverse body axes.

heart. The fetal head is usually out of view at this level. The frontal plane provides a view of the right and left ventricles (see Fig. 3b), and the interventricular septum (IVS), which is optimal for determining ventricular dimensions in M-mode.

3. Transverse plane (see Fig. 3c): In this cross-sectional view, the heart and arms are in the same plane. As with the 4-chamber apical view in the adult heart, this provides a long-axis view of the left and right ventricles and atrioventricular valves. Thus, this plane can be used to obtain ejection fraction, tricuspid, and mitral inflow velocities, as well as right and left ventricular ejection via the right ventricular outflow tract (RVOT) and left ventricular outflow tract (LVOT), respectively. Color Doppler can be used to assist in locating the inflow and outflow tracts of the heart. Also, like the human fetal heart, RVOT and LVOT can be seen crossing each other at 90° (see Subheading 3.12).

3.5. Use of Color and Pulse Doppler to Identify the Left and Right Ventricles

The concept of color and pulsed-wave Doppler ultrasound is derived from the Doppler effect, which is based on the apparent variation in frequency of a sound wave as its source approaches or moves away, relative to an observer. When ultrasound waves with a given transmitted frequency insonate a blood vessel, the reflected frequency or frequency shift is directly proportional to the velocity of the red blood cells. The frequency shift is also proportional to the cosine of the angle that the ultrasound beam interrogates the vessel and the frequency of the insonating ultrasound. To maintain accuracy, the interrogation angle should be made as close to 0° as possible.

With regard to the fetal mouse heart, it is imperative to be able to discern between the left and right ventricles. This is especially important in genetically modified animals which may have defects in one of the ventricles. In 2D imaging, the left and right cardiac ventricles are relatively similar in size and structure throughout embryonic development. It is only after birth that the mass of the left ventricle becomes significantly greater than the right ventricle. In addition to repositioning the transducer and/or mother, using color Doppler and PW Doppler in combination with 2D imaging is very effective in determining left-to-right orientation of the heart. Increasing either the transmitted power of the instrument or the receiver gain will result in a larger jet, as weaker echoes on the periphery of the jet are detected. In general, color gain should be increased until random color pixels begin to appear in the tissue and then the gain reduced just slightly. It is preferable to first use 2D imaging and color Doppler to obtain a view of both ventricles in the long axis. Both mitral inflow and ejection from the left ventricle (LVOT) can be readily observed using pulse Doppler. This is in contrast to the right ventricle, in which the tricuspid inflow and outflow through the RVOT are not simultaneously visualized using pulse Doppler, unless the sample volume is too wide. Below are key aspects of distinguishing between LVOT and RVOT using color and PW Doppler.

1. Depending on orientation of the transducer, color jets through the mitral inflow and LVOT may be displayed in red or blue. Mitral flow can be readily identified by synchronizing a particular flow with the relaxation of the heart (diastole) that can be seen in the background to the color Doppler.
2. Location of the LVOT is readily discernable during systole. However, aliasing might occur if the pulse-rate frequency (PRF) is low. The PRF should be optimized to identify areas of maximum flow velocities.
3. The RVOT can be readily identified as a branching vessel underneath the aortic arch.
4. Pulmonary vein flow can be identified by manipulating the *X*–*Y* plane of the echo stage while reducing the PRF. Pulmonary vein flow can be estimated by identifying the aliasing vessel posterior to the left atria. Once identified, the PRF can be increased such that the aliasing is diminished and the presence of the A wave can be identified. The Vevo 2100 allows the use of color Doppler to locate blood flow and thus aid in performing PW Doppler. This is especially important in analyzing blood flow in the pulmonary vein.

3.6. Determination of Cardiac Dimensions and Systolic Function Using M-Mode

Similar to echocardiography of adult mouse hearts, M-mode images can be used to obtain ventricular dimensions, ventricular fractional shortening (FS), ejection fraction (EF), and ventricular mass in fetal mice (see Fig. 4). Although M-mode images can be obtained for fetal mice as early as E10.5, scanning both ventricles at this stage in either the long- or short-axis of the heart is technically challenging, due to the small heart size (~1 mm) and limited ability to orient and maintain the embryo stationary. The following are key aspects of scanning fetal hearts in M-mode (see Fig. 5):

1. In the adult mouse, scanning in both long- and short-axis is carried out at the level of the papillary muscles, which serve as landmarks. Because the papillary muscles are difficult to detect in early fetal hearts (E10.5–13.5), scanning can be performed close to the mitral annulus, which is highly echogenic. In later stages of development (≥16.5), M-mode images of the papillary muscle are more visible making it easier to obtain ventricular measurements.
2. Ensure that the sample volume is sufficiently wide to encompass the area of the heart to be scanned, as well as some surrounding static tissue.
3. The mother's position can be manipulated to help orient the fetal heart across the M-mode sample gate.

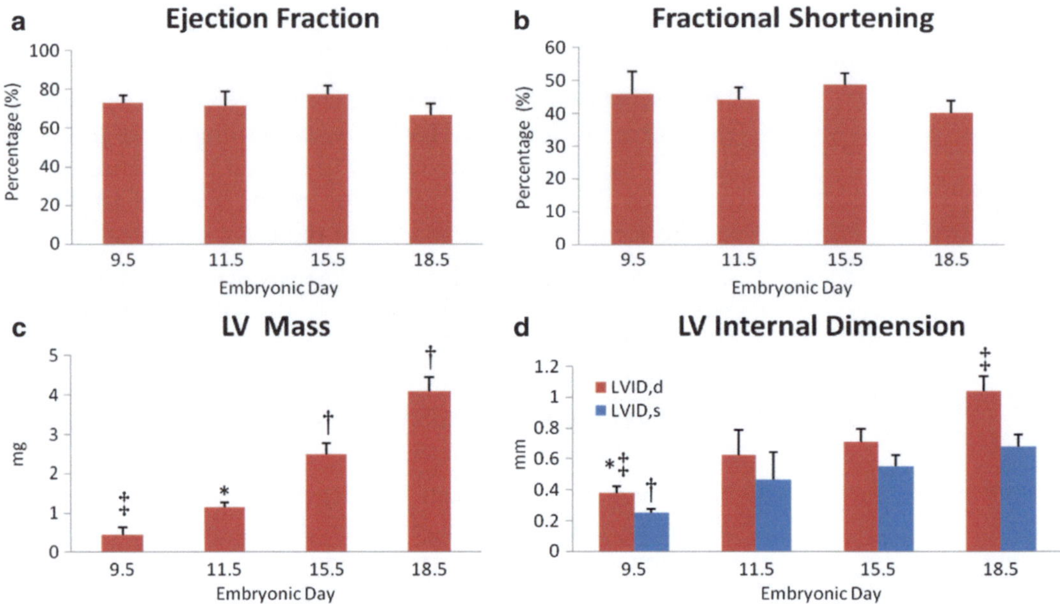

Fig. 4. Measurements of LV dimensions and function using M-mode. (**a**) Ejection fraction, (**b**) fractional shortening, and (**c**) LV mass (*$P<0.05$ vs. E15.5; **$P<0.01$ vs. E9.5; ***$P<0.001$ vs. E18.5) were calculated using the VisualSonics software package, based on LV volume measurements during five cardiac cycles. Both fractional shortening and ejection fraction are maintained relatively constant during fetal mouse development (E9.5–18.5), although LV mass significantly increases. (**d**) LV internal dimensions during diastole (LVID,d) and systole (LVID,s) also significantly increase with development (*$P<0.05$ vs. E18.5; **$P<0.01$ vs. E18.5; s vs. d, ***$P<0.05$). LVID is measured as the width of the LV from the base of the interventricular septal wall to the LV posterior wall (see Fig. 5). $N=6$–11 embryos per group.

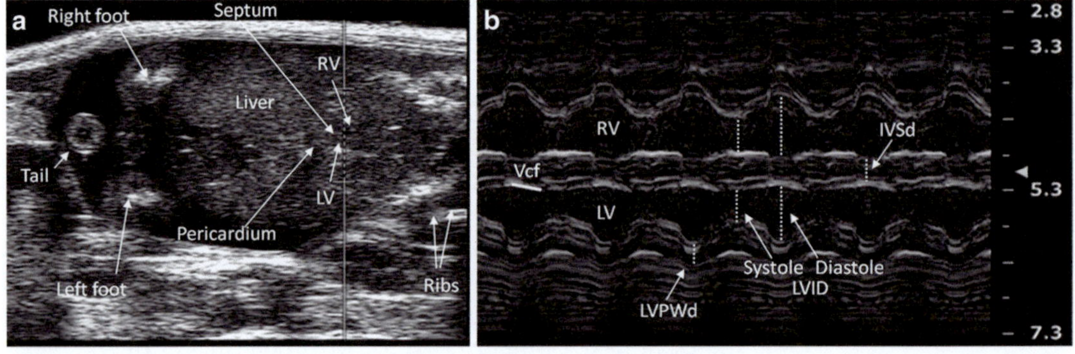

Fig. 5. Determination of dimensions and systolic function in the fetal mouse heart. (**a**) A 2D image in the frontal plane showing the sample volume gate across the heart used to obtain M-mode tracing in an E16.5 mouse embryo. (**b**) M-mode tracing with *lines* indicating end-systolic and end-diastolic diameters in the right and left ventricles. Note that the blood in the ventricular chambers is highly echogenic, due to the presence of nuclei in the red blood cells. *RV* right ventricle; *LV* left ventricle; *Vcf* velocity of circumferential fiber shortening; *IVSd* interventricular septal wall thickness during diastole; *LVPWd* left ventricular posterior wall thickness during diastole; *LVID* left ventricular internal dimension.

4. Unlike the adult mouse heart, in which ventricular chambers appear as "black," fetal heart chambers are highly reflective due to the presence of nuclei in the red blood cells.

3.7. Blood Flow Measurements Using Color and Pulse Doppler

Pulse Doppler is important for determining diastolic and systolic function of the myocardium. Peak systolic velocity and time-to-peak velocity are the most commonly used indices for quantification via PW Doppler. These indices reflect ventricular contractility, arterial pressure, and afterload. In the aorta and pulmonary artery, peak systolic velocity and time-to-peak velocity increase with advancing gestation in the mouse. Assessment of left ventricular diastolic function requires an integrated approach involving flow through the mitral valve (MV) and pulmonary vein (PV), as well as tissue Doppler of the mitral annulus. Pulse Doppler interrogation of the ventricular outflow tract provides stroke volume (SV) and cardiac output (SV × HR), which are important systolic parameters.

In the human and mouse, circulation is different in the fetus compared to adult in several respects. The fetal circulation through the heart (see Fig. 6) is in parallel, rather than in series, in which the foramen ovale and ductus arteriosus allow blood to flow from the right side of the heart to the left, bypassing the underdeveloped fetal lung, which has high resistance to blood flow. Thus, the majority of blood ejected from the right ventricle is directed through the ductus arteriosus into the thoracic aorta, with a small volume entering the lungs through the right and left pulmonary arteries. Because of this shunt, stroke volume in the right ventricle is greater than the left ventricle. Procedures for optimizing the sample area for interrogation with PW Doppler are as follows:

1. In color Doppler mode, focus on the region of interest.
2. Slowly reduce the PRF until a small portion of color flow jet appears to have flow reversal. For example, if the color jet is "red," blue pixels will start to appear in the regions with highest velocity and is referred to as "aliasing" (see Fig. 7a). Further reduction of the PRF will enlarge the color jet and thus decrease resolution of the area being interrogated.
3. Minimize the pulse sample volume and place the sample volume across the area of highest aliasing.
4. Increase the PRF until aliasing is resolved (see Fig. 7b).
5. The sample volume should be placed distal to targeted valves and the insonating angle should be less than 20° from the direction of blood flow.
6. Optimal flow measurements should be laminar, at maximal flow velocities, and interrogated using the proper sample volume.

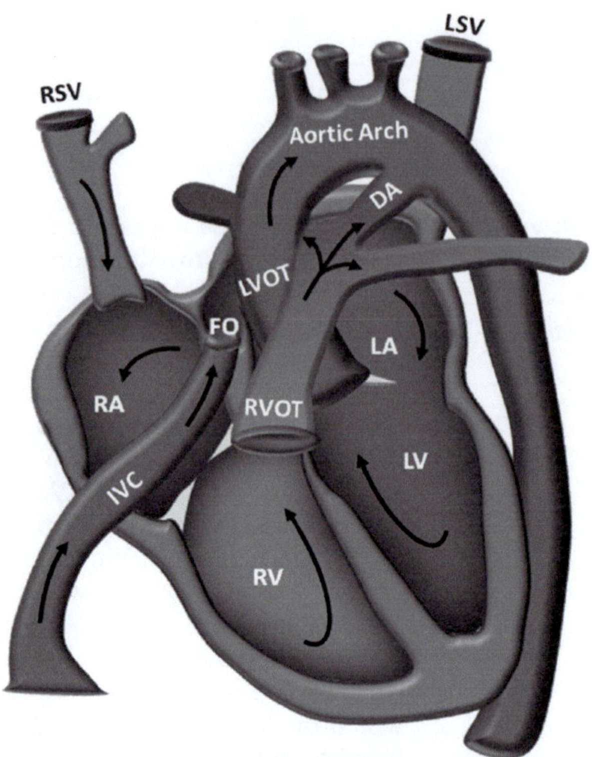

Fig. 6. Blood flow through the fetal mouse heart. Maternal blood from the inferior vena cava (IVC) enters the right atrium (RA), and guided by the valve of the IVC, passes through the foramen ovale (FO) into the left atrium (LA), where it mixes with a small quantity of blood returned from the lungs by the pulmonary veins. Blood in the LA passes into the left ventricle (LV) and then from the LV into the aorta and is subsequently distributed to the head, upper extremities, and other parts of the body via the descending aorta. From the head and upper extremities, the blood is returned by the right superior vena cava (RVC) to the RA, where it mixes with a small portion of the blood from the IVC. From the RA, it descends into the right ventricle (RV) and passes into the pulmonary artery through the right ventricular outflow tract (RVOT). Since the lungs of the fetus are relatively inactive, these organs receive only a small quantity of the blood from the pulmonary artery, which is returned by the pulmonary veins to the LA. The majority of blood from the RV passes through the ductus arteriosus (DA) into the aorta, where it mixes with a small quantity of the blood transmitted by the LV into the aorta.

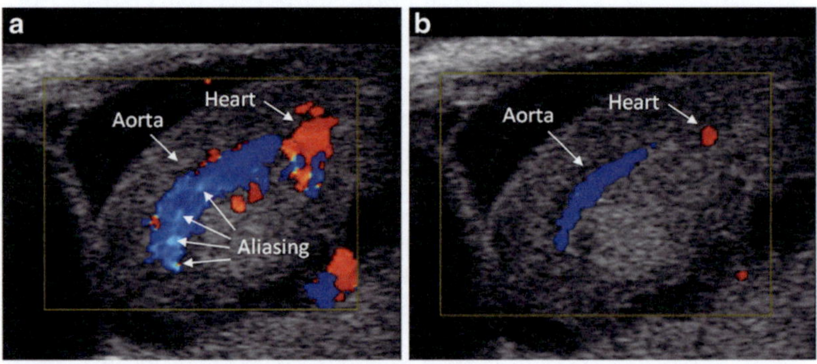

Fig. 7. Example of aliasing to locate the region of highest blood flow. (**a**) Sagittal view of an E16.5 fetus showing aliasing of flow through the abdominal aorta. The region of highest flow velocity results in pixels which suggest that flow is reversing (see *arrows*). (**b**) Nonaliasing is corrected by increasing the pulse-rate frequency (PRF) of the transducer.

3.8. Pulsed-Wave Doppler Assessment of Mitral and Tricuspid Inflow

PW Doppler assessment of mitral and tricuspid inflow can be obtained in the frontal plane of the embryo (see Fig. 8a). The Doppler waveforms across the atrioventricular valves are bicuspid in shape (see Fig. 8b). The first peak (E wave) corresponds to early ventricular filling of diastole, and the second peak (A wave) corresponds to atrial systole (i.e., "atrial kick"). Unlike in postnatal life, velocity of the A wave is higher than that of the E wave (see Figs. 8b and 9e), highlighting the importance of atrial systole in ventricular filling in the fetus. Other functional indicators derived from pulsed Doppler of transmitral flow include deceleration time of the E wave, mitral interval duration, and isovolumic relaxation time (IVRT), which are primary indicators of diastolic function (see Fig. 9).

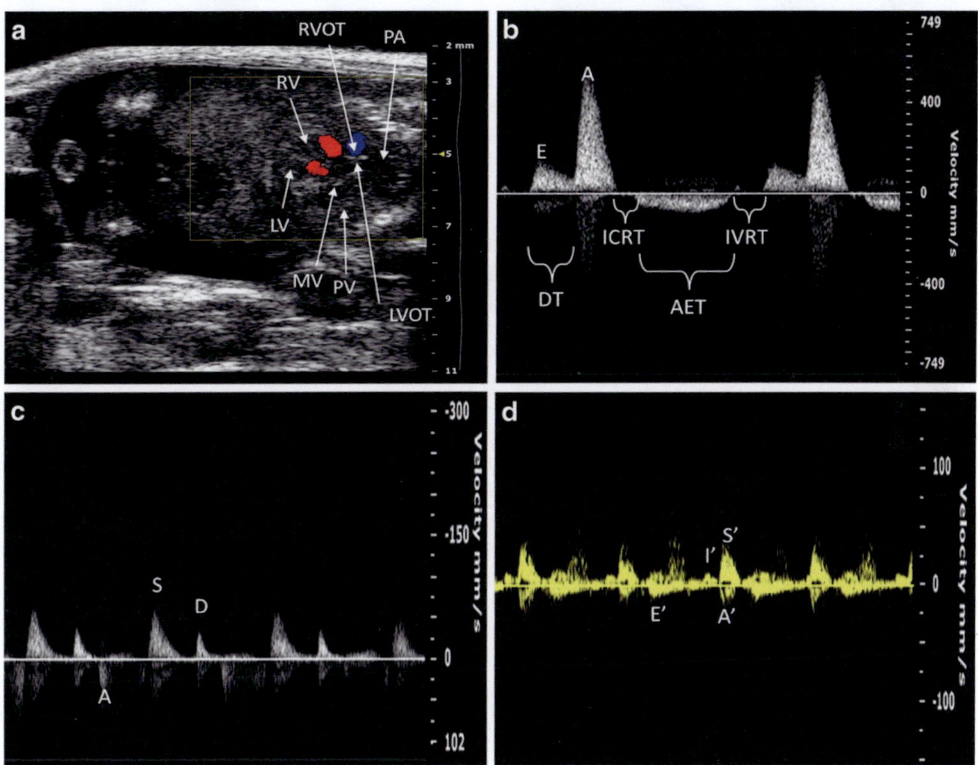

Fig. 8. Acquisition of diastolic and systolic function measurements in the fetal heart using pulsed-wave and tissue Doppler. (**a**) Representative 2D view of a fetal heart at E16.5. *Arrows* show locations of the right and left ventricular walls, and atrioventricular valves. (**b**) PW Doppler recording of mitral valve leaflet tips provides mitral inflow velocity patterns from which early diastolic velocity, late diastolic velocity with diastolic contraction (**a**), and the *E/A* ratio can be derived. The Isovolumic relaxation time (IVRT) is also a useful variable to characterize diastolic function and filling pressures. Aortic ejection time (AET) indicates left ventricular ejection time. (**c**) Tracings of the pulmonary vein, in which the systolic wave (S), diastolic wave (D), and atrial wave (A) are shown. (**d**) PW Doppler recording of tricuspid valve leaflet tips provides mitral inflow velocity patterns similar to that obtained from the mitral valve. However, ventricular ejection waves are not observed as with interrogation of the mitral inflow.

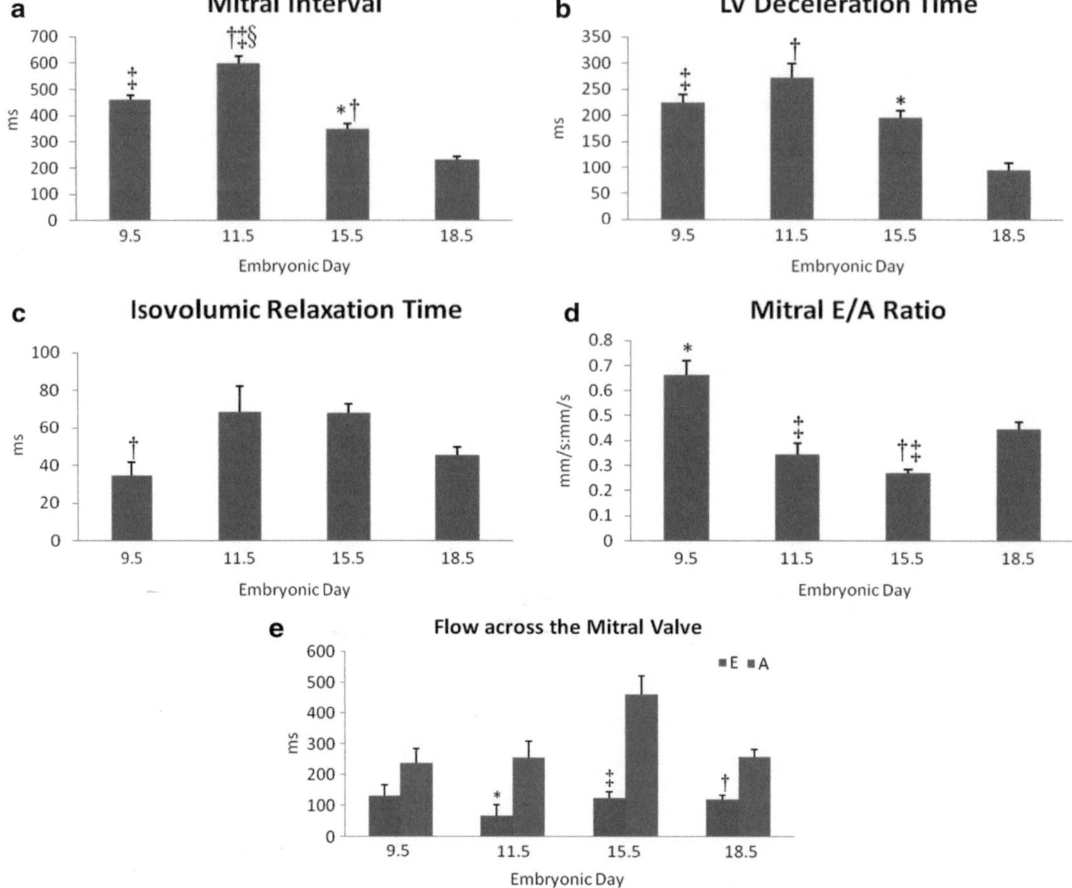

Fig. 9. Diastolic functional measurements in the fetal heart. Diastolic function becomes significantly more efficient during the later stages of fetal mouse development (E15.5–18.5), as reflected by changes in diastolic functional parameters including (**a**) mitral interval duration (*$P<0.05$ vs. E18.5; **$P<0.01$ vs. E9.5; ***$P<0.001$ vs. E18.5; ****$P<0.001$ vs. E15.5), (**b**) LV deceleration time (*$P<0.05$ vs. E18.5; **$P<0.01$ vs. E18.5; ***$P<0.001$ vs. E18.5), (**c**) IVRT (**$P<0.01$ vs. E15.5), (**d**) mitral *E/A* ratio (*$P<0.05$ vs. E18.5; **$P<0.01$ vs. E18.5; **$P<0.001$ vs. E9.5), and (**e**) Flow across the mitral valve during early and late diastolic filling measured as the E and A waves, respectively (s vs. d: *$P<0.05$; **$P<0.01$; ***$P<0.001$). $N=6$–11 embryos per group.

1. In color Doppler mode, the mitral and tricuspid inflows are readily visible as the ventricles fill during relaxation (see Fig. 8a). In the absence of color, the papillary muscle (later stages) and leaflets should be visible in B-mode.
2. Once the mitral flow and the mitral valve are identified, the pulse sample volume can be placed across the papillary muscles of the mitral valve.
3. The velocity, PRF, and baseline can be adjusted as needed.
4. On B-mode, the papillary muscle of the mitral valve can be readily identified.

5. On the same echo plane, obtain a color Doppler. Mitral inflow and the LVOT outflow jets can be identified at the same plane and temporally differentiated (see Fig. 8b).
6. The sample volume can be placed across the area where the mitral flow and the LVOT flow can be identified. Placement of the sample volume of pulse Doppler slightly downstream of the mitral leaflets allows a better estimation of the IVRT and IVCT. This view is unique in that it can identify systolic and diastolic function at the same time.

3.9. Pulse Doppler of the Pulmonary Vein

Towards the end of cardiac development, blood flow is increased through the pulmonary vein due to increased stroke volume from the right ventricle, decreased resistance to blood flow through the lung, and closing of the ductus arteriosus and foramen ovale. Although technically challenging, it is possible to assess pulmonary venous flow which is a useful adjunct in the characterization of mitral E and A waves and reflects the degree of lung development. The PV and Tissue Doppler imaging (TDI) measurements are most easily performed in transverse plane of the fetus. The mouse pulmonary vein enters the left atrium via a solitary opening, which is in contrast to the human heart which has four openings. The pulmonary vein consists of the S wave, D wave, and the A wave, which correspond to ventricular systole, passive filling of the left ventricle, and left atrial contraction, respectively. As shown in Fig. 8c, the S wave is normally larger than the D wave and the A wave is well pronounced in the fetal heart.

1. Pulmonary vein flow is more easily detectable in later gestational stages, when the lungs are more fully developed.
2. The left atria is superior-dorsal to the left ventricle. The blood flow in the left atria can be visualized on the color Doppler.
3. Postero-lateral to the left atria is the pulmonary vein. Lower the PRF until aliasing is noticed in the vessels attached to the atria.
4. Place the sample volume on the highest flow region of the pulmonary vein and use pulse Doppler to obtain the upright S wave and D wave and inverted A wave.

3.10. Tissue Doppler Imaging of the Mitral Annulus

TDI is a modification of conventional blood-flow Doppler to image tissue-derived, high-amplitude, and low-velocity Doppler signals (4). Tissue Doppler has proven useful as a quantitative index of regional ventricular systolic function, dP/dt (5). In diastolic dysfunction studies, TDI is relatively independent of preload (6), and therefore less likely to show the pseudonormalization pattern of transmitral flow. When focused on the mitral annulus, TDI consists of a systolic wave (S′), as well as an E′ and A′ wave which correspond to the E and A waves on mitral inflow (see Fig. 8d).

Other parameters such as isovolumic relaxation time (IVRT) and isovolumic contraction time (ICRT) can be obtained as well. Though not previously reported, the ability to measure these parameters with UBM provides another modality for assessing systolic and diastolic function in fetal mouse hearts.

3.11. Pulse Doppler of the Left Ventricular Outflow Tract

Stroke volume of the LV is calculated using the LVOT diameter and the amount of blood flowing through the LVOT needs to be measured. The volume of blood passing through the LVOT during ventricular ejection is given by the VTI (velocity time integral) of the flow, which is obtained from tracing the outline of the pulsed-Doppler wave. Stroke volume is calculated using the equation SV = CSA × VTI, where CSA is the cross-sectional area (area = π(LVOT diameter/2]^2) of the outflow tract. The cardiac output (CO) is calculated by multiplying the SV times HR. As shown in Fig. 10, systolic function progressively improves during fetal mouse development. Below are procedures for obtaining LVOT measurements in the fetal heart.

1. Using procedures described above in Subheading 3.5, use color Doppler to identify the LVOT (see Fig. 11a).

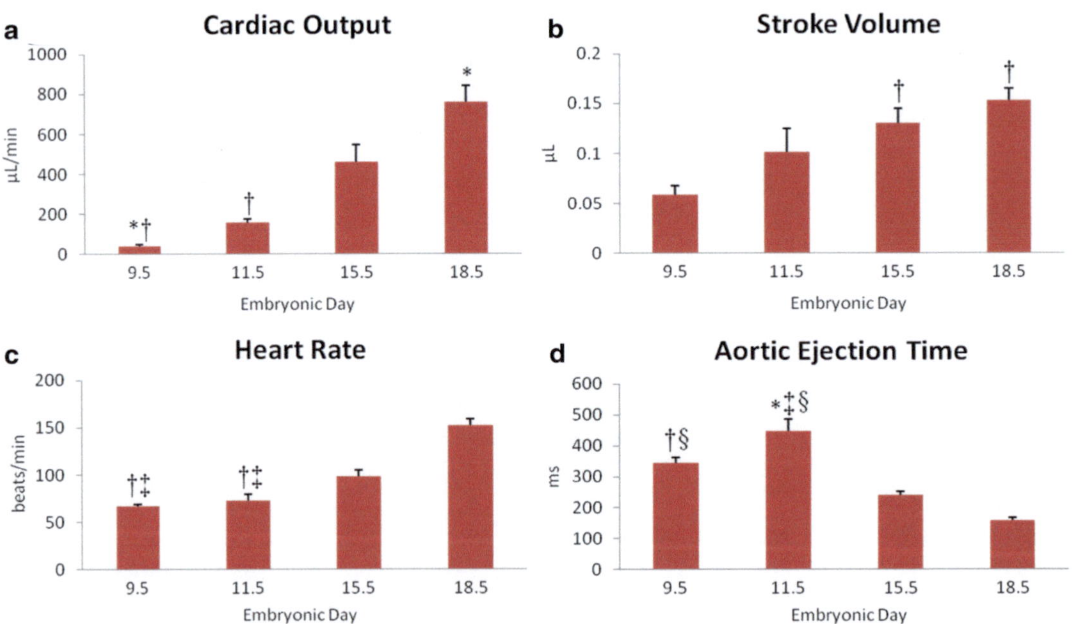

Fig. 10. Systolic functional measurements in the fetal heart. During fetal mouse development, (**a**) cardiac output (**P*<0.05 vs. E15.5; ***P*<0.001 vs. E18.5), (**b**) stroke volume (***P*<0.01 vs. E9.5), and (**c**) heart rate (***P*<0.01 vs. E15.5; ****P*<0.001 vs. E18.5) significantly improve. (**d**) The pattern of AET (**P*<0.05 vs. E9.5; ***P*<0.01 vs. E15.5; ****P*<0.001 vs. E15.5; *****P*<0.001 vs. E18.5), similar to the duration of the mitral interval, also becomes more efficient in the later stages of development. *N*=6–11 embryos per group.

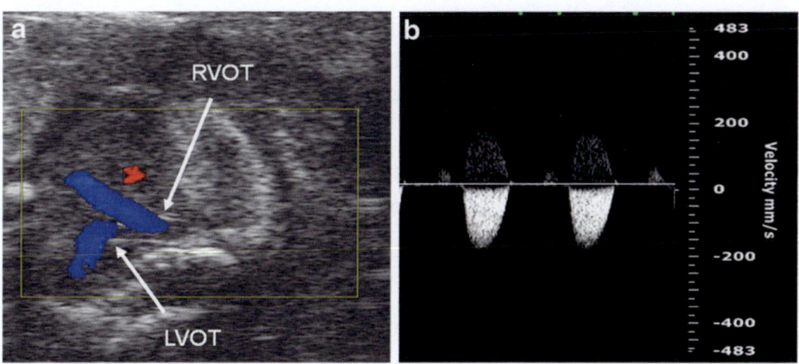

Fig. 11. Acquisition of blood flow velocity through the left ventricular outflow tract (LVOT) using Color Doppler. (**a**) Transverse section through the fetal (E16.5) thorax, in which color Doppler shows blood flow through the LVOT and RVOT. (**b**) Example of pulsed-Doppler flow through the LVOT.

2. Identify the highest flow velocity of the color jet at the base of the aortic valve by manipulating the PRF, as described in Subheading 3.7.
3. Place the pulsed-Doppler sample volume within the aorta, distal to the valve annulus at the brightest colors of the blood flow to obtain the aortic ejection jet (see Fig. 7b). Traces of the mitral inflow (E and A waves), as well as ICRT and IVRT, may be visible in pulsed-Doppler trace.
4. Trace the outline of the aortic ejection wave to obtain the VTI.
5. Heart rate can be obtained by measuring the distance between peaks of the aortic ejection trace.
6. Once the LVOT outflow tract has been identified using color Doppler, its diameter can be measured.
7. As described above, these measurements are sufficient to calculate both the SV and CO.

3.12. Pulse Doppler of the Right Ventricular Outflow Tract

The presence of right-to-left shunts at the level of the foramen ovale and ductus arteriosus has a significant impact on cardiac flow patterns. The shunting of flow from the right ventricle to the aorta ensures delivery of blood with high oxygen content to the coronary and cerebral circulation. As a result of shunting, the right ventricular flow exceeds the LV flow volume in the fetal heart. Below are procedures for obtaining RVOT measurements in the fetal heart.

1. Using procedures described above in Subheading 3.5, use color Doppler to identify the RVOT (see Fig. 11). In the transverse plane of the embryo, both the RVOT and LVOT can be located using color Doppler. The RVOT is the vessel present underneath the aortic arch and typically crosses the LVOT at ~90°.

2. Identify the highest flow velocity of the color jet at the base of the pulmonary valve by manipulating the PRF, as described in Subheading 3.7.
3. Place the pulse Doppler sample volume within the pulmonary artery, distal to the valve annulus at the brightest colors of the blood flow to obtain the pulmonary artery ejection trace.
4. Trace the outline of the pulmonary artery wave to obtain the VTI.
5. Heart rate can be obtained by measuring the distance between peaks of the aortic ejection trace.
6. Once the RVOT outflow tract has been identified using color Doppler, its diameter can be measured.
7. The above information can be used to calculate both the SV and CO.

4. Notes

1. The probe should only be inserted about 8–10 mm into the rectum to prevent the risk of rupturing the colon.
2. It is important to standardize the level of anesthesia, body temperature, and heart rate within a cohort of mice to facilitate the comparison between different groups or genotypes of mice, as even moderate changes in temperature and heart rate affect cardiac function in mice.
3. The vital functions of the mother must be closely observed in order to prevent hemodynamic failure and death.
4. Insure that all residual epilator is removed in order to prevent chemical burns of the skin.
5. Compared to magnetic resonance imaging, ultrasound is a very inefficient method for fetal counting. This is because the use of the high frequency probe (40 MHz) restricts exploration to a limited range (around 10 mm in area and depth), thus some conceptuses will not be detected as the probe is moved over the maternal abdomen.
6. Ultrahigh frequency probes have low penetrance (5–10 mm), which can result in suboptimal structural resolution and the appearance of artifacts, such as reflections in the fluid-filled compartments in the scans.
7. Obtaining measurements at different cardiac cycles will help ensure reproducibility of results.

Acknowledgments

This work was supported by the National Institutes of Health (5R01-HL068838-06) and Scott and White Hospital.

References

1. Petiet, A. E., Kaufman, M. H., Goddeeris, M. M., Brandenburg, J., Elmore, S. A., and Johnson, G. A. (2008) High-resolution magnetic resonance histology of the embryonic and neonate mouse: a 4D atlas and morphologic database. Proc Natl Acad USA, **34**, 12331–12336.
2. Phoon, C. K., Ji, R. P., Aristizabal, O., Worrad, D. M., Zhou, B., Baldwin, H. S. and Turnbull, D. H. (2004) Embryonic heart failure in NFATc1−/− mice: novel mechanistic insights from in utero ultrasound biomicroscopy. Circ Res, **95**, 92–99.
3. Srinivasan, S., Baldwin, H. S., Aristizabal, O., Kwee, L., Labow, M., Artman, M. and Turnbull, D. H. (1998) Noninvasive, in utero imaging of mouse embryonic heart development with 40-MHz echocardiography. Circulation, **98**, 912–918.
4. Hatle, L. and Sutherland, G. R. (2000) Regional myocardial function-a new approach. Eur Heart J, **21**, 1337–1357.
5. Wilkenshoff, U. M., Sovany, A., Wigstrom, L., Olstad, B., Lindstrom, L., Engvall, J., Janerot-Sjoberg, B., Wranne, B., Hatle, L. and Sutherland, G. R. (1998) Regional mean systolic myocardial velocity estimation by real-time color Doppler myocardial imaging: a new technique for quantifying regional systolic function. J Am Soc Echocardiogr, **11**, 683–692.
6. Sohn, D. W., Chai, I. H., Lee, D. J., Kim, H. C., Kim, H. S., Oh, B. H., Lee, M. M., Park, Y. B., Choi, Y. S., Seo, J. D. and Lee, Y. W. (1997) Assessment of mitral annulus velocity by Doppler tissue imaging in the evaluation of left ventricular diastolic function. J Am Coll Cardiol, **30**, 474–480.

Chapter 24

Isolation and Preparation of RNA from Rat Blood and Lymphatic Microvessels for Use in Microarray Analysis

Eric A. Bridenbaugh

Abstract

DNA microarray methodologies have proven to be an indispensable tool for genome-wide transcriptional profiling of organs, tissues, and cells. Here, we present a protocol for the optimized isolation and preparation of RNA from rat microvessels (including arteries, veins, and lymphatics) for subsequent use in two-color microarray analysis. The investigation of wide-ranging vessel sizes from all three vessel lineages necessitates an RNA isolation strategy that can effectively isolate high-quality RNA from varying and often very small quantities (<1 mg) of fibrous vessel tissue. Additionally, the lack of sample biomass necessitates the use of amplification strategies to generate enough RNA for use in microarray analysis. While the methods presented here were developed for use with two-color microarray analysis, the procedures and general concepts are applicable to most fluorescence-based microarray platforms.

Key words: Microarray, Gene expression, RNA isolation, Lymphatic, Artery, Vein

1. Introduction

From a transcriptional perspective, DNA microarray methodologies (1, 2) provide expression analysis of thousands of genes simultaneously, thus facilitating the identification of gene expression patterns that may provide clues to the cellular mechanisms underlying a tissue's biological activity. Microarray techniques have been successfully utilized to identify the unique transcriptional patterns of several basic mammalian tissues such as the central nervous system (3), olfactory mucosa (4), and lymphoid organs (5). In addition, these techniques have been used to identify the regional variability in gene expression present within an organ or organ system such as the individual transcriptional patterns of the four chambers of the heart (6) or the organs of the gastrointestinal system (7). These observations collectively demonstrate the power of microarray

Xu Peng and Marc Antonyak (eds.), *Cardiovascular Development: Methods and Protocols*, Methods in Molecular Biology, vol. 843, DOI 10.1007/978-1-61779-523-7_24,

technology for gene expression profiling and provide a model for the application of this technique to the transcriptional comparison of the mammalian vascular and lymphatic systems. Here, we present a protocol for the optimized isolation and preparation of RNA from rat microvessels (including arteries, veins, and lymphatics) for subsequent use in two-color microarray analysis. Because many investigators choose to utilize the services of a microarray core facility and/or company for microarray production and hybridization, the focus of this chapter will be the generation of high-quality, fluorescently labeled RNA samples ready for microarray hybridization.

The desire to investigate wide-ranging vessel sizes from all three vessel lineages requires an RNA isolation strategy that can effectively isolate high-quality RNA from varying and often very small quantities (<1 mg) of carefully dissected fibrous vessel tissue. To accomplish this, special attention is paid to choosing a disruption/homogenization method that is stringent enough to disrupt the fibrous architecture of these vessels while also preserving as much cellular lysate as possible. Additionally, the total lysate volume should be kept as small as possible to enhance RNA recovery. Finally, the isolation method must yield full-length (i.e., nondegraded) RNA free of impurities that would inhibit subsequent enzymatic reactions. For our experiments, we selected an electrical rotor-stator homogenizer with a 7-mm generator. When specifically used in combination with 2-mL microcentrifuge tubes and 0.5 mL lysate volumes, the rotor-stator homogenizer provided near complete tissue disruption/homogenization and excellent sample recovery. This resulted in consistently high RNA yields across all of the vessel sizes tested. The use of a rotor-stator homogenizer did limit our selection of RNA isolation methods, however, since aqueous detergent-based homogenization buffers produced excessive foaming with the small lysate volumes preferred for these small vessel samples (<1 mg of tissue). We thus selected a phenol-based RNA isolation procedure that is an improvement to the single-step RNA isolation method developed by Chomczynski and Sacchi (8) and provides excellent sample recovery due to minimal sample handling and limited lysate retention by the homogenizer (see Note 1). The RNA isolation technique presented here was developed and optimized for rat vessels; however, it should be equally applicable to any small (<~2 mm diameter) mammalian blood or lymphatic vessel that can be surgically isolated via microdissection.

The lack of sample biomass necessitates the use of amplification strategies to generate enough RNA for use in microarray analysis. While there are several commercially available microarray platforms (Affymetrix GeneChip, Agilent DNA microarrays, Codelink Bioarrays, Operon OpArrays, etc.), most can successfully be used in conjunction with a linear RNA amplification protocol based on the technique originally developed by the Eberwine laboratory (9).

Briefly, mRNA is reverse transcribed to form cDNA containing a T7 promoter. After conversion of cDNA to double-stranded DNA, T7 RNA Polymerase is used to generate numerous antisense copies of each mRNA. This method of RNA amplification is preferred over other methods (e.g., polymerase chain reaction) because RNA polymerase activity is generally insensitive to template sequence and concentration, and thus, linear amplification does not significantly distort the relative abundance of individual mRNA species within an RNA population (9–11). Linear amplification can be applied sequentially in a nested format, thereby greatly reducing the amount of starting RNA required to perform a successful microarray experiment. To facilitate dye-labeling of the amplified RNA (aRNA), 5-(3-aminoallyl)-UTP (aaUTP) is utilized during the final amplification step. aaUTP contains a reactive primary aminogroup that can be chemically coupled to *N*-hydroxysuccinimidyl ester-derivatized reactive dyes (NHS ester dyes). The use of aaUTP during amplification only minimally affects reaction efficiency, and since aaUTP incorporation is theoretically identical in all samples, there is no sample bias introduced by differential dye-labeling in two-color microarray applications (12). While the following RNA labeling and microarray hybridization protocols were specifically optimized for two-color microarray analysis, the procedures and general concepts are applicable to most fluorescence-based microarray platforms.

2. Materials

2.1. RNA Isolation

1. Dulbecco's Phosphate-Buffered Saline (DPBS) (Invitrogen, equivalent formulation from another company is okay).
2. Dissection dish: petri dish or similar dish large enough to store the tissue containing the vessels of interest (see Note 2).
3. RNA*later* (Ambion).
4. 0.5-mL Microcentrifuge tubes: RNase-free polypropylene.
5. 1.5-mL Microcentrifuge tubes: RNase-free polypropylene.
6. 2.0-mL Microcentrifuge tubes: RNase-free polypropylene with flat- or conical-bottoms (the bottom of the tube should be shaped to allow the 7-mm rotor-stator generator to reach as close as possible to the bottom of the tube).
7. RNase-free aerosol-resistant (i.e., barrier filter) pipette tips.
8. TRIzol Reagent (Invitrogen), toxic—wear appropriate PPE particularly during homogenization: store at 4°C (see Note 3).
9. Electric rotor-stator homogenizer with 7-mm stainless steel generator (a variable-speed homogenizer with a maximum speed of ~30,000 rpm is preferred—e.g., Fisher PowerGen 125).

10. 5-mL Tubes: round-bottomed polypropylene.
11. RNase-free water (commercially available product is generally preferred).
12. 2.0 mL Phase Lock Gel—Heavy (5 Prime, Hamburg, Germany): store at room temperature (RT).
13. Chloroform: RNase-free, ACS grade or better.
14. Isopropanol: RNase-free, ACS grade or better.
15. 50% Isopropanol: prepare as 1:1 mixture of RNase-free isopropanol (item 14) and RNase-free water (item 11).
16. Linear acrylamide (Ambion): store at –20°C.
17. 100% Ethanol: RNase-free, ACS grade or better.
18. 75% Ethanol: prepare as 3:1 mixture of RNase-free 100% ethanol (item 17) and RNase-free water (item 11).
19. DNA-*free* (Ambion): store at –20°C (do NOT use a "frost-free" freezer).
20. 2100 Bioanalyzer and RNA6000 *Pico* LabChip Kit (Agilent Technologies) or Experion Automated Electrophoresis System and Experion RNA *HighSens* Analysis Kit (Bio-Rad Laboratories).

2.2. RNA Amplification and Labeling

1. Amino Allyl MessageAmp II with Cy3/Cy5 (Ambion): all kit components supplied in microcentrifuge tubes (i.e., ≤2.0 mL; except Nuclease-free Water) should be stored at ≤–20°C (do NOT use a "frost-free" freezer); enzyme solutions should be subjected to as few freeze–thaw cycles as possible; Nuclease-free Water, all reagents supplied in containers >2 mL, and all tubes, filters, etc. should be stored at RT (see Notes 4–6).
2. Thermal cycler with temperature-adjustable heated lid (compatibility with 0.5-mL tubes is preferred).
3. PCR tubes: 0.5-mL thin-walled RNase- and DNase-free microcentrifuge tubes ("non-stick" tubes are preferred) compatible with the above thermal cycler (0.2-mL tubes may be used if a compatible thermal cycler is not available; however, this may require the transfer of the contents to a 0.5-mL microcentrifuge tube prior to the cDNA Binding Buffer addition step).
4. 37°C Air incubator (e.g., temperature-calibrated cell/tissue culture incubator or hybridization oven).
5. Vacuum centrifuge concentrator (e.g., Savant DNA 120 SpeedVac Concentrator, Thermo Fisher Scientific, Waltham, MA).
6. 2100 Bioanalyzer and RNA6000 *Nano* LabChip Kit (Agilent Technologies) or Experion Automated Electrophoresis System and Experion RNA *StdSens* Analysis Kit (Bio-Rad Laboratories).
7. RNA Fragmentation Reagents (Ambion): store at RT.
8. Stop Solution (Ambion).

3. Methods

3.1. RNA Isolation

1. Rapidly dissect the tissue containing the vessels of interest from an anesthetized animal (see Note 7) and quickly rinse the tissue in DPBS. If the presence of RNA from blood or lymph-borne cells is not desired, then the lumens of the vessels of interest should be purged or flushed of their luminal contents during this rinsing step as it will be much more difficult to clean the lumen after the following step.
2. Immediately transfer the tissue/s to a dissection dish filled with RT RNA*later*. The volume of RNA*later* should be greater than tenfold the mass of tissue (e.g., >10 μL/1 mg of tissue) and sufficient to completely cover the tissue in the dissection dish (e.g., 1–2 mL for a 35-mm petri dish). The tissue must be less than 5 mm in at least one dimension (see Note 8).
3. Equilibrate the tissue in RNA*later* for at least 30 min at RT (see Note 9).
4. Using stereomicroscopy and microsurgical instruments, isolate the vessels of interest from the RNA*later*-equilibrated tissue. Care should be taken to keep the tissue submerged in RNA*later* at all times during the dissection process (see Note 10). Unless otherwise desired, the vessels should be cleaned of ALL extravascular tissue to ensure that the data generated during subsequent steps are specific to the cells of the vascular wall. For large vessel segments, the vessel should be cut axially and/or laterally into smaller pieces to permit the vessel to fit into the side windows of the 7-mm generator used in step 6 (see Note 11).
5. After dissection, the cleaned vessels should each be transferred to a 0.5-mL microcentrifuge tube containing 200–400 μL of fresh RNA*later* (the volume must be sufficient to thoroughly cover the vessel sample throughout storage) and stored at 4°C until the next step (see Note 12).
6. Transfer each vessel from RNA*later* to a 2.0-mL microcentrifuge tube containing 500 μL chilled TRIzol Reagent and *immediately* homogenize the tissue at 30,000 rpm for 20–30 s using a rotor-stator homogenizer with a 7-mm stainless steel generator (see Notes 13–17). Immediately place and leave the sample on ice until next step (see Notes 18 and 19).
7. To increase the aqueous volume of the lysate prior to phase separation, add 100 μL RNase-free water to each sample, vortex thoroughly, and incubate 10 min at RT.
8. Transfer each sample to 2.0 mL Phase Lock Gel—Heavy (spin gel 1 min at 12,000 × *g* prior to use), add 100 μL Chloroform, and mix 1 min by repeated inversion (do NOT vortex).

9. Incubate samples 5 min at RT and then spin 5 min at 12,000 × *g* at 4°C (see Notes 20 and 21).
10. For each sample, carefully transfer the upper aqueous phase to a new 1.5-mL microcentrifuge tube (see Note 22), add 400 μL isopropanol and 3 μL linear acrylamide (15 μg), vortex, and incubate overnight at –20°C (see Note 23).
11. Spin samples 15 min at 12,000 × *g* at 4°C and remove supernatants by aspiration (see Notes 24 and 25).
12. To each RNA pellet, add 500 μL of cold (–20°C) 75% EtOH, vortex gently for 10 s (see Note 26), and spin tube 5 min at 7,500 × *g* at 4°C (see Note 27).
13. Remove supernatants by aspiration and air dry pellets (lay open tubes on their sides) for 10 min at RT.
14. To each RNA pellet, add 15 μL 75°C RNase-free water and gently vortex several times to resuspend pellet.
15. To each sample, add 1.5 μL 10× DNase I Buffer and 1 μL DNase I (from DNA-*free* kit), mix by gently flicking, and incubate 20 min at 37°C.
16. To each sample, add 2 μL DNase Inactivation Reagent (from DNA-*free* kit; vortex reagent immediately before pipetting to resuspend slurry) and incubate 2 min at RT (flick all tubes frequently during incubation to keep reagent suspended in solution).
17. Spin samples 1.5 min at 10,000 × *g* to pellet DNase Inactivation Reagent.
18. Transfer each sample to a new 0.5-mL microcentrifuge tube. Do not transfer inactivation reagent to subsequent reactions (see Note 28). Place the sample on ice and proceed immediately to the next step or store the sample at –80°C (see Notes 29 and 30).
19. Analyze the total RNA integrity and quantity for each sample using a 2100 Bioanalyzer and RNA6000 *Pico* LabChip Kit OR Experion Automated Electrophoresis System and Experion RNA *HighSens* Analysis Kit according to the manufacturers' instructions (see Notes 31–33). Assess the integrity of the RNA by examining the RNA integrity number (RIN) calculated by the system software (see Note 34).

3.2. RNA Amplification and Labeling (See Notes 35–41)

1. For each sample, place up to 1 μg of total RNA into a PCR tube and adjust total volume to exactly 10 μL using Nuclease-free Water and/or concentration via vacuum centrifugation (see Note 42). Generally, the same approximate mass of total RNA is utilized for all samples to be amplified within a given experiment to ensure consistent amplification.
2. Prepare Reverse Transcription Master Mix in a 0.5-mL microcentrifuge tube at RT: for each sample, add (in the indicated

order) 1.05 μL Nuclease-free Water, 1.05 μL T7 Oligo(dT) Primer, 2.1 μL 10× First Strand Buffer, 4.2 μL dNTP Mix, 1.05 μL RNase Inhibitor, and 1.05 μL ArrayScript.

3. Add 10 μL of Reverse Transcription Master Mix to each sample, gently mix, briefly centrifuge, incubate 2 h at 42°C (50°C lid temperature) in a thermal cycler (see Note 43), and then proceed immediately to step 5. Step 4 below should be completed during the final several minutes of the 2-h incubation.
4. Prepare Second Strand Master Mix in a 1.5-mL microcentrifuge tube on ice: for each sample, add (in the indicated order) 66.15 μL Nuclease-free Water, 10.5 μL 10× Second Strand Buffer, 4.2 μL dNTP Mix, 2.1 μL DNA Polymerase, and 1.05 μL RNase H.
5. Briefly centrifuge samples (~5 s) and then place them on ice. Immediately add to each sample 80 μL of Second Strand Master Mix, gently mix, briefly centrifuge, incubate 2 h at 16°C (heated lid off) in a thermal cycler, and proceed immediately to step 6. Preheat Nuclease-free Water to 55°C during the 2-h incubation.
6. To each sample, add 250 μL of cDNA Binding Buffer and thoroughly mix by repeated pipetting and gently flicking the tube. Briefly centrifuge the sample and immediately transfer the sample to the center of a cDNA Filter Cartridge firmly seated in its wash tube (see Note 44). Centrifuge the cDNA Filter Cartridges 1 min at 10,000 × *g* and discard flow-through.
7. Add 500 μL of Wash Buffer to the center of each cDNA Filter Cartridge, centrifuge 1 min at 10,000 × *g*, discard flow-through, and centrifuge 1 additional minute to remove trace amounts of Wash Buffer from the cDNA Filter Cartridges.
8. Transfer the cDNA Filter Cartridges to the cDNA Elution Tubes, add 18 μL of 55°C Nuclease-free Water to the center of each cDNA Filter Cartridge, incubate 2 min at RT, and then centrifuge 1 min at 10,000 × *g*. Place samples on ice. This step should yield ~16 μL of double-stranded cDNA.
9. Prepare In Vitro Transcription Master Mix in a 0.5-mL microcentrifuge tube at RT: for each sample, add (in the indicated order) 12.6 μL ATP, CTP, GTP Mix, 6.3 μL UTP Solution (50 mM), 4.2 μL T7 10× Reaction Buffer, and 4.2 μL T7 Enzyme Mix (see Note 45).
10. Add 26 μL of In Vitro Transcription Master Mix to each sample, gently mix, briefly centrifuge, incubate 14 h at 37°C in a calibrated temperature air incubator (cell culture incubator is ideal). Stop the in vitro transcription reaction by adding 58 μL of Nuclease-free Water to each sample and gently mixing (total sample volume should now be exactly 100 μL). Preheat additional Nuclease-free Water to 55°C for the following steps.

11. For each sample, add 350 μL of aRNA Binding Buffer, immediately add 250 μL of 100% ethanol, mix by pipetting up and down exactly three times (do NOT vortex and do NOT centrifuge), and immediately transfer the mixture to the center of an aRNA Filter Cartridge placed firmly into an aRNA Collection Tube. Repeat for remaining samples and centrifuge 1 min at 10,000 × *g*. Discard flow-through and replace aRNA Filter Cartridges into the aRNA Collection Tubes.
12. Add 650 μL of Wash Buffer to the center of each aRNA Filter Cartridge, centrifuge 1 min at 10,000 × *g*, discard flow-through, and centrifuge 1 additional minute to remove trace amounts of Wash Buffer from the aRNA Filter Cartridges.
13. Transfer each aRNA Filter Cartridge to a new aRNA Collection Tube and add 200 μL of 55°C Nuclease-free Water to the center of each aRNA Filter Cartridge. Incubate samples 10 min at 55°C in a heat block and then centrifuge 1.5 min at 10,000 × *g*. This step should yield ~200 μL of unlabeled aRNA. Place the aRNA on ice and proceed to the next step (see Notes 46 and 47).
14. Analyze the aRNA distribution profile and quantity for each sample with a 2100 Bioanalyzer and RNA6000 *Nano* LabChip Kit OR Experion Automated Electrophoresis System and Experion RNA *StdSens* Analysis Kit following the manufacturers' instructions for mRNA analysis. The expected aRNA profile is a distribution of sizes ranging from ~250 to 5,500 nt with a peak centered around ~1,000–1,500 nt. A greater proportion of longer (i.e., more nucleotides) products is indicative of greater fidelity during the amplification process. Size distributions heavily skewed towards 0 nt with a peak less than 500 nt are generally indicative of a failed or poor amplification reaction. In this case, the sample should be discarded and not used for subsequent steps. Use the estimated aRNA concentration measured during this analysis for the following steps (see Notes 48–50).
15. For each sample, place up to 2 μg of first round aRNA (see Notes 51 and 52) into a PCR tube and adjust the total volume to exactly 10 μL using Nuclease-free Water and/or concentration via vacuum centrifugation (see Note 53). Use the same quantity of first round aRNA for all samples to be analyzed within a given experiment.
16. Add 2 μL of Second Round Primers, gently vortex, briefly centrifuge, and incubate 10 min at 70°C in a thermal cycler (set lid to default temperature or 100–105°C). Briefly centrifuge (~5 s) and cool the samples on ice before proceeding to step 18. Step 17 below should be started during the 10-min incubation above.
17. Prepare Second Round Reverse Transcription Master Mix in a 0.5-mL microcentrifuge tube at RT: for each sample, add (in the indicated order) 2.1 μL 10× First Strand Buffer, 4.2 μL dNTP Mix, 1.05 μL RNase Inhibitor, and 1.05 μL ArrayScript.

18. Add 8 μL of Second Round Reverse Transcription Master Mix to each sample, gently mix, briefly centrifuge, incubate 2 h at 42°C (50°C lid temperature) in a thermal cycler (see Note 42). Centrifuge briefly after incubation and proceed immediately to the next step.
19. Add 1 μL of RNase H to each sample, gently mix, centrifuge briefly, and incubate 30 min at 37°C in a calibrated temperature air incubator (cell culture incubator is ideal). Proceed immediately to step 20.
20. To each sample, add 5 μL of T7 Oligo(dT) Primer, gently vortex, briefly centrifuge, and incubate 10 min at 70°C in a thermal cycler (set lid to default temperature or 100–105°C). Briefly centrifuge (~5 s) and cool the samples on ice before proceeding to step 22. Step 21 below should be started during the 10-min incubation above.
21. Prepare Second Round Second Strand Master Mix in a 1.5-mL microcentrifuge tube on ice: for each sample, add (in the indicated order) 60.9 μL Nuclease-free Water, 10.5 μL 10× Second Strand Buffer, 4.2 μL dNTP Mix, and 2.1 μL DNA Polymerase.
22. To each sample, add 74 μL of Second Round Second Strand Master Mix, gently mix, briefly centrifuge, immediately incubate 2 h at 16°C (heated lid off) in a thermal cycler. Immediately following this incubation, repeat steps 6–8 above. Preheat Nuclease-free Water to 55°C during the 2-h incubation.
23. Prepare Second Round In Vitro Transcription Master Mix in a 0.5-mL microcentrifuge tube at RT: for each sample, add (in the indicated order) 12.6 μL ATP, CTP, GTP Mix, 3.15 μL UTP Solution (50 mM), 3.15 μL aaUTP (50 mM), 4.2 μL T7 10× Reaction Buffer, and 4.2 μL T7 Enzyme Mix.
24. Repeat steps 10–14 above (see Notes 54 and 55). Place the purified amino allyl aRNA on ice and proceed immediately to the dye coupling reactions in the following steps. Alternatively, the purified amino allyl aRNA can be stored at −80°C for several months.
25. Resuspend one tube of Cy3 dye and/or Cy5 dye for each sample to be labeled (as appropriate for the specific experimental design) by adding 11 μL of DMSO to each tube, thoroughly vortexing, and briefly centrifuging (see Note 56). Once resuspended, the Cy dyes must be used within 1 h. Only prepare those tubes of Cy dye that you can use within 1 h. Store the resuspended tubes of dye in the dark at RT until use (see Note 57).
26. For each sample to be labeled, add 5–20 μg of purified amino allyl aRNA (from step 24) to a PCR tube and dry using vacuum centrifugation with medium or low heat. Check the progress of drying frequently and remove the sample(s) from the vacuum centrifuge as soon as they are dry (do NOT overdry).

The quantity of purified aRNA used at this step is critical since it will determine the concentration of the labeled aRNA following the dye coupling reaction, which will subsequently be used for the microarray hybridization. Use the exact same quantity of aRNA for all experimental samples (see Notes 58 and 59).

27. To label the amino allyl aRNA samples, resuspend the dried aRNA samples in 9 μL of Coupling Buffer, vortex thoroughly, add 11 μL of dye (from step 25) to each sample, vortex thoroughly, and incubate 30 min at RT in the dark (see Note 60).
28. To quench the coupling reactions, add 4.5 μL of 4 M Hydroxylamine to each sample, vortex thoroughly, and incubate 15 min at RT in the dark. Add 5.5 μL of Nuclease-free Water to each sample to bring the total volume to 30 μL and proceed to the next step. Preheat Nuclease-free Water to 55°C during the above incubation.
29. For each sample, add 105 μL of aRNA Binding Buffer, immediately add 75 μL of 100% ethanol, mix by pipetting up and down exactly three times (do NOT vortex and do NOT centrifuge), and immediately transfer the mixture to the center of an aRNA Filter Cartridge placed firmly into an aRNA Collection Tube. Repeat for remaining samples and centrifuge 1 min at 10,000 × *g*. Discard flow-through and replace the aRNA Filter Cartridges into the aRNA Collection Tubes.
30. Add 500 μL of Wash Buffer to the center of each aRNA Filter Cartridge, centrifuge 1 min at 10,000 × *g*, discard flow-through, and centrifuge 1 additional minute to remove trace amounts of Wash Buffer from the aRNA Filter Cartridges. Transfer each aRNA Filter Cartridge to a new aRNA Collection Tube.
31. For each sample, add 10 μL of 55°C Nuclease-free Water to the center of the aRNA Filter Cartridge, incubate 2 min at RT in dark, and then centrifuge 1.5 min at 10,000 × *g*. Repeat one additional time. This step will yield ~20 μL of labeled aRNA. Place the aRNA on ice in the dark and proceed to the next step or store the sample at –80°C protected from light for up to several days (prolonged storage of labeled aRNA is not recommended).
32. For each pair of samples to be hybridized to the same array, add equal quantities of each sample (see Note 61) to a 0.5-mL PCR tube (generally 1–5 μg of labeled aRNA is used per sample per array) (see Note 62). Use vacuum centrifugation and/or the addition of Nuclease-free Water to adjust the volume of the mixture to exactly 9 μL (see Note 63).
33. Add 1 μL of 10× Fragmentation Buffer to each aRNA sample mixture, vortex briefly, centrifuge briefly, and incubate 15 min at 70°C in a thermal cycler (set lid to default temperature or 100–105°C). Add 1 μL of Stop Solution to each aRNA sample

mixture, vortex briefly, centrifuge briefly, and place on ice (see Notes 64 and 65).

34. Proceed immediately to microarray hybridization. If the samples must be transported to another facility for microarray hybridization, freeze the samples at –80°C and transport the samples to the facility on dry ice.

3.3. Microarray Hybridization

General Considerations: Consistency of data between microarray platforms (Affymetrix GeneChip, Agilent DNA microarrays, Codelink Bioarrays, Operon OpArrays, etc.) has been demonstrated (13), and thus, the investigator may select any microarray platform based on the availability of platform-specific equipment and/or the needs of the experiment. Every microarray manufacturer and/or microarray facility has optimized, platform-specific microarray hybridization procedures that are beyond the scope of this chapter. Consult with your microarray manufacturer/facility to determine the optimum format and quantity of labeled aRNA (sometimes also referred to as "cRNA") to be used with each array as well as the appropriate buffer in which to suspend your samples prior to hybridization. Additional considerations include the pre- and post-hybridization wash strategies for the arrays as well as the hybridization time and temperature. As with the steps above, consistency between samples is paramount, and thus, arrays should be processed in small batches to ensure uniform handling through the prehybridization, hybridization, posthybridization, and scanning/imaging steps.

4. Notes

1. A bead mill homogenizer may produce similar disruption/homogenization results with much higher throughput and allow for the use of aqueous or organic homogenization buffers; however, optimization of homogenization conditions and subsequent RNA isolation will be required.
2. The dissection dish should be sized large enough to allow adequate access to the tissue to dissect the vessels of interest while also being as small as possible to minimize the volume of RNA*later* required. In some circumstances, it may be advantageous to coat the bottom of the dissection dish with silicone elastomer (Dow Corning Sylgard 184 or similar) to facilitate pinning of the tissue or to provide a softer surface against which the tissue can be dissected. Under most circumstances, a 35-mm petri dish is very convenient for microvessel dissection.
3. This RNA isolation protocol is specifically optimized for this reagent. Use of similar commercially available monophasic solutions of phenol and guanidine isothiocyanate will likely result

in undesirable results during the phase separation step of the following RNA isolation protocol.

4. At the time of this publication, the instruction manuals for the Ambion MessageAmp kits provide very thorough detailed protocols as well as extensive descriptions of various concerns, considerations, and tips pertinent to the successful completion of an RNA amplification and labeling experiment. These manuals are freely available online and should be considered a valuable resource for any linear RNA amplification and labeling experiment.

5. The use of amino allyl-modified UTP for the subsequent fluorescent labeling of aRNA is compatible with many fluorescence-based microarray platforms and numerous commercially available fluorescent dyes, and it is the preferred labeling method for two-color microarray analysis. The manufacturers of some one-color microarray platforms, however, recommend the use of biotinylated-UTP and subsequent labeling using streptavidin-conjugated fluorescent dyes. Consult with your microarray manufacturer/facility regarding the compatibility of fluorescently labeled aRNA produced via the amino allyl method with your selected microarray platform. If the use of the biotin-streptavidin labeling system is strictly recommended, alternative MessageAmp kits that use biotinylated-UTP are available from Ambion. In most cases, these alternate amplification kits utilize a protocol very similar to the one described below with the exception of the dye-labeling procedure.

6. This kit is supplied with Cy3 and Cy5 dyes for use with two-color microarray analysis using a compatible scanner. This kit is also available with individual Cy3 or Cy5 dye as well as without dye to best meet the needs of the investigator (e.g., one- vs. two-color arrays, alternate dyes, etc.). If the Amino Allyl MessageAmp II kit without dye is selected, the investigator may select any fluorescent dye(s) to label the aRNA provided that an NHS ester of the dye is commercially available and the selected microarray imager/scanner is compatible with the spectral properties of the selected dye(s). For instance, Alexa Fluor 555 and Alexa Fluor 647 (Cat. #A-20009 & #A-20006, respectively, Invitrogen) may be used in place of Cy3 and Cy5, respectively.

7. If the tissues will be isolated postmortem, efforts should be made to perform the dissection as soon as possible after euthanasia to minimize the opportunity for RNA degradation.

8. RNA*later* rapidly permeates cells and preserves cellular RNA. The goal is to transfer the tissue from the in vivo state to RNA*later* as rapidly as possible to capture the in vivo RNA profile before significant RNA turnover or degradation is

induced by the surgical processes. Care should be taken to process the tissue as rapidly as possible after the initiation of the surgical procedure and/or the euthanasia of the animal. For this reason, the tissue is initially only grossly dissected prior to equilibration in RNA*later* with subsequent dissection to be performed in the presence of RNA*later*.

9. This step may be extended for several hours with no effects on the tissue; however, prolonged storage will increase the likelihood of RNA*later* precipitation, which will increase the difficulty of dissection. This is an excellent opportunity to isolate and/or process additional samples.

10. Following equilibration in RNA*later*, the mechanical disruption of the tissue introduced by the dissection process will not harm the RNA. Significant disruption of the tissue, however, could potentially cause RNA to diffuse out of the cells and into the RNA*later* thus reducing subsequent RNA yield.

11. During the dissection process, the repeated introduction and removal of the surgical instruments into the RNA*later* bath will eventually initiate precipitant formation. This process will significantly affect the visual clarity of the solution thus impeding microdissection. To minimize and slow RNA*later* precipitation, the surgical instruments should be rinsed in distilled water following each removal from the RNA*later* solution (rapidly swirling the instrument in a beaker of distilled water is a convenient way to accomplish this task). If the RNA*later* solution becomes too cloudy to complete dissection, transfer the tissue to a new dissection dish with fresh RNA*later* and resume dissection.

12. Samples may be stored in RNA*later* at 4°C for 1–2 weeks following this step. If longer storage is desired, the samples may be stored in RNA*later* at –20°C indefinitely (incubate the samples for 24 h at 4°C before transferring to –20°C; do NOT use a "frost-free" freezer).

13. Excessive RNA*later* carryover into the RNA isolation procedure will prevent effective precipitation of the RNA. To prevent this, transfer the samples from RNA*later* to TRIzol Reagent using microforceps that have been cleaned with ethanol and dried prior to each vessel transfer. Upon removing the vessel from the RNA*later*, touch it to the side or lid of the RNA*later* tube to wick some of the excess RNA*later* off of the vessel and forceps. Often (particularly after long storage) the vessel will be partially encapsulated in crystallized RNA*later*. In this case, attempt to carefully break off excess crystals before proceeding.

14. Run the homogenizer for ~1 min in a 5-mL round-bottom polypropylene tube containing ~2 mL of TRIzol Reagent prior to homogenizing the first sample so the generator will be clean

of any contaminants that it may have picked up during storage and handling.

15. Rotor-stator homogenizers work by sucking fluid in through the side windows of the generator and shearing it between the rotor and stator (much to the surprise of many people, the teeth on the bottom of many generators are only for manually smashing and tearing large tissue so it can make its way up to the windows—if you put a microvessel under the teeth, it will just spin in circles). In order to effectively homogenize blood and lymphatic vessels, you must ensure that the vessels enter one of the generator windows immediately upon the onset of homogenization. To do this, simply stick the vessel to the side of the 2.0-mL microcentrifuge tube above the level of the TRIzol Reagent. Then, insert the generator into tube, and press it against the vessel on the side of the tube such that the vessel becomes trapped inside one of the windows. Push the generator into the TRIzol Reagent keeping the vessel stuck in the generator window, and then immediately begin homogenization after the window is completely submerged.
16. To maximize sample homogenization, the generator should be submerged into the TRIzol Reagent until the side windows are fully covered and immediately turned to high speed. Move the generator around in the solution during homogenization to encourage full circulation of the sample particles through the generator; however, care should be taken to keep the generator windows fully submerged in the solution. To maximize sample recovery following homogenization, the homogenizer should be adjusted to the lowest speed setting for 1–2 s *before* removing the generator from the sample solution. Raise the generator to just above the solution surface and turn off the homogenizer. Before completely removing the generator from the tube, touch the generator to the inner sidewall of the tube to wick any remaining solution off the side of the generator. After briefly cooling the samples on ice, inspect the solution for any remaining large vessel fragments and homogenize, if necessary, for an additional 15–20 s at 30,000 rpm before being placed back on ice.
17. Cleaning the generator with soap and water between samples can be very tedious and time-consuming. To increase sample throughput, fill four 5-mL round-bottom polypropylene tubes with ~2 mL of TRIzol Reagent. After homogenizing each sample, run the homogenizer for ~1 min in each of the four tubes. Number the tubes so you go in the same order after each sample. After every ~5–6 samples, discard the first tube and add a new last tube so that the final rinse remains relatively clean. This cleaning strategy is only effective for small samples such as the vessels described above (large samples will very quickly

contaminate all of the tubes of TRIzol). Clean the generator with soap and water after all samples have been homogenized.

18. From this step forward through *ALL* subsequent steps (including RNA isolation, RNA amplification and labeling, and microarray hybridization), basic RNA handling procedures should be strictly followed to prevent RNA degradation. This includes the strict use of RNase- and DNase-free pipette tips (with aerosol-resistant barrier filters), tubes, and solutions (particularly water). *Clean* gloves should be worn at all times (gloves that have touched any surface contaminated by biological material including skin, hair, door handles, etc. should be replaced). Work surfaces, tube racks, pipettes, etc. should be clean and, ideally, not used for other non-RNA related procedures during the course of this protocol (it may be advantageous to use a product such RNase*Zap* from Ambion to eliminate RNase activity from work surfaces, pipette barrels, tube racks, etc.).
19. For all RNA samples to be isolated in a single day, process all samples through this step before proceeding. The RNA*later*-immersed samples should be kept at 4°C until immediately prior to homogenization. Homogenized samples should be kept on ice until all samples are homogenized. For the remaining steps of this RNA isolation protocol, several samples can be easily processed simultaneously without ill effects on the success of the experiment.
20. A refrigerated centrifuge is preferred to maintain sample temperature at or below RT during centrifugation.
21. The volume of TRIzol Reagent, RNase-free water, and chloroform as well as the centrifugation time and speed is specifically optimized to facilitate the even distribution of the Phase Lock Gel between the organic and aqueous layers. Depending upon the composition of the vessel samples, the volume of RNase-free water and chloroform may need be adjusted. If after centrifugation some Phase Lock Gel is distributed above the clear aqueous phase, carefully disrupt the Phase Lock Gel with a pipette tip, and then using a fresh pipette tip, transfer all aqueous and organic liquid to a new 1.5-mL RNase-free microcentrifuge tube. Repeat steps 7–9 of section 3.1 (for future samples of similar composition, simply increase the volume of RNase-free water added in step 7 of section 3.1 until the Phase Lock Gel is consistently distributed under the clear aqueous phase following step 9 of section 3.1). If after centrifugation some of the pink organic phase is distributed above the Phase Lock Gel, carefully disrupt the Phase Lock Gel with a pipette tip, and then using a fresh pipette tip, transfer all aqueous and organic liquid to a new 2.0 mL Phase Lock Gel—Heavy (spin gel 1 min at 12,000 × *g* prior to use), add 100 μL Chloroform, and mix 1 min by repeated inversion. Repeat step 9 of section 3.1

(for future samples of similar composition, simply increase the volume of chloroform added in step 8 until the Phase Lock Gel is consistently distributed above the pink organic phase following step 9 of section 3.1).

22. When removing the upper aqueous phase, care should be taken to place the pipette tip as close to the Phase Lock Gel as possible to maximize sample recovery; however, the pipette tip should not be allowed to touch the Phase Lock Gel to prevent pipette tip clogging as well as contamination of subsequent steps with Phase Lock Gel.
23. For convenience, incubation in isopropranol at –20°C may be extended to up to 1 week. Do NOT use a "frost-free" freezer.
24. Pay close attention during this step. After precipitation from isopropanol, the RNA pellet will be very small and nearly clear. It is nearly impossible to see the pellet. During aspiration, tilt the tube away from the side of the tube that was outboard during centrifugation to aid in drawing the solution away from the pellet. Do not place the pipette tip near the bottom outboard side of the tube to prevent pellet disruption. The liquid in the tube should be uniform in appearance. If there are any signs of two phases of liquid in the tube (the phase separation line would generally be very near the bottom of the tube), this is a sign of excessive RNA*later* carryover from step 6 of section 3.1 (see Note 25).
25. If a pellet fails to form due to RNA*later* carryover, add 700 μL cold 50% Isopropanol, vortex, incubate at least 2 h at –20°C, and repeat step 11 of section 3.1. If a second phase is still visible after the second isopropanol precipitation, vortex the solution, transfer to a larger tube, add as much 50% isopropanol as possible, and repeat the incubation and centrifugation steps.
26. The RNA pellet can be stored in 75% ethanol for ~1 month at –20°C (do not use a "frost-free" freezer).
27. After the ethanol wash, the RNA pellet will become white and much easier to see; however, it will no longer stick to the side of the tube. Be cautious while removing the supernatant to avoid accidental aspiration.
28. The DNase Inactivation Reagent is a slurry of beads coated with chelating agents. If any of these beads are carried over into subsequent steps, the presence of the chelating agents will dramatically reduce the efficiency of the subsequent enzymatic reactions. For this reason, absolute care should be taken to not disturb the pellet of DNase Inactivation Reagent during this step. It is preferred to leave some sample remaining in this DNase Inactivation Reagent rather than risk transferring the reagent to subsequent steps.

29. The RNA solution may be stored at −80°C following this step; however, freezing and subsequent thawing of RNA is very detrimental to RNA integrity. It is thus preferred, if possible, that the RNA be immediately utilized in subsequent procedures following this step. If storing the RNA sample at −80°C is selected, first remove a 1 μL aliquot of each sample for use in the next step. This aliquot may be analyzed immediately or stored at −80°C for future analysis. By separately aliquoting the volume to be analyzed, it prevents an otherwise unnecessary thawing of the main sample volume.
30. Following this step, the total RNA sample is ideally suited for all downstream analytical techniques including microarray, PCR, etc.
31. These kits only utilize 1 μL of sample to examine the quantity and quality of the total RNA. Because the volumes utilized are so small, very careful sample pipetting is imperative. Add all other reagents to the wells of the analysis "chips" prior to adding the RNA sample or the ladder. When aspirating your 1 μL of RNA or ladder from your RNA or ladder sample tube, do not submerge the pipette tip into the solution, but rather draw your sample with the pipette tip on or just below the sample surface to prevent the accumulation of sample on the outside of the pipette tip. When dispensing your 1 μL of RNA or ladder, be sure to place your pipette tip in the very center of the well on the analysis chip and dispense the sample with the pipette tip on or just below the surface of the solution in the well. Also when dispensing, the pipette plunger should only be advanced beyond the first stop a small amount to ensure full sample delivery while preventing the introduction of bubbles into the analysis chip (i.e., do not do a full blow-out by pushing the pipette plunger all the way to the second stop).
32. It is our experience that the RNA6000 Pico LabChip/Experion RNA HighSens Analysis Kits provide the best results with approximately 1–4 ng of total RNA. If upon analysis, your RNA concentrations are calculated to be above this 1–4 ng/μL, it may be advantageous to dilute a small aliquot of sample down to this range and analyze again. If your samples are above 25 ng/μL, you may use the RNA6000 Nano LabChip or Experion RNA StdSens Analysis Kits. There is no practical lower limit to the amount of RNA that can be successfully amplified for microarray in the following protocol (single cell microarrays are possible (14)); however, RNA quality/quantity analysis with less than 1 ng of total RNA, in our experience, becomes increasingly less informative with decreasing RNA quantity (i.e., the estimated RNA quality/quantity may not reflect the actual quality/quantity).

33. In all cases, the RNA concentration calculated using these microfluidic analysis chips should be considered an estimate of the actual concentration. If a more accurate and reproducible measurement of actual RNA concentration is desired, the NanoDrop 1000A Spectrophotometer (NanoDrop products, Wilmington, DE) is recommended.

34. Generally a RIN≥8 is sufficient for microarray analysis of rat microvessels isolated using the above protocol. Use of different species, vessels, and/or isolation protocols may change the minimum effective RIN for microarray analysis. The minimum effective RIN for microarray analyses in your system may need to be determined empirically (for a detailed description of the RIN, see ref. 15). Failure to obtain expected RNA concentrations at this step is usually related to homogenization; revisit step 6 and all associated notes. Failure to obtain high-quality (i.e., nondegraded) RNA at this step is usually related to isolation and/or handling. Be sure to remove the vessel tissue from the animal as quickly as possible (and before the animal is euthanized or as quickly as possible thereafter) and transfer the tissue to RNA*later* as quickly as possible. From step 5 of section 3.1 forward, be sure to adhere strictly to RNase-free lab practices including *clean* gloves and work surfaces at all times as well as RNase-free pipette tips, tubes, instruments, and solutions. In some circumstances, it may be beneficial to perform all RNA isolation steps following step 6 in a dedicated RNA workspace or hood.

35. Preparation of RNA samples for microarray analysis is a long process with numerous time-sensitive steps. The amplification and labeling protocol should be reviewed several times before beginning, and a detailed procedural plan for how the samples will be processed should be developed. For large microarray experiments with large sample sizes and/or multiple samples groups, careful consideration must be given to sample handling to ensure that ALL incubation and processing times are precise and consistent across all samples (failure to accomplish this may skew the final data outcome). When processing samples through the following protocol, it is important to divide the RNA samples into sufficiently small batches (generally 6–12 samples) such that the technician(s) performing the procedures can uniformly apply the exact same treatment to all samples. Since the possibility of day-to-day and technician variance is always present, it is beneficial to have even representation of all sample groups in each sample processing batch. In this regard, any technical bias introduced will be applied evenly across all sample groups, thus not distorting the final data in favor of any particular sample group.

36. Utilizing an external, arbitrary reference RNA sample in each sample processing batch and subsequent microarray analysis of

the reference RNA samples is an additional mechanism to control for any technical variance that may be present. Since transcriptional profiling using microarray analysis is a comparative technique in which gene expression in one sample/group is always expressed relative to another sample/group, the use of an arbitrary reference RNA sample has the added benefit of being a consistent entity against which all samples can be normalized. In this regard, statistical analysis of multigroup comparisons is simplified and sample size can be increased at future time points by processing new RNA samples with fresh aliquots of reference RNA. The criteria for a reference RNA sample are: (1) no experimental interest in the sample's gene expression, (2) broad representation of gene expression across all genes expected in the experimental samples, and (3) large quantity of uniform RNA sample to allow its use throughout entire experiment(s). The reference RNA sample could be experimentally derived such as a mixture of extra RNA from all experimental conditions. In this format, all genes present in your experimental samples will be guaranteed in your reference sample; however, this reference becomes specific to the given experiment and, thus, does not permit comparison of data between experiments. Commercially available reference RNAs (such as the Universal Reference RNAs available from Agilent Technologies) provide broad representation of gene expression across the entire genome and function as a uniform reference that can permit normalization between experiments and even between labs; however, a small percentage of genes within an organism's genome will likely not be found in the commercially available reference RNA (usually a mixture of RNA derived from several cell lines), thus limiting the utility of the reference sample for the study of these particular genes.

37. Unless otherwise indicated in the Subheading 2 above, all reagents listed are included in the Amino Allyl MessageAmp II with Cy3/Cy5 kit.

38. All reaction components except enzymes should be completely thawed, thoroughly vortexed, and stored on ice. Enzymes should be thawed, mixed by gently flicking the tube, and then stored on ice. For master mix preparation, all reaction components except enzymes should be added and thoroughly vortexed. Enzymes are then added, the complete mixture is mixed by gently flicking, and the mixture is briefly centrifuged before being stored on ice. When adding the master mix to the samples, mix briefly by pipetting up and down, and then gently flicking the tube several times. Briefly centrifuge the samples (~5 s) to collect the volume at the bottom of the tube. Repeated freezing and thawing of enzyme solutions should be avoided as much as possible. It is important to follow these instructions consistently to ensure precise preparation of reaction mixtures

without reducing enzyme activity through mechanical damage. These procedures are applicable to ALL steps of this protocol.

39. All reaction master mix recipes already include a 5% overage to account for pipetting error.

40. While there are several points indicated in the Amino Allyl MessageAmp II protocol where the samples can be frozen or placed on ice and the procedure temporarily stopped, it is best to proceed continuously through the entire protocol with the samples only being placed on ice during the RNA quality/quantity analysis steps (or frozen during the RNA analysis steps only if the RNA analysis equipment is not readily available for immediate access). In this regard, the investigator should plan for 3 consecutive days of experimentation beginning with step 11 or 12 of section 3.1 of the above RNA isolation protocol early on day 1 and continuing through the first round of amplification with the in vitro transcription step proceeding overnight. Day 2 will include purification of aRNA from round one and aRNA quality/quantity analysis followed by the second round of amplification with the in vitro transcription step proceeding overnight. Day 3 will include purification of aRNA from round two and aRNA quantity/quality analysis followed by dye-coupling and final sample purification.

41. The following protocol utilizes two sequential rounds of linear amplification, which is generally preferred when less than 100 ng of starting total RNA is available. Generally, 10–100 ng of total RNA is available from rat microvessels and subsequently used for linear amplification. If greater than 100 ng of starting total RNA is available for all samples to be analyzed, the investigator may elect to do one round of amplification. If greater than 1 μg of starting total RNA is available for all samples, then use 1 μg.

42. If the desired quantity of total RNA is present in a volume greater than 10 μL, first add the desired quantity of total RNA to a PCR tube and dry the sample using vacuum centrifugation. Then add 10 μL of Nuclease-free Water to the dry RNA sample and mix by gentle vortexing (note: it may be necessary to incubate the sample at 55°C for several minutes with intermittent gentle vortexing to aid the rehydration of the RNA sample).

43. If an adjustable temperature heated lid is NOT available, then the heated lid function of the thermal cycler should be turned off during this incubation.

44. Upon addition of the cDNA Binding Buffer, each sample should be mixed and transferred to the cDNA Filter Cartridge before cDNA Binding Buffer is added to the next sample. The cDNA Binding Buffer will sometimes form precipitants during storage. If precipitants are evident, heat the solution to

37°C and vortex vigorously until all precipitants are dissolved. Cool to room temperature before use.

45. If only one round of amplification will be used (i.e., when greater than 100 ng of starting total RNA is available for all samples), reduce UTP (50 mM) volume to 3.15 μL/sample and add 3.15 μL of aaUTP (50 mM)/sample. Additionally, skip steps 15–24.
46. Alternatively, the purified aRNA can be stored at −80°C for several months. If storage at −80°C is selected, first prepare a 1 μL aliquot of each sample for use in the next step to prevent an unnecessary thawing of the main sample volume. This aliquot may be used immediately or stored at −80°C for future analysis.
47. The aRNA produced from this first round of linear amplification does not contain any modified nucleotides and is thus suitable for other downstream applications. Since the first round of amplification often produces much more aRNA than is required for input into the second round of amplification, it may be advantageous to reverse transcribe the remaining aRNA to cDNA for use in real-time or traditional PCR. In this regard, aRNA from the same samples used in the microarray analysis can also be used for the subsequent PCR validation of the microarray results.
48. The author has successfully used the estimated RNA, aRNA, and amino-allyl aRNA concentrations provided by these microfluidic RNA analyses for subsequent steps. If a more accurate and reproducible measurement of actual aRNA concentration is desired, the NanoDrop 1000A Spectrophotometer (NanoDrop products, Wilmington, DE) is recommended.
49. Using 10–100 ng of starting total RNA isolated from rat blood and lymphatic vessels via the above RNA isolation technique, the author routinely averages 80–100 ng of aRNA produced per 1 ng of starting total RNA during the first round of amplification
50. Failure to obtain an aRNA distribution profile with a peak at ≥500 nt can be caused by several factors. To alleviate, consider the following: (1) A higher RIN threshold may be needed for microarray analysis of your total RNA in your experimental system. Partially degraded total RNA will not produce full-length aRNA. Furthermore, mRNA with degraded poly-A tails will not effectively prime with the oligo(dT) primers used during reverse transcription. (2) Be sure that you are not disturbing the Phase Lock Gel during the phase separation step of the RNA isolation and/or be sure that the Phase Lock Gel is effectively separating the organic and aqueous phases. Residual phenol from the TRIzol Reagent would inhibit the enzymatic processes of RNA amplification. (3) Be sure you are not carrying

over ANY of the DNase Inactivation Reagent. (4) Be sure that there is no residual Wash Buffer in the cDNA or aRNA Filter Cartridges before the 55°C Nuclease-free Water is added to elute the cDNA/aRNA. The Wash Buffer contains ethanol, which may inhibit subsequent reactions. (5) Adhere strictly to the indicated incubation temperatures and times—they are all critical. (6) Adhere strictly to the stated method of temperature control. For 37°C incubations, a cell culture incubator or calibrated temperature hybridization oven should be used. For all other incubations, a thermal cycler must be used. All other methods of maintaining temperature do not bring the reaction to the appropriate temperature fast enough and/or maintain the appropriate temperature stably enough. Follow the stated heated lid temperature instructions specifically to avoid condensation formation in the tubes (which would alter the reaction composition) and/or avoid the lid temperature increasing the reaction temperature. (7) Adhere strictly to RNase-free lab practices including *clean* gloves and work surfaces at all times as well as RNase-free pipette tips, tubes, instruments, and solutions. (8) The enzymes used in this protocol are very sensitive to mechanical damage. Adhere strictly to the handling and mixing guidelines stated for enzymes in Note 38.

51. Only aRNA synthesized with unmodified UTP can be utilized for the second round of amplification. Amino allyl aRNA synthesized with amino allyl-modified UTP is not compatible with a second round of amplification.

52. Generally, 250 ng of first round aRNA is used for the second round of amplification when working with rat microvessel samples reserving the remaining first round aRNA for other applications such as real-time PCR validation of the microarray results.

53. If the desired quantity of aRNA is present in a volume greater than 10 μL, first add the desired quantity of aRNA to a PCR tube and reduce the sample volume to less than 10 μL using vacuum centrifugation. Do NOT dry the sample completely as this could impede reverse transcription. Then add Nuclease-free Water to the aRNA sample to increase the volume to exactly 10 μL and mix by gentle vortexing.

54. In the author's experience, 250 ng of input aRNA will yield approximately 100 μg of amino allyl aRNA following the second round of amplification. The amino allyl-modified aRNA is NOT compatible with other downstream enzymatic applications such as PCR and is generally used for microarray analysis only.

55. When examining the second round aRNA profile (i.e., 2100 Bioanalyzer/Experion Automated Electrophoresis System), be aware that the aRNA distribution will usually consist of shorter (i.e., less nucleotides) products compared to the first

round results. In the author's experience, a successful second round amplification will generally have a distribution centered around ~600–1,000 nt. Once again, if the size distribution is heavily skewed towards 0 nt with a peak less than 500 nt, the sample should be discarded and not used for subsequent steps.

56. Each tube of dye included in the Amino Allyl MessageAmp II kits contains enough dye for exactly one dye coupling reaction. Thus, if you plan (for instance) to label one sample with Cy3 and eight samples with Cy5, prepare one tube of Cy3 dye and eight tubes of Cy5 dye.
57. If performing two-color microarray analysis using an arbitrary reference RNA sample (see Note 36), label your reference aRNA sample with Cy3 and all of your experimental samples with Cy5. The intensity of the Cy3 signal is generally more robust than the Cy5 signal, and thus, Cy3 is best used with the reference sample. Because all experimental samples are labeled with the same dye (Cy5; likewise, all arrays have the same Cy3-labeled reference sample), dye bias between samples is eliminated by distributing any dye-dependent differences in fluorescent intensity evenly across all samples and sample groups. Thus, in this experimental design, dye swaps are not necessary.
58. Consult your microarray manufacturer/facility regarding the appropriate quantity of fluorescently label aRNA to use with your selected microarray platform, and adjust your input aRNA quantity for this reaction accordingly (staying within the recommended range of 5–20 μg). Generally, 1–5 μg of labeled aRNA is used per sample per array.
59. While you must use the same quantity of aRNA for all experimental samples, you may use a different quantity of reference sample aRNA if desired (if performing a reference sample-based experimental design). If the microarray samples are processed and labeled in batches (as recommended in Note 35), it is important that the exact same quantity of experimental sample aRNA and reference sample aRNA be consistently used across all sample preparation batches.
60. From this point forward, the samples will be labeled with the fluorescent dyes. Thus, every effort should be made to keep the samples protected from light as much as possible to prevent sample photobleaching. Perform all subsequent incubations in the dark and store the samples in containers that protect them from light.
61. The concentration of each sample can be estimated as the quantity of aRNA input into step 26 of section 3.2 divided by the volume of aRNA eluted during step 31 of section 3.2. If desired, a very accurate-labeled aRNA concentration can be calculated

using the A_{260} value measured via spectrophotometry in the presence of TE buffer following standard protocols for calculating RNA concentration.

62. This step is preparing the exact solution that will be hybridized to each array. A separate tube should be prepared for each array to be hybridized. Consult your microarray manufacturer/facility regarding the specific recommended quantity of labeled aRNA to be used per sample per array.
63. Cover the vacuum centrifuge lid with aluminum foil, if necessary, to protect the samples from light during the drying step. Do NOT overdry the samples. Inspect them frequently during the vacuum centrifugation process and remove them as soon as the volume is ≤9 μL or as soon as they become dry.
64. This step utilizes RNA hydrolysis to fragment the aRNA into the 60–200 nt size range for use with arrays printed with oligonucleotides. Consult with your microarray manufacturer/facility regarding whether this step is appropriate for your selected microarray platform.
65. This step yields an 11 μL-labeled aRNA sample (in Nuclease-free Water) ready for addition of hybridization buffer and subsequent microarray hybridization. Depending upon the recommendations of your microarray manufacturer/facility, it may be necessary to adjust this volume via vacuum centrifugation and/or addition of Nuclease-free Water prior to the addition of hybridization buffer.

Acknowledgments

These protocols were developed and optimized with the support of NIH HL070308 and HL071599.

References

1. Pease, A. C., Solas, D., Sullivan, E. J., Cronin, M. T., Holmes, C. P., and Fodor, S. P. (1994) Light-generated oligonucleotide arrays for rapid DNA sequence analysis, *Proc Natl Acad Sci U S A* ***91***, 5022–5026.
2. Schena, M., Shalon, D., Davis, R. W., and Brown, P. O. (1995) Quantitative monitoring of gene expression patterns with a complementary DNA microarray, *Science* ***270***, 467–470.
3. Zhang, J., Moseley, A., Jegga, A. G., Gupta, A., Witte, D. P., Sartor, M., Medvedovic, M., Williams, S. S., Ley-Ebert, C., Coolen, L. M., Egnaczyk, G., Genter, M. B., Lehman, M., Lingrel, J., Maggio, J., Parysek, L., Walsh, R., Xu, M., and Aronow, B. J. (2004) Neural system-enriched gene expression: relationship to biological pathways and neurological diseases, *Physiol Genomics* ***18***, 167–183.
4. Genter, M. B., Van Veldhoven, P. P., Jegga, A. G., Sakthivel, B., Kong, S., Stanley, K., Witte, D. P., Ebert, C. L., and Aronow, B. J. (2003) Microarray-based discovery of highly expressed olfactory mucosal genes: potential roles in the various functions of the olfactory system, *Physiol Genomics* ***16***, 67–81.
5. Hutton, J. J., Jegga, A. G., Kong, S., Gupta, A., Ebert, C., Williams, S., Katz, J. D., and Aronow, B. J. (2004) Microarray and comparative

genomics-based identification of genes and gene regulatory regions of the mouse immune system, *BMC Genomics 5*, 82.

6. Tabibiazar, R., Wagner, R. A., Liao, A., and Quertermous, T. (2003) Transcriptional profiling of the heart reveals chamber-specific gene expression patterns, *Circ Res 93*, 1193–1201.
7. Bates, M. D., Erwin, C. R., Sanford, L. P., Wiginton, D., Bezerra, J. A., Schatzman, L. C., Jegga, A. G., Ley-Ebert, C., Williams, S. S., Steinbrecher, K. A., Warner, B. W., Cohen, M. B., and Aronow, B. J. (2002) Novel genes and functional relationships in the adult mouse gastrointestinal tract identified by microarray analysis, *Gastroenterology 122*, 1467–1482.
8. Chomczynski, P., and Sacchi, N. (1987) Single-step method of RNA isolation by acid guanidinium thiocyanate-phenol-chloroform extraction, *Anal Biochem 162*, 156–159.
9. Van Gelder, R. N., von Zastrow, M. E., Yool, A., Dement, W. C., Barchas, J. D., and Eberwine, J. H. (1990) Amplified RNA synthesized from limited quantities of heterogeneous cDNA, *Proc Natl Acad Sci U S A 87*, 1663–1667.
10. Pabon, C., Modrusan, Z., Ruvolo, M. V., Coleman, I. M., Daniel, S., Yue, H., and Arnold, L. J., Jr. (2001) Optimized T7 amplification system for microarray analysis, *Biotechniques 31*, 874–879.
11. Baugh, L. R., Hill, A. A., Brown, E. L., and Hunter, C. P. (2001) Quantitative analysis of mRNA amplification by in vitro transcription, *Nucleic Acids Res 29*, E29.
12. t Hoen, P. A., de Kort, F., van Ommen, G. J., and den Dunnen, J. T. (2003) Fluorescent labelling of cRNA for microarray applications, *Nucleic Acids Res 31*, e20.
13. Shi, L., Reid, L. H., Jones, W. D., Shippy, R., Warrington, J. A., Baker, S. C., Collins, P. J., de Longueville, F., Kawasaki, E. S., Lee, K. Y., Luo, Y., Sun, Y. A., Willey, J. C., Setterquist, R. A., Fischer, G. M., Tong, W., Dragan, Y. P., Dix, D. J., Frueh, F. W., Goodsaid, F. M., Herman, D., Jensen, R. V., Johnson, C. D., Lobenhofer, E. K., Puri, R. K., Schrf, U., Thierry-Mieg, J., Wang, C., Wilson, M., Wolber, P. K., Zhang, L., Amur, S., Bao, W., Barbacioru, C. C., Lucas, A. B., Bertholet, V., Boysen, C., Bromley, B., Brown, D., Brunner, A., Canales, R., Cao, X. M., Cebula, T. A., Chen, J. J., Cheng, J., Chu, T. M., Chudin, E., Corson, J., Corton, J. C., Croner, L. J., Davies, C., Davison, T. S., Delenstarr, G., Deng, X., Dorris, D., Eklund, A. C., Fan, X. H., Fang, H., Fulmer-Smentek, S., Fuscoe, J. C., Gallagher, K., Ge, W., Guo, L., Guo, X., Hager, J., Haje, P. K., Han, J., Han, T., Harbottle, H. C., Harris, S. C., Hatchwell, E., Hauser, C. A., Hester, S., Hong, H., Hurban, P., Jackson, S. A., Ji, H., Knight, C. R., Kuo, W. P., LeClerc, J. E., Levy, S., Li, Q. Z., Liu, C., Liu, Y., Lombardi, M. J., Ma, Y., Magnuson, S. R., Maqsodi, B., McDaniel, T., Mei, N., Myklebost, O., Ning, B., Novoradovskaya, N., Orr, M. S., Osborn, T. W., Papallo, A., Patterson, T. A., Perkins, R. G., Peters, E. H., Peterson, R., Philips, K. L., Pine, P. S., Pusztai, L., Qian, F., Ren, H., Rosen, M., Rosenzweig, B. A., Samaha, R. R., Schena, M., Schroth, G. P., Shchegrova, S., Smith, D. D., Staedtler, F., Su, Z., Sun, H., Szallasi, Z., Tezak, Z., Thierry-Mieg, D., Thompson, K. L., Tikhonova, I., Turpaz, Y., Vallanat, B., Van, C., Walker, S. J., Wang, S. J., Wang, Y., Wolfinger, R., Wong, A., Wu, J., Xiao, C., Xie, Q., Xu, J., Yang, W., Zhong, S., Zong, Y., and Slikker, W., Jr. (2006) The MicroArray Quality Control (MAQC) project shows inter- and intraplatform reproducibility of gene expression measurements, *Nat Biotechnol 24*, 1151–1161.
14. Esumi, S., Wu, S. X., Yanagawa, Y., Obata, K., Sugimoto, Y., and Tamamaki, N. (2008) Method for single-cell microarray analysis and application to gene-expression profiling of GABAergic neuron progenitors, *Neurosci Res 60*, 439–451.
15. Schroeder, A., Mueller, O., Stocker, S., Salowsky, R., Leiber, M., Gassmann, M., Lightfoot, S., Menzel, W., Granzow, M., and Ragg, T. (2006) The RIN: an RNA integrity number for assigning integrity values to RNA measurements, *BMC Mol Biol 7*, 3.

Chapter 25

Visual Data Mining of Coexpression Data to Set Research Priorities in Cardiac Development Research

Vincent VanBuren

Abstract

Over the past decade, an immense amount of biomedical data have become available in the public domain due to the development of ever-more efficient screening tools such as expression microarrays. To fully leverage this important new resource, it has become imperative to develop new methodologies for mining and visualizing data to make inferences beyond the scope of the original experiments. This need motivated the development of a new freely available web-based application called StarNet (http://vanburenlab.medicine.tamhsc.edu/starnet2.html). Here we describe the use of StarNet, which functions primarily as a query tool that draws correlation networks centered about a gene of interest. To support inferences and the development of new hypotheses using the resulting correlation network, StarNet queries all genes in the correlation network against a database of known interactions and displays the results in a second graph and provides a statistical test of Gene Ontology term enrichment (keyword enrichment) to provide tentative summary functional annotations for the correlation network. Finally, StarNet provides additional tools for comparing networks drawn from two different selected data sets, thus providing methods for making inferences and developing new hypotheses about differential wiring for different regulatory domains.

Key words: Microarray, Transcriptional regulatory network, Correlation network, Development, Differential wiring

1. Introduction

This protocol describes the use of StarNet, a free web-based tool for visually mining coexpression data. The method used here for the development of new hypotheses for setting research priorities will be introduced by establishing a rationale for using visualization techniques combined with data mining of published microarray data.

Xu Peng and Marc Antonyak (eds.), *Cardiovascular Development: Methods and Protocols*,
Methods in Molecular Biology, vol. 843, DOI 10.1007/978-1-61779-523-7_25,

1.1. The Limitations of Standard Microarray Analysis

Microarray analysis is normally conducted to identify a list of genes whose expressions differ between a control condition and an experimental condition. To identify the genes whose expression is different between these two conditions, microarrays are used to measure the fluorescence intensity that results from a surface hybridization of fluorescently tagged mRNA from the samples with complementary oligos preimmobilized to a rigid surface. The amount of fluorescence thus measured is taken to be proportionate to the amount of transcript encoded by a particular gene. This technology, and emerging technologies with a similar strategy for measuring gene expression, can assess expression profiles for thousands of genes in a sample simultaneously. Microarrays and similar emerging technologies have thus been extremely popular screening tools in molecular biology.

The standard approach to microarray analysis is to conduct null hypothesis testing for the expression of each gene between two groups of samples, each group comprising several biological replicates of some biologically interesting condition (e.g., control samples and experimental treatment samples). The null hypothesis to be tested is that, for a particular transcript whose expression is assessed, the mean expression of that transcript in the two groups of samples is the same. Because thousands of transcripts are measured simultaneously, multiple test corrections are often employed.

Null hypothesis significance tests (NHST), however, have some important shortcomings: (1) They don't really allow biologists to make the type of assertions they would like to make about their hypothesis, and (2) when employed to test for a difference between groups, whether or not a difference is found is related to the number of samples used. Cohen made these points more than 15 years ago in his landmark exposition, "The Earth is Round ($p < 0.05$)" (1), and his remarks echo the remarks made by numerous others in the preceding decades. The first problem is made poignantly clear in the following excerpt from Cohen's paper, where he shows a flaw in the logic typically applied to the results of NHST that arises from the inappropriate application of probabilistic thinking:

If a person is an American, then he is probably not a member of Congress (TRUE, RIGHT?).

This person is a member of Congress.

Therefore, he is probably not an American Refrence (12).

This is formally exactly the same as

If *Ho* is true, then this result (statistical significance) would probably not occur.

This result has occurred.

Then *Ho* is probably not true and therefore formally invalid (1).

The problem with this logic applied to null hypothesis testing is that it is an invalid Bayesian interpretation. Formulated in absolute terms, the logic holds:

If *Ho* is true, then this result would not occur.

This result has occurred.

Then *Ho* is not true and therefore formally invalid (1).

The appropriate interpretation of the null hypothesis test is that a statistically significant result gives evidence that the null hypothesis is false, as the ***data is unlikely, given the hypothesis.*** The *p*-value does not give the probability that the null hypothesis is correct given the data, which is the interpretation that we would like to make, and is sometimes made incorrectly. The first problem above is thus a general problem of the interpretation of any NHST.

The second problem is specific to NHSTs applied to detect differences between groups. Anyone who is asked, "which is better for statistical testing, a large number of samples, or a small number of samples?," will undoubtedly reply that a large number of samples is better. Herein lies the issue with testing for differences between groups: Given a sufficiently large number of samples, there will always be a statistically significant difference. Therefore, finding a difference is only a matter of using enough samples. So the list of differentially expressed genes (DEG) that one gets from a typical microarray experiment really reflects those genes whose combination of effect size and low variance allowed them to cross a threshold for statistical significance. Using enough samples, we would find that all genes are differentially expressed. The only thing that NHST grants us directly is the direction of the difference. However, because we know that getting a statistically significant result is influenced by effect size and variance, DEGs will tend to have a large effect size. These drawbacks of the NHST suggest that it must be used and interpreted cautiously, and that it emphasizes the wrong thing (looking for any detectable difference, regardless of biological significance).

There is no single test that replaces NHST with something that does exactly what we want (i.e., identify biologically significant differences between two groups), but Cohen gives some suggestions to better approach the kind of results that are of interest to us (1). These include the use of confidence intervals, data visualizations, and meta analysis that combines the findings of several experiments. Cohen (1) and Abelson (2) have both remarked that statistics should not supplant expert judgment, only act as a tool to aid that judgment. Cohen's advice was followed in the creation of a new visual data mining tool called StarNet.

1.2. Leveraging Published Data

Scientific progress builds upon yesterday's findings. High-throughput experimentation over the previous decade, however, has greatly changed the landscape of "yesterday's findings." High-throughput experimentation produces many more results than can be thoughtfully considered in their respective published reports. It is therefore imperative that we develop new methodologies, such as we describe here, to leverage these vast resources. The cost of conducting a high-throughput experiment is considerable, and the increased efficiency that will result from the effective mining of already published data will both greatly reduce the cost of biomedical science, as well as make powerful screening tools available to a wider swath of scientific investigators. StarNet addresses this imperative by providing free web-based visual data mining of correlation matrices derived from numerous published microarray experiments.

1.3. Guilt by Association

Popular clustering techniques are all motivated by the notion of "guilt by association." Similar measurements of biologically important characteristics, such as gene expression profiles, are frequently used to infer relationships between biological entities, or to infer similar biological functions for those entities. These techniques are usually applied to individual experiments, and the results are typically given as nonoverlapping groups of biological entities, or *clusters.* In the context of microarray experiments, many techniques have been applied for this purpose, including K-means clustering, hierarchical clustering, self-organizing maps, and principal component analysis. The main shortcoming of these methods is that they typically do not produce a resource that can be easily queried, and that they generally do not preserve much detail about which genes are most similar to a particular gene of interest. StarNet enhances the notion of "guilt by association" by using numerous microarray experiments to draw correlation networks that radiate from a gene of interest in a query-based analysis.

1.4. An Aid to Expert Inference

StarNet was created as an aid to expert reasoning, not as a substitute for that reasoning. This underlying philosophy means that StarNet will not readily supply explicit predictions of functional interactions. Instead, by querying coexpression data in an intuitive way, ideas for the formation of strong hypotheses are brought forward with data visualization and supporting analysis. The important point here is that although StarNet draws edges between nodes that represent gene transcripts, the edges do not indicate that there is a predicted functional relationship between the connected genes. The edges are merely drawn between genes that have a high magnitude correlation of their expression profiles (see Note 1). Although there are tools that integrate several types of data to make an explicit prediction of functional relationships, we leave that to the expert user here. The trade-off is between complete automation and the applied judgment of an expert user in assessing easily understood relationships.

StarNet draws Pearson correlation networks derived from a large collection of preselected microarray experiments. Insofar as transcript expression is the only aspect of transcriptional regulatory plans that is assessed in a correlation network, it should be understood that many uncharacterized regulatory circuits are expected to have controls at the level of posttranscriptional, translational, or posttranslational activation. Thus, differences in the transcript abundance of a transcription factor may not be closely related to the transcript abundance of a target of that transcription factor. This is an important limitation of StarNet analysis and it underscores a need to supply supporting information for the interpretation of a correlation network. StarNet provides two ways to support such interpretations: (1) Members of the correlation network are searched against a database of documented biomolecular interactions, and any known interactions involving genes in the correlation network are drawn in a separate graph associated with the correlation network, and (2) members of the correlation network are assessed for enrichment of Gene Ontology terms (keywords describing gene function, pathway membership, and localization), as compared with the background of all the genes on the array platform that the data were derived from. The latter analysis tells us if any terms, such as "cell cycle," "cytoskeleton," "apoptosis," etc., are enriched in the set of genes in the correlation network with respect to the complete set of genes on the array. If such enrichments are identified, it provides a provisional annotation for inferring possible related functional roles of other genes in the correlation network.

2. Materials

2.1. The StarNet Web-Based Application

StarNet is a web-based interface for querying precomputed Pearson correlation matrices derived from selected published microarray data (3, 4). Microarray data used for computing correlation matrices were retrieved from the Gene Expression Ominbus database of microarray data. Ten different organisms are supported by StarNet. For four of these organisms (mouse, human, rat, and *Drosophila*), additional "Developmental" data subsets were formed from samples derived from early embryonic, cardiac embryonic, and adult heart tissues. For each organism represented in StarNet, a single array platform was selected, and a collection of raw microarray data was selected for computing Pearson correlations. After normalizing and scaling with justRMALite (5), Pearson correlation coefficients were computed for all pairs of genes within a data set, and the results were stored in a MySQL database along with other supporting information retrieved from NCBI. A web-based interface is used to query this database and create new analyses and returns linked figures and linked text as a result. For full details on how StarNet was developed, see Jupiter and VanBuren (4) and Jupiter et al. (3). Table 1 lists the array platforms, the number of gene features on each platform, and the number of arrays included in each of the 14 data sets that users can chose from in StarNet queries. StarNet is freely available at http://vanburenlab.medicine.tamhsc.edu/starnet2.html and does not require user registration.

Table 1
Data sets available for visual data mining across ten different species in StarNet at http://vanburenlab.medicine.tamhsc.edu/starnet2.html

Species	Affymetrix platform name	GEO ID	Number of gene features on array	Number of arrays in full array set	Number of arrays in Developmental array set
Homo sapiens	Human Genome U133 Plus 2.0 Array	GPL570	17,726	3,763	372
Mus musculus	Mouse Genome 430 2.0	GPL1261	16,331	2,145	239
Rattus norvegicus	Rat Genome 230 2.0 Array	GPL1355	11,427	1,982	247
Gallus Gallus	Chicken Genome Array	GPL3213	12,491	164	–
Danio rerio	Zebrafish Genome Array	GPL1319	6,838	222	–
Drosophila melanogaster	*Drosophila* Genome 2.0 Array	GPL1322	13,060	454	195
Caenorhabditis elegans	*C. elegans* Genome Array	GPL200	15,015	381	–
Oryza sativa Japonica Group	Rice Genome Array	GPL2025	23,419	148	–
Arabidopsis thaliana	*Arabidopsis* ATH1 Genome Array	GPL198	21,281	3,249	–
Saccharomyces cerevisiae	Yeast Genome 2.0 Array	GPL2529	5,566	254	–

Each of the ten “Full” array sets contains a heterogeneous set of experiments covering multiple tissue types and was conducted in multiple labs. The four “Developmental” array sets are subsets of the respective “Full” sets, where the samples come from early embryonic tissues, embryonic heart, or adult heart. A complete list of the sample IDs used can be found in the StarNet Documentation at: http://vanburenlab.medicine.tamhsc.edu/starnet2_doc.html

2.2. Gene ID for the Query

To get started using StarNet, all that is required from the user is an Entrez Gene ID, official Entrez Gene Symbol, or unofficial (but unique) Entrez Gene Synonym for a gene of interest. If one of these is not known for a particular gene of interest, then a provided lookup tool should be helpful in obtaining one of these IDs: http://vanburenlab.medicine.tamhsc.edu/gene_lookup.html .

3. Methods

3.1. Quick Start

StarNet is equipped with default settings to make it easy to become acquainted with using this tool for visually mining gene coexpression data. Figure 1 shows the StarNet web interface (http://vanburenlab.medicine.tamhsc.edu/starnet2.html) and gives an overview of the essential steps for making a query.

3.1.1. Select a Data Set for Analysis

There are 14 data sets to choose from in a drop-down menu for a StarNet query (Table 1) (see Note 2). Note that each data set is composed of a different number of arrays, with a different contribution from different types of experiment and different types of samples, and that the experiments were conducted by a number of different groups. Although our intent was to try to be as representative

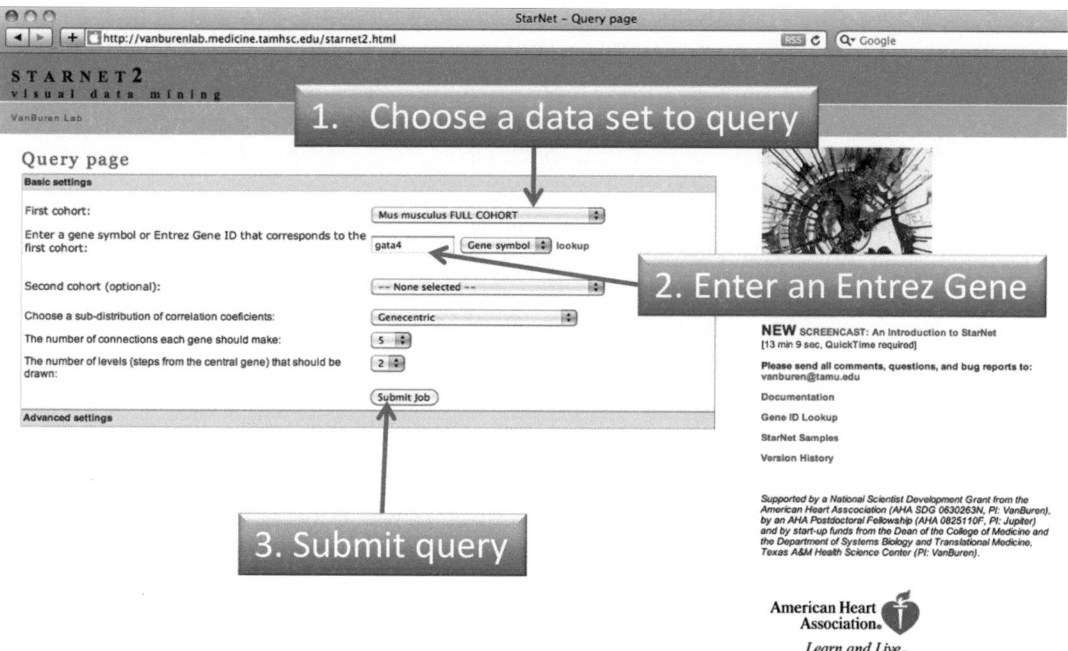

Fig. 1. Quick start procedure for using StarNet (http://vanburenlab.medicine.tamhsc.edu/starnet2.html). Queries using default parameters will quickly produce an easily comprehensible result. The number of genes in the resulting correlation network (≤31) is also a suitable number of genes for applying Bayesian inference techniques to predict causal networks.

as possible in our selections, the above factors must be considered when interpreting StarNet results. No effort on our part to select representative samples could ever truly reflect a sampling of the biology of a group of organisms. It is better to think of the population we sample from as the "population of tissues and experimental conditions that scientists have used microarrays to investigate."

3.1.2. Enter a Query Gene

StarNet performs gene-level queries to produce a graph of highly correlated gene expression profiles. The expected gene ID is either an official Entrez Gene Symbol or Entrez ID number. Unofficial gene synonyms that uniquely identify a gene are also acceptable, and StarNet will automatically replace these with the official Entrez Symbol and ID in the subsequent analysis. The Symbol or ID must correspond to the organism represented by the selected data set (see Subheading 3.1.1 above).

3.1.3. Submit the Query

Clicking "Submit" begins a new on-the-fly analysis that produces a graph of correlations radiating from the query gene. Using the default settings, StarNet will typically return a result in 1 or 2 min. Run time is influenced by the size of the networks drawn. The resulting size of the correlation network is controlled by parameters for the number of connections to draw for each gene and the number of levels to radiate from the query gene. For each gene in the correlation network, a search is performed in a database of documented biomolecular interactions, and the resulting network(s) are also drawn. The size of resulting network of known interactions is thus influenced indirectly by the size of the correlation network and by the number of known interactions for a given set of genes. As the number of known interactions for a given set of genes varies, so does the run time of StarNet. For example, there are many more documented interactions for human than there are for mouse, so analyses made with the same network parameters generally take much longer for human data because of the increased time required for drawing the larger network of known interactions.

The upper left panel of Fig. 2 shows the main result of StarNet analysis using the default parameters for the query "Gata4" against the data set "Mouse full cohort." The magnitude of correlations is encoded by edge color, where darker color indicates a higher magnitude, as given by the scale bar. The default behavior is to retrieve the five highest magnitude correlations for the query gene and expand the network to two levels radiating from the query gene. This means that for each of the top-ranking genes correlated with the query gene, the top five ranking correlations will also be retrieved. The resulting network is drawn accordingly, such that the tail of each edge (the "from" end) is unmarked and the head of head edge (the "to" end) is marked with a large dot. This indicates that the gene on the dotted end (head) of the edge is among the top five correlates of the gene at the unmarked end (tail).

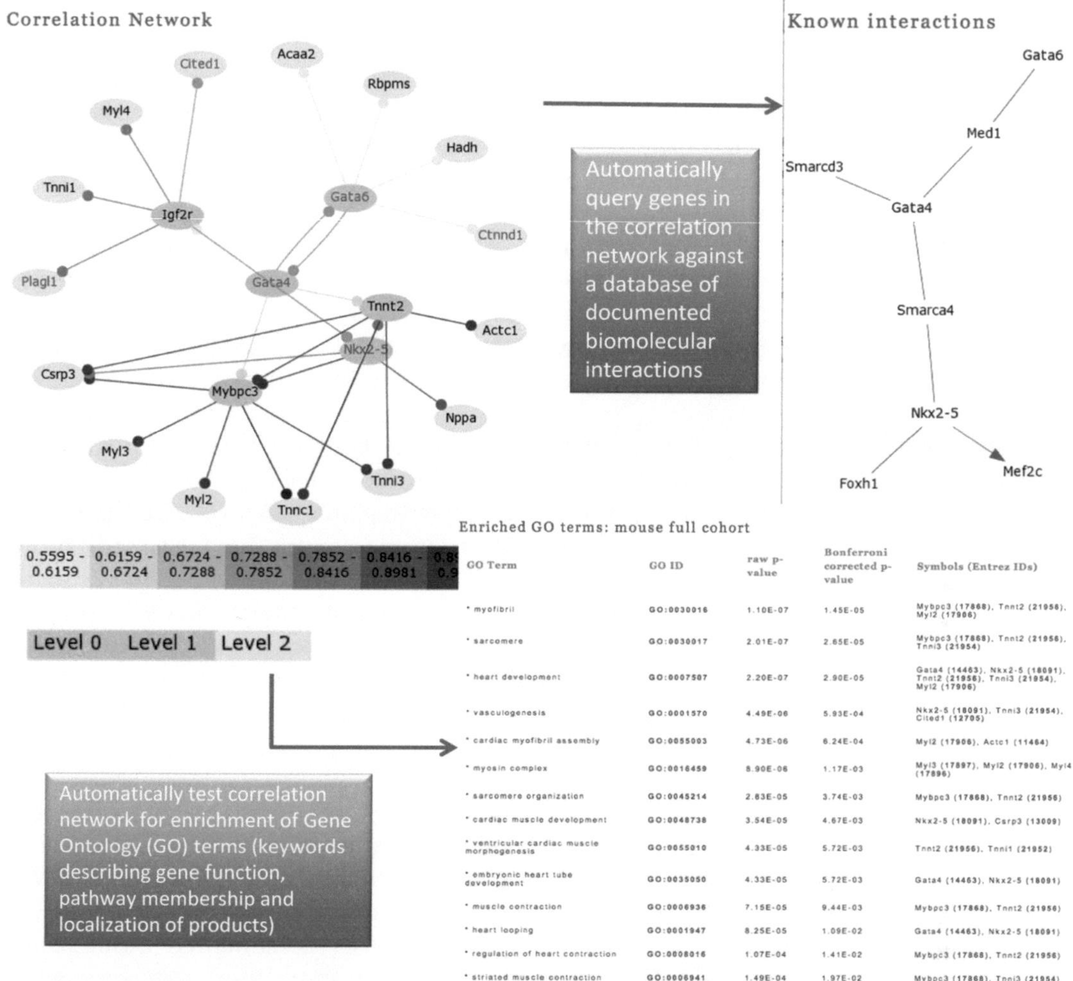

Enriched GO terms: mouse full cohort

GO Term	GO ID	raw p-value	Bonferroni corrected p-value	Symbols (Entrez IDs)
• myofibril	GO:0030016	1.10E-07	1.45E-05	Mybpc3 (17868), Tnnt2 (21956), Myl2 (17906)
• sarcomere	GO:0030017	2.01E-07	2.65E-05	Mybpc3 (17868), Tnnt2 (21956), Tnni3 (21954)
• heart development	GO:0007507	2.20E-07	2.90E-05	Gata4 (14463), Nkx2-5 (18091), Tnnt2 (21956), Tnni3 (21954), Myl2 (17906)
• vasculogenesis	GO:0001570	4.49E-06	5.93E-04	Nkx2-5 (18091), Tnni3 (21954), Cited1 (12705)
• cardiac myofibril assembly	GO:0055003	4.73E-06	6.24E-04	Myl2 (17906), Actc1 (11464)
• myosin complex	GO:0016459	8.90E-06	1.17E-03	Myl3 (17897), Myl2 (17906), Myl4 (17896)
• sarcomere organization	GO:0045214	2.83E-05	3.74E-03	Mybpc3 (17868), Tnnt2 (21956)
• cardiac muscle development	GO:0048738	3.54E-05	4.67E-03	Nkx2-5 (18091), Csrp3 (13009)
• ventricular cardiac muscle morphogenesis	GO:0055010	4.33E-05	5.72E-03	Tnnt2 (21956), Tnni1 (21952)
• embryonic heart tube development	GO:0035050	4.33E-05	5.72E-03	Gata4 (14463), Nkx2-5 (18091)
• muscle contraction	GO:0006936	7.15E-05	9.44E-03	Mybpc3 (17868), Tnnt2 (21956)
• heart looping	GO:0001947	8.25E-05	1.09E-02	Gata4 (14463), Nkx2-5 (18091)
• regulation of heart contraction	GO:0008016	1.07E-04	1.41E-02	Mybpc3 (17868), Tnnt2 (21956)
• striated muscle contraction	GO:0006941	1.49E-04	1.97E-02	Mybpc3 (17868), Tnni3 (21954)

Fig. 2. The main result returned by StarNet is a Pearson correlation network centered about the query gene. The highest magnitude correlations (default = 5 highest magnitude correlations) are retrieved for the query gene and the network radiates a specified number of levels (default = 2 levels). *Edge color* shows the magnitude of the correlation between two gene expression profiles, as indicated by the *scale bar*. With the default settings, known transcription factors are shown with *red text*. StarNet automatically produces additional analyses to support interpretation of the correlation network, including a query of all genes in the correlation network against a database of documented biomolecular interactions, and an enrichment test of GO terms. Genes in the "known interactions" graph that are also in the correlation network are shown in *blue* text. *Black edges* in the interactions graph represent known protein–protein interactions, and *red arrows* represent known protein–DNA interactions.

The default behavior is to find top-ranking correlates even if they are already in the network, so we can see that sometimes lines are drawn between genes at the same level (e.g., *from* Nkx2-5 *to* Mybpc3) and sometimes lines may be drawn in both directions between the same pair (e.g., *from* Gata4 *to* Gata6 and *from* Gata6 *to* Gata 4). The latter example of the association between Gata4 and Gata6 indicates that each of them is among the top five correlates of the other, which may suggest an especially strong coexpression relationship.

Upon returning a result, StarNet produces graphs that may be reduced from their original size. Clicking on a graph redirects the user to a page with full-size graphs that are graphically linked to Entrez Gene. Clicking on any node then redirects the user to the Entrez Gene entry for that gene at NCBI. In addition to the graph of the correlation network, tabular output is also returned to the user, including a list of the genes in the network with brief descriptions and links to Entrez Gene and a list of all edges with links to Entrez Gene together with a list of the corresponding Pearson correlation coefficients and their 95%- and 99%-confidence intervals.

3.2. Supporting Analyses

Interpretation of the correlation network that is returned in a StarNet analysis is supported by additional analyses. The key questions addressed by these supporting analyses are, "Are there genes or gene products in the correlation network that are already known to have some biomolecular interaction with other genes in the network, either directly or through an intermediate?," and "Are the genes or gene products in the correlation network enriched for any Gene Ontology terms (annotation keywords) that can be used to assign a putative functional summary annotation to all or part of the network?"

3.2.1. Known Interactions

NCBI maintains a database called Gene Reference Into Function (GeneRIF), which is a knowledgebase of gene characterizations where each functional reference is supported by evidence from a PubMed entry. A subset of this database, which is supplied by NCBI as a separate downloadable text file, lists documented biomolecular interactions. StarNet leverages this interaction database, which includes data from four major interaction databases (BIND (6), BioGRID (7), HPRD (8), and EcoCyc (9)). For the development of the StarNet application, the interaction file was retrieved from NCBI, processed, and deposited as a local MySQL database that is queried to support interpretation of StarNet analysis.

For each gene in a StarNet correlation network, an automated query is performed against the associated interaction database. All interactions identified in this process are listed as tabular output with links to the respective Entrez Gene entries and PubMed references. The interactions are also combined into a single graph, which may or may not be connected (Fig. 2, upper right panel). For ease of identification, genes from the correlation network are shown in blue text in the interaction network. The example output in the upper right panel of Fig. 2 shows an interaction network that corresponds to the StarNet correlation network in the upper left panel.

The rationale for providing known interactions involving genes and gene products from the StarNet correlation network is to provide a basis for judging the biological relevance of genes sharing membership in the correlation network. A highly connected network may provide some measure of confidence that the correlation network as a whole may be useful for uncovering functional relationships between members. A similar rationale motivates testing for enrichment of Gene Ontology terms that annotate the genes in the correlation network.

3.2.2. Gene Ontology Enrichment

The Gene Ontology (GO) is a controlled vocabulary of keywords for annotating genes (10). GO term enrichment testing asks if a given GO term annotates members of a group of genes more frequently than one would expect if the selection of genes was made randomly. The purpose of using this test is to identify GO terms that may provide provisional annotation of putative functional roles for members of the correlation network as a group or cluster. StarNet employs the Hypergeometric statistical test in order to make this assessment for each of the GO terms annotating any gene in the StarNet correlation network (11, 12) (Fig. 2, lower right panel). Because a separate test is employed for each GO term, StarNet uses the Bonferroni multiple test correction to reduce the chance of false positive results. The Bonferroni correction is generally considered the strictest form of multiple test correction.

3.2.3. Gene Ontology Term Tagging

By default, StarNet highlights genes annotated with any Gene Ontology (GO) term containing the word "transcription," with red text in its resulting correlation network. This should be useful for establishing hypotheses about the direction of regulatory influences between members of the correlation network, where genes previously annotated as transcription factors are highlighted as good candidates for influencing the expression of other genes in the correlation network (see Note 3). The term to highlight can also be supplied by the user to similarly tag any GO term of interest. Under "Basic settings" in the StarNet interface, a text box labeled "Highlighted GO Terms" is provided for this purpose and multiple terms separated by commas may also be provided. The gene lookup tool (click "lookup" next to the text box) may be useful for identifying appropriate GO terms to tag.

3.3. Exploratory Analysis: Selection of Parameters

Here we will confine our attention to the "Basic settings" parameters for StarNet analysis. The basic parameters are "sub-distribution of correlation coefficients," "the number of connections each gene should make," and "number of levels (steps from the central gene) that should be drawn."

The number of connections and the number of levels affect the size and topology of the resulting network. The default selections (connections = 5, levels = 2) will produce a network that contains less than or equal to 31 genes (nodes). These parameters were chosen to produce a network of tractable size for visually exploring and interpreting the results. The number of genes in the resulting network is also a reasonable number of genes for causal inference techniques such as Bayesian network analysis, so StarNet can be used to provide a list of candidate genes for further analysis. Increasing the number of connections (up to a maximum of 10) and levels (up to a maximum of 4) will greatly increase the number of genes returned in the resulting correlation network. Changing these parameters to something other than the default values is a major part of the exploratory nature of the analysis provided by StarNet. Increasing these parameters will provide more complicated results that may make interpretation more difficult. On the other hand, increasing the network size may be useful for investigators who wish to do a very broad screen for genes with possible functional relationships with a gene of interest.

There are four subdistributions to choose from when conducting a StarNet query: "100K highest magnitude correlations from the tails," "Gene-centric," "Transcription Gene-centric," and "Transcription an Signal Gene-centric." The default subdistribution is "Gene-centric," which includes the ten highest magnitude positive correlations and ten highest magnitude negative correlations for every gene on the respective array platform. The 100K highest magnitude subdistribution is made by identifying the 100,000 highest magnitude positive correlations and the 100,000 highest magnitude negative correlations from the entire distribution derived from the respective array platform, regardless of the genes involved. There is much "cliquishness" among very highly correlated genes, so the 100K highest magnitude subdistribution does not contain coverage of all genes on the array platform. The Genecentric distribution is thus the default choice because it contains complete coverage of all genes. For example, there are over 16,000 genes represented on the mouse array platform, all of which are represented in the Genecentric distribution, but less than 4,000 are present in the 100K highest magnitude subdistribution. The latter distribution is therefore only suggested to users who have a special interest in identifying gene pairs that have very high magnitude correlations.

The "Transcription Genecentric" and "Transcription and Signal Genecentric" subdistributions are versions of the Genecentric subdistribution that have been filtered for GO terms that contain the word "transcription," or the words "transcription" and "signal," respectively. This filtering requires that the submitted query gene also satisfies the requirement for being annotated in this way. The utility of these subdistributions is that they allow the user to drill down to only those genes that may be of central importance in transcription regulation or transcription regulation and signaling.

3.4. Differential Wiring: Comparing Two Networks

StarNet analyses can be performed in parallel to produce side-by-side results for two different data sets (Fig. 3). To achieve this, the user simply selects a second data set from the optional drop-down menu. The Gene ID or Symbol provided by the user should correspond

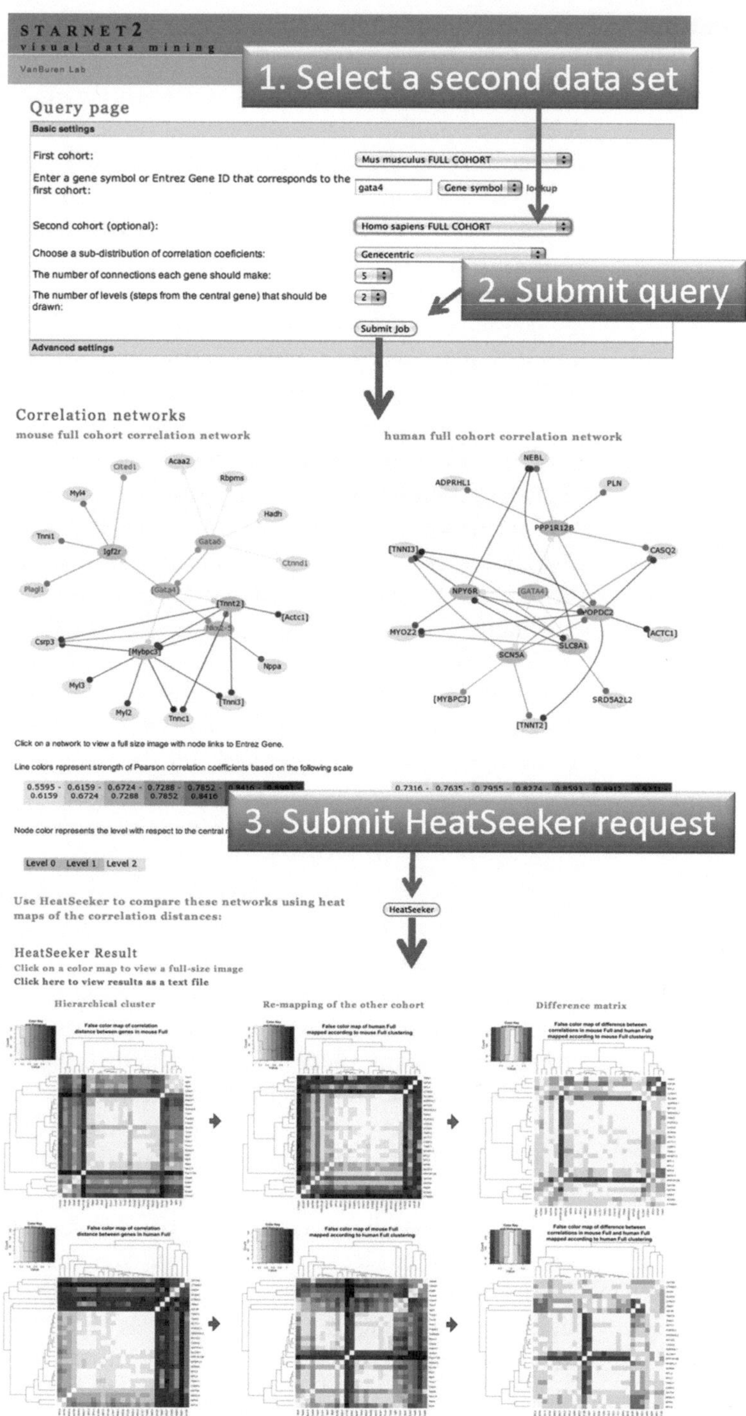

Fig. 3. Exploratory analysis of differential wiring using StarNet. Selecting a second data set in a StarNet Query will produce side-by-side results for each data set (if the query gene can be found in both sets). Orthologous genes found in both correlation networks are indicated with *square brackets* around the Entrez Symbol or ID. It should be noted that the manner in which the correlation networks are created causes arbitrary differences in the networks, so a direct comparison may not lead to useful inferences. However, invoking the HeatSeeker module allows for unbiased comparisons between the groups of genes created by making a superset of both networks from those genes where data are available for each ortholog. Hierarchical clustering is then combined with false color maps to show differences and similarities between the entire correlation matrices derived from the two data sets (see text).

to the first data set. The most straightforward comparative analysis is between a "full" data cohort and its respective "developmental" data cohort on the same array platform. As long as there is coverage of the selected gene on the platform, the analysis should proceed. Cross-species analysis can also be performed, although these comparisons require that the query gene has a known ortholog in the second species, and that each ortholog is represented on their respective array platforms. In either case, genes that are common to both networks are identified by default with square brackets around the appropriate gene symbols in the resulting networks.

Although simple identification of the genes common to two networks may be useful if the networks are highly similar, it is not likely to be useful for inferring possible differential wiring between two networks. The reason for this is that the assembly of the correlation networks is done in a manner that will produce arbitrary differences between two networks, and these differences are thus not likely to be biologically meaningful. Let's consider an example *Gene X* that we query against the mouse full data set and the mouse developmental data set in parallel and request five connections (the five highest magnitude correlations). Now suppose that *Gene Y* is returned in the analysis of full data set, but not for the developmental set. Can we infer anything from this difference? This difference cannot be used for inference because it may be arbitrary: suppose it was the fifth highest magnitude correlate in the first case, but the sixth highest magnitude correlate in the second case. That would produce a result where it was returned in the first result, but not the second. Moreover, the correlations between pairs from different data sets do not necessarily have to be different at all in order to achieve a different ranking (other correlations could change to outrank them). Finally, the fifth highest-ranking correlation might not be statistically different from the sixth highest-ranking correlation, so even the ordering may be arbitrary. The possibility of such arbitrary differences between correlation networks sharply limits their usefulness for making inferences about differential wiring.

To address the need to support inferences about differential wiring, the HeatSeeker module was created to augment StarNet. To perform HeatSeeker analysis, the user first performs a parallel StarNet analysis with two data sets as described above, and then clicks on the "HeatSeeker" button that appears on the results page below the correlation networks (Fig. 3). Briefly, HeatSeeker combines the lists of genes resulting from two parallel StarNet analyses to make a superset of the two lists, where each member of the list has an ortholog in the other species and is covered by the parallel platform (if the networks are derived from different platforms). The original data are then used to compute a complete correlation matrix of the superset for each platform. The results are viewed using false color maps, where white indicates a correlation of one and darker colors (red or blue) indicate lower correlations.

The data are organized by pattern using hierarchical clustering. In the first series of graphs, hierarchical clustering is performed on the first data set correlation matrix, and the second data set correlation matrix is reordered according to this clustering. Then the difference is taken between the reordered first and second correlation matrices, and this is also shown as a false color map (Fig. 3, lower panel, upper row of false color images). In the second series of graphs, hierarchical clustering is performed on the second data set correlation matrix, and the first data set correlation matrix is reordered according to this clustering. As with the first series of graphs, the difference between the two matrices is taken and shown as a false color map (Fig. 3, lower panel, lower row of false color images). Tabular HeatSeeker data are also available for download, and the tabular data indicate all statistically significant differences between the two superset correlation matrices.

3.5. Conclusion

StarNet is a free web-based tool for visually mining coexpression data across ten different species. The correlations are derived from numerous microarray experiments covering a variety of tissues and different experimental conditions. The powerful visual data mining enabled by StarNet provides a highly cost-efficient way for investigators to develop new hypotheses by leveraging existing data to intuitively aid their expert judgment.

4. Notes

1. Edges in the correlation network produced by StarNet only represent the highest magnitude correlations for a gene and do not imply any direct functional association. We leave it to the investigator to judge whether specific edges or comembership in a particular correlation network is useful for predicting functional associations. Automated queries of a database of documented biomolecular interactions and automated assessment of Gene Ontology enrichment are provided to assist the investigator's judgment in the formation of new hypotheses for setting research priorities.
2. Although StarNet has general applicability across numerous tissues for each of the organisms represented, several of the data sets were created to focus on cardiac development research. For four organisms (human, mouse, rat, and *Drosophila*), there were enough developmental samples available in the selected full cohort of data to create a subset of developmental samples.
3. We have found on anecdotal basis that the full data cohort often produces stronger GO enrichments for gene queries on known cardiac development genes than the corresponding

developmental data. This result may be surprising, as one might expect the developmental data cohort to be better suited for identifying functional associations related to development. There are different possible explanations for this type of occurrence, and we have not yet made a systematic effort to determine the best explanations. Here are two competing explanations we are currently considering: (1) The lower magnitude correlations between developmentally related genes in the developmental data cohort may be spurious and may be simply explained by the lower number of samples in this data subset, and (2) the lower magnitude correlations between developmentally related genes in the developmental data cohort may be expected, as conditioning on the factor "developmental sample" will have the effect of lowering the rank of correlations between "developmental" genes. Recall that StarNet returns a graph of the highest magnitude correlations, so that although the magnitude of correlation for a pair of genes may not be very different between the two data sets, in one graph the pairing may be absent due to an increase in magnitude of another gene pair that arises due to the conditioning on developmental samples. Correlations that increase in magnitude (in the developmental data cohort) for gene pairs not previously characterized as "developmental" genes may thus advance ahead of developmental genes in the ranking of correlations, which could then replace them in the resulting graph. If this second explanation is correct, it suggests that gene pairs that improve in their correlation ranking for the developmental data cohort may have a developmental functional association that was previously uncharacterized because it is more subtle than the associations previously characterized. It is thus reasonable that the developmental data cohort yields correlation data that offer a higher level of resolution for assessing functional associations related to development, and that StarNet analysis with this data set could uncover subtle associations that have not been previously characterized. This idea is consistent with the logic of statistical conditioning, but remains to be shown with systematic analysis and experimental validation.

Acknowledgments

This work was supported by a National Scientist Development Grant from the American Heart Association (AHA SDG 0630263N, PI: VanBuren) and by start-up funds from the Dean of the College of Medicine and the Department of Systems Biology and Translational Medicine, Texas A&M Health Science Center (PI: VanBuren).

References

1. Cohen, J. (1994) The Earth Is Round (p < .05), *American Psychologist* **49**, 997–1003.
2. Abelson, R. P. (1995) *Statistics as Principled Argument*, Psychology Press, New York.
3. Jupiter, D., Chen, H., and VanBuren, V. (2009) STARNET 2: a web-based tool for accelerating discovery of gene regulatory networks using microarray co-expression data, *BMC Bioinformatics* **10**, 332.
4. Jupiter, D. C., and VanBuren, V. (2008) A visual data mining tool that facilitates reconstruction of transcription regulatory networks, *PLoS One* **3**, e1717.
5. Irizarry, R. A., Hobbs, B., Collin, F., Beazer-Barclay, Y. D., Antonellis, K. J., Scherf, U., and Speed, T. P. (2003) Exploration, normalization, and summaries of high density oligonucleotide array probe level data, *Biostatistics* **4**, 249–264.
6. Willis, R. C., and Hogue, C. W. (2006) Searching, viewing, and visualizing data in the Biomolecular Interaction Network Database (BIND), *Curr Protoc Bioinformatics* **Chapter 8**, Unit 8 9.
7. Breitkreutz, B. J., Stark, C., Reguly, T., Boucher, L., Breitkreutz, A., Livstone, M., Oughtred, R., Lackner, D. H., Bahler, J., Wood, V., Dolinski, K., and Tyers, M. (2008) The BioGRID Interaction Database: 2008 update, *Nucleic Acids Res* **36**, D637–640.
8. Keshava Prasad, T. S., Goel, R., Kandasamy, K., Keerthikumar, S., Kumar, S., Mathivanan, S., Telikicherla, D., Raju, R., Shafreen, B., Venugopal, A., Balakrishnan, L., Marimuthu, A., Banerjee, S., Somanathan, D. S., Sebastian, A., Rani, S., Ray, S., Harrys Kishore, C. J., Kanth, S., Ahmed, M., Kashyap, M. K., Mohmood, R., Ramachandra, Y. L., Krishna, V., Rahiman, B. A., Mohan, S., Ranganathan, P., Ramabadran, S., Chaerkady, R., and Pandey, A. (2009) Human Protein Reference Database–2009 update, *Nucleic Acids Res* **37**, D767–772.
9. Keseler, I. M., Bonavides-Martinez, C., Collado-Vides, J., Gama-Castro, S., Gunsalus, R. P., Johnson, D. A., Krummenacker, M., Nolan, L. M., Paley, S., Paulsen, I. T., Peralta-Gil, M., Santos-Zavaleta, A., Shearer, A. G., and Karp, P. D. (2009) EcoCyc: a comprehensive view of Escherichia coli biology, *Nucleic Acids Res* **37**, D464–470.
10. Ashburner, M., Ball, C. A., Blake, J. A., Botstein, D., Butler, H., Cherry, J. M., Davis, A. P., Dolinski, K., Dwight, S. S., Eppig, J. T., Harris, M. A., Hill, D. P., Issel-Tarver, L., Kasarskis, A., Lewis, S., Matese, J. C., Richardson, J. E., Ringwald, M., Rubin, G. M., and Sherlock, G. (2000) Gene ontology: tool for the unification of biology. The Gene Ontology Consortium, *Nat Genet* **25**, 25–29.
11. Rivals, I., Personnaz, L., Taing, L., and Potier, M. C. (2007) Enrichment or depletion of a GO category within a class of genes: which test? *Bioinformatics* **23**, 401–407.
12. Pollard, P., and Richardson, J. T. E. (1987) On the probability of Making Type I Errors, *Psychological Bulletin* **102**, 159–163.

Chapter 26

High-Speed Confocal Imaging of Zebrafish Heart Development

Jay R. Hove and Michael P. Craig

Abstract

Due to its optical clarity and rudimentary heart structure (i.e., single atrium and ventricle), the zebrafish provides an excellent model for studying the genetic, morphological, and functional basis of normal and pathophysiological heart development in vivo. Recent advances in high-speed confocal imaging have made it possible to capture 2D zebrafish heart wall motions with temporal and spatial resolutions sufficient to characterize the highly dynamic intravital flow-structure environment. We have optimized protocols for introducing fluorescent tracer particles into the zebrafish cardiovasculature, imaging intravital heart wall motion, and performing high-resolution blood flow mapping that will be broadly useful in elucidating flow-structure relationships.

Key words: High-speed confocal microscopy, CLSM, *Danio rerio*, Velocimetry, PTV, PIV, Shear

1. Introduction

The developing heart undergoes a series of dramatic structural changes as it transforms from a primordial tube to a valveless unidirectional pump, and finally to its mature valved conformation. A combination of genetically preprogrammed signals and fluid forces undoubtedly drive these conformational changes, but the contextual cues (i.e., pressure thresholds, bed resistance, etc.) that trigger specific events are not well understood. High-speed confocal laser scanning microscopy (CLSM) is being used to gain insight into the forces, both genetic and physical, that shape cardiac development and disease. CLSM studies utilizing heart-specific transgenic and mutant zebrafish have already revealed that early heart tube blood flow results not from peristalsis but from suction due to elastic wave propagation stemming from the naturally occurring heterogeneity in vascular wall compliance (1). Additionally, CLSM studies

Xu Peng and Marc Antonyak (eds.), *Cardiovascular Development: Methods and Protocols*,
Methods in Molecular Biology, vol. 843, DOI 10.1007/978-1-61779-523-7_26,

have identified that only the caudal and medial cardiomyocytes are active in the developing heart tube (2). An off-axis image acquisition version of CLSM called selective plane illumination microscopy (SPIM) has been used to show that atrioventricular valve leaflets form through a process of invagination and not through a transient endocardial cushion structure (3). This technology is not commercially available and will not be addressed further herein as the approach is not widely available to the scientific community. Instead we will focus on confocal imaging, in its many forms, as it is the imaging tool for advancing our understanding of the highly dynamic intravital flow-structure environment that drives complex cardiac developmental processes.

Moving beyond the historical limitations of visualizing largely static structures, we have pioneered protocols for introducing fluorescent tracer particles into the zebrafish cardiovasculature, imaging intravital heart wall motion (1), and performing high-resolution blood flow mapping. Combined with a range of available mutant and transgenic animals, these tools are proving to be invaluable in facilitating a more "systems biology" approach for understanding the many genetic and mechanical factors that guide heart development.

2. Materials

2.1. Embryo Mounting and Anesthesia

1. Wild-type, mutant, transgenic, or morphant zebrafish to be imaged. Most broadly useful are the tie2:GFP, fli:GFP, and flk:GFP available from ZFIN (Eugene, OR) which have fluorescent heart valves, vascular endothelia, and angioblasts, respectively.
2. E3 egg medium (60×): 300 mM NaCl, 10.2 mM KCl, 19.8 mM $CaCl_2$, 19.8 mM $MgCl_2$ (4). Adjust pH to mirror the water pH for the adult breeding population (typically pH 7.0–7.8). Refrigerate at 4–8°C. Add 10^{-5}% methylene blue (Fisher Scientific, Waltham, MA) to 1× E3 egg medium if fungal growth is observed.
3. Diurnal Incubator (VWR, West Chester, PA) (see Note 1).
4. Prefabricated glass-bottom 35 × 10 mm petri dishes (Mat Tek Corporation, Homer Avenue, Ashland) (see Note 2, Fig. 1a).
5. 1.2% agarose (type IX ultra-low gelling temperature, Sigma-Aldrich, St. Louis, MO) prepared in E3 egg medium (see Note 3). Apply an overlay of E3 to leftover solid agarose to keep agarose moist for extended refrigerated storage (not to exceed 3 months).
6. 0.4% (4 mg/mL) phosphate buffered stock solution of Tricaine anesthetic (ethyl 3-aminobenzoate methanesulfonate salt, Sigma-Aldrich) prepared in double-distilled water with 1% dibasic sodium phosphate (350 mM) (see Note 4). Dilute 1:20

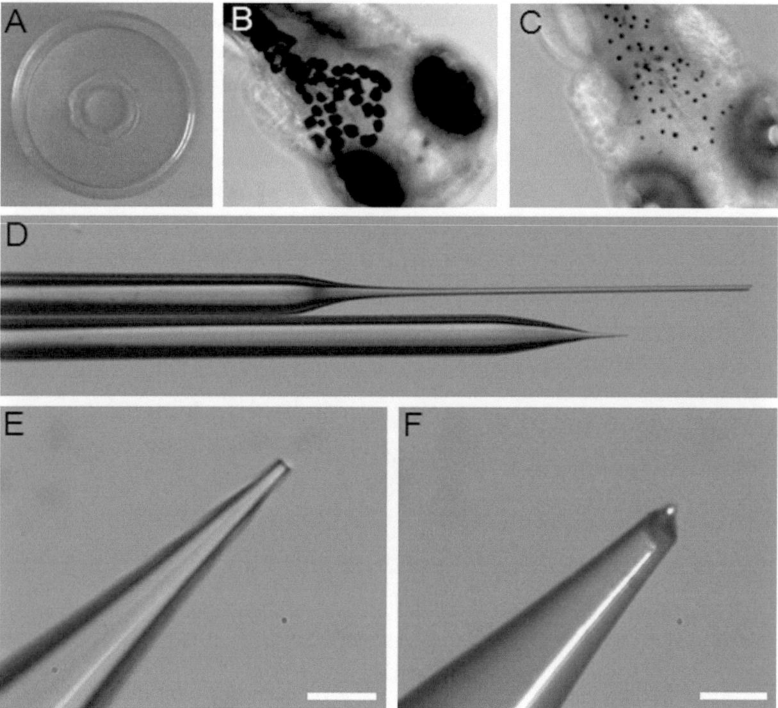

Fig. 1. Setup. (**a**) Lab-fabricated glass-bottom petri dish. (**b**) Normally pigmented 5-dpf wild-type zebrafish and (**c**) an animal from the same clutch treated with 0.003% PTU treatment to block pigment formation. (**d**) Standard injection pipettes for aqueous solution (*top*) and microsphere injections (*bottom*). (**e**) Unbeveled borosilicate tip and (**f**) beveled tip for deep-tissue microinjection. (*Scale bars* indicate 10 μm).

to 1:100 and adjust the pH to between 7.0 and 7.5 for use. Store refrigerated in an amber glass bottle for up to 3 months. Aliquot the 0.4% stock for long-term frozen storage (–20°C).

7. 1-Phenyl-2-thiourea (PTU, Sigma-Aldrich) 10× stock at a concentration of 0.03% in egg water.
8. Fine-point forceps (e.g., Dumont #5).
9. Dissecting stereomicroscope for observing mounting orientation and embryo placement.

2.2. Microinjection Needle Preparation

1. Micropipette puller (e.g., horizontal laser puller model S-2000, Sutter Instruments, Novato, CA) for pipette fabrication (see Note 5). Horizontal or vertical-style pullers may be used (as available).
2. Pressure microinjector (e.g., Harvard Apparatus, Holliston, MA) (see Note 6).

2.3. Tracer Particle Microinjection for Blood Flow Mapping

1. Light mineral oil for calibration of injection volume.
2. 34-gauge MicroFil needles for backfilling microinjection pipettes (optional) (World Precision Instruments, Sarasota, FL).

3. Pipette beveler (e.g., BV-10, Sutter Instruments) for micropipette beveling to facilitate microinjections in fish over 3 weeks of age (see Note 7).
4. 1 mm OD, 0.58 mm ID borosilicate glass tubing (World Precision Instruments). Other glass types and dimensions may be utilized to meet specific project requirements.
5. Danieau buffer for dilution of microspheres. Prepare Danieau buffer (58 mM NaCl, 0.7 mM KCl, 0.4 mM $MgSO_4$, 0.6 mM $Ca(NO_3)_2$, 5.0 mM HEPES, pH 7.1–7.3) as a 50× refrigerated stock solution (4).
6. Upright widefield fluorescence microscope for performing microinjections (see Note 8).
7. 3-axis, Huxley-type high-resolution micromanipulator (e.g., MP-85, Sutter Instruments) (see Note 9).
8. Fluorescent carboxylated microspheres (0.02 μm for angiographic structural mapping, 0.2–1.0 μm for blood flow mapping) (see Note 10).
9. Bath sonicator (e.g., model 2510, Branson Ultrasonic Corporation, Danbury, CT).

2.4. High-Speed Confocal Imaging of the Zebrafish Heart

1. Inverted fluorescence microscope (preferred) or an upright microscope with dipping objectives (see Note 11). Imaging midline structures in the embryonic zebrafish (i.e., vasculature) at or near the working distance of the objective raises the risk that the objective will compress the fish body and disrupt normal physiology.
2. Temperature control unit set at desired experimental temperature (usually near 28.5°C) (see Note 12).
3. High numerical aperture 25, 40, or 63× water-immersion objectives (see Note 13).
4. High-speed confocal scanner capable of 30 full frames per second (fps) or greater (see Note 14). This includes spinning disc, line-scanning, and other resonant scanning confocal systems.
5. Immersion medium appropriate for the objective used.

2.5. Angiography

1. Side- or back-mounted embryos.
2. 0.02 μm carboxylate-modified red fluorescent (580 nm λ_{EX}, 605 nm λ_{EM}) diluted 1:10 for a final 0.2% working dilution of microspheres (see Note 15).

2.6. 3D Imaging of Heart Wall Motions

1. Fli:GFP or Flk:GFP embryos mounted in agarose.
2. A confocal system capable of greater than ten times the heart rate of the fish (e.g., 30 fps for a 3 Hz heart beat) (see Note 16).

2.7. Negative-contrast Particle Tracking Velocimetry

1. Bodipy-FL C5-Ceramide (Invitrogen) diluted to 0.001% (10 μg/mL) in 2% DMSO, aliquoted into 50–100 μL volumes, and stored at −20°C.
2. Tracking software such as ImageJ (open-source, US National Institutes of Health, Bethesda, MD), Improvision Volocity (PerkinElmer, Waltham, MA), Metamorph (Molecular Devices, Sunnyvale, CA), or Bitplane with the Imaris Match subsystem (Bitplane Scientific Software, Geneva, Switzerland). While these are the most commonly used packages in confocal microscopy applications, others specific to the biofluidics discipline are acceptable.

2.8. Microsphere-Based PTV

1. Fluorescent carboxylated microspheres with a diameter of 0.2–1.0 μm and any of the software packages listed above.

2.9. Digital Particle Image Velocimetry

1. Fluorescent carboxylated microspheres, 0.02-μm diameter.
2. Pixel Flow (PixelFlow, General Pixels Inc., Arcadia, CA) software.

2.10. Image Analysis

1. The selection of software for image processing and analysis is application-specific and will be left to the discretion of the end-user. (Note: Analysis methodologies are not addressed in Subheading 3 that follows). The following list of useful utilities and software packages is by no means comprehensive, but simply represents a suite of tools that have proven indispensible in handling the large data files typical of high-speed imaging applications (see Note 17):
   (a) File conversion freeware or shareware utilities: Image J, VLC Media Player, Bink, and Smacker.
   (b) Intensity measurement, particle tracking, and image segmentation: Improvision Volocity, Metamorph, Bitplane, and Image-Quant.
   (c) Fluid dynamics analysis software: PixelFlow (no longer commercially available), URAPIV, PyPIV, JPIV, OSIV, and Gpiv.
   (d) Statistical and Mathematical Analysis: TecPlot, MatLab.

3. Methods

3.1. Embryo Mounting and Anesthesia

1. Normally pigmented zebrafish lines older than 5 days of fertilization (dpf) require the addition of PTU to the egg medium to block pigmentation. Add 0.003% PTU (1:10 of the prepared stock) during the first day of age to facilitate unimpeded optical access to the heart and vasculature. Preference should be given to lowly pigmented lines such as *casper*, *albino*, or *blingless* to

circumvent the need for chemical melanophore and iridophore inhibition (Fig. 1b, c).

2. Mount up to four embryos per petri dish keeping experimental and control animals mounted side-by-side (as accommodated by the experimental design) (see Note 18).
3. Place embryos in the center well of a glass-bottom petri dish using a 3-mL transfer pipette.
4. Discard water overlay from 1.2% agarose stock (if present) and heat in the microwave until melted but not boiling.
5. Prepare a mix of agarose and MS-222 to 0.01–0.02% (a 1:20–1:40 dilution of the stock). A 125 mg/L final concentration (1:32) consisting of 484 μL agarose and 16 μL of MS-222 is recommended. Pipette to mix.
6. Remove residual water from the embryos and add 80–100 μL of agarose /MS-222 mixture. The agarose mixture should just fill the depressed well of the petri dish.
7. View the suspended embryos on a dissecting stereoscope and orient them using dissecting forceps. Chill the petri dish briefly in a refrigerator or on wet ice to solidify the agarose (not to exceed 30 s). Monitor agarose gelling by dragging forceps across the mount surface. The embryonic heartbeat may slow or stop temporarily, but should recover within a minute. Chilling too long can cause a loss of peripheral flow, especially in the intersegmental vessels, or euthanize the embryos.
   (a) General imaging of heart morphology is best performed with fish mounted ventral side down and tails elevated so that the pericardium is resting against the coverglass. This orientation can be difficult to maintain since embryos tend to roll onto their sides. Alternating back and forth between briefly chilling the dish (for about 10 s at a time) and correcting fish orientation on the microscope stage provides the opportunity to tweak fish orientation before final agarose gelling.
   (b) Gross heart tube morphology and wall motion can be viewed laterally, so most imaging projects involving flow mapping during early developmental events (20–48 h post fertilization) can be performed by both microinjecting and viewing fish mounted on their sides. It is frequently necessary, however, to utilize different mounting orientations for microinjecting and imaging fish. In these instances, fish should be mounted on their sides or backs for microinjection, gently removed from the agarose mount with forceps, and remounted in an orientation that facilitates imaging.
8. Apply an overlay of embryo medium (3 mL) containing MS-222 at the same concentration used in the agarose mount to keep the mount from drying out and accelerate the acclimation of the mounted embryos to experimental temperature.

9. Place mounted embryos in an incubated chamber or on a slide warmer to maintain the desired experimental temperature. Allow the embryos to acclimate for 30 min before physiological measurements are made.

3.2. Microinjection Needle Preparation

1. Obtain glass tubing of the desired wall thicknesses (e.g., quartz, borosilicate, or aluminosilicate) with or without a filament. 1 mm OD × 0.75 mm ID borosilicate glass is recommended (see Note 19).
2. The injection site and age of the fish greatly affect the optimal tip design and puller performance varies slightly from day to day making it difficult to predict reasonable puller settings. For that reason, it is recommended that pipettes be prepared a few at a time on the day of the experiment until the right tip shape is determined.
3. Let the puller warm up for a minimum of 30 min to ensure that the instrument heating unit (laser or peltier-controlled) has stabilized for consistent tip manufacture.
4. For dye, DNA, morpholino, or other aqueous injections, microinjection pipettes should be needle-like with a 1-µm tip diameter (Fig. 1d). Filamented borosilicate glass tubing measuring 1 mm OD × 0.75 mm ID pulled on a Sutter P-2000 puller may be pulled to the desired dimensions using heat 800, pull 30, filament 4, velocity 120, and delay 210.
5. Microsphere injections performed during flow mapping or angiography applications are best performed using pipettes with a slightly shorter taper and a larger (2–4 µm) tip diameter. Suitable injection needle may be prepared using filamented borosilicate glass tubing measuring 1 mm OD × 0.75 mm ID pulled on a Sutter P-2000 puller using heat 340, pull 0, filament 4, velocity 32, and delay 200. The resulting tip ID of approximately 3 µm works well for injection of microspheres up to 0.5 µm in diameter. Injecting larger microspheres requires larger tip diameters of around 4–5 µm which can be obtained by decreasing HEAT to 280.
6. Pipette beveling is beneficial when injecting fish older than a month of age or when attempting to access deep-tissue injection sites (e.g., the primordial hindbrain channel or the basilar artery). Grind tips to a 30° bevel according to manufacturer guidelines. Beveling progress is monitored either by changes in tip resistance or optically with an 80–100× magnification microscope attachment. Grinding typically takes less than 30 s per borosilicate tip using a fine grit diamond abrasive plate.

3.3. Tracer Particle Microinjection for Blood Flow Mapping

1. Most microsphere stocks are provided in suspensions of 2% solids. A tenfold dilution of this stock is sufficient to minimize injection pipette clogging and maximize the number of particles

introduced into the bloodstream. Adjust the dilution as needed to fulfill experimental needs.

2. Sonicate diluted microsphere suspensions for 5–10 min prior to each injection session. Centrifuge the sonicated suspension at 12,000 × *g* for 2 min to remove large particulates or nondispersed clumps of microspheres (see Note 20).
3. Perform microinjections on an upright microscope with a stand-mounted high-resolution micromanipulator. Alternatively, inverted microscopes and basic micromanipulator models may be used. The following description assumes optimal equipment availability.
4. Fill the microinjection pipette by vacuum suction through the tip as follows (see Note 21): Deliver a pressure pulse to clear tip debris picked up in handling. Submerge the tip in the sonicated bead suspension and apply a short (1 s) vacuum in short (1 s) pulses until about 15–20 μL of solution enters the tip. Note: The rate of tip filling can be used as a crude metric of expected tip performance. Broken tips that fill too quickly or tips that are too small or clogged that don't fill should be discarded.
5. Set the microinjection pressure between 2 and 4 psi. The balance pressure should be 0.2–0.4 psi to prevent suction of liquid into the tip or premature expulsion of pipette contents. Injection duration should be approximately 50 ms. Caution: Any change to injection pressure or duration alters the volume delivered. If these values are changed, a follow-up measure of injected volume should be performed.
6. Perform micropipette volume measurement by injecting a series of 10–15 boluses into a capillary glass tube of known internal diameter (see Note 22). The height of the filled portion of the capillary tube is measured to calculate the total contained volume ($\pi r^2 h$). This volume is divided by the number of boluses to obtain the volume of a single-injection bolus.
7. Select an injection target location. Injections into the bloodstream of fish younger than 2 dpf may be made directly into the confluence of blood flow over the yolk. The posterior cardinal vein and dorsal aorta are optimal for fish between 2 and 5 dpf. The common collecting duct is preferred after 5 dpf and through the first month of development. The common collecting duct is accessed through the developing gill slit (just anterior to the cleithrum) by placing the tip just inside the gill operculum and moving it toward the tail (forcing the operculum backward) so that it is directly over the common collecting duct.
8. Place the fish to be injected on the microscope stage and center the injection target in the field of view.
9. Position the loaded pipette near the fish body while under low magnification. Gradually increase magnification as needed as

the tip is moved closer to the target injection site. Advance the injection pipette through the body wall and into the target vessel. Final tip placement performed under fluorescent illumination allows visualization of the influx of red blood cells that frequently occurs when the tip enters the target vessel. (This event is difficult to discern under brightfield illumination).

10. Inject the first bolus of tracer particles at a low starting injection pressure (2–4 psi). If the tip appears plugged as a result of transit through the body wall, withdraw and reinsert the tip to try and clear debris.
11. A clog caused by a mass of microspheres is viewed as a brightly fluorescent tip. These clogs frequently require discarding the pipette and loading of a new one. Withdrawing the tip from the petri dish completely and pressing the "eject" button clears a small portion of these clogs to salvage the tips for another attempt.
12. Once fluorescent uptake into the blood is observed, continue injecting the desired number of boluses at a rate of approximately one every 10 s. Observations of gross blood flow patterns should be used as a guide for injection volume and frequency to verify that the injection parameters are appropriate. Too much injection volume administered too quickly causes immediate hypertrophy, reduced heart rate, and loss of some peripheral flow (predominantly observed in the intersegmental vessels). Microinjection of multiple 2 nL boluses (e.g., five boluses over a 1-min period) is well accommodated by 2-dpf or older fish. (The 2 nL volume is approximated by a 3 psi injection pressure using a 3-μm diameter tip and a 50 ms injection pulse).

3.4. High-Speed Confocal Imaging of the Zebrafish Heart

1. The following procedural guidelines are designed for spinning disc users since those systems are designed specifically for high-speed imaging and are widely used, although the theoretical components apply more broadly.
2. Full laser power is frequently required when recording at peak frame rates, so age-related declines in laser performance directly impact the maximum achievable frame rate of these systems. A starting laser output reference measurement and annual follow-up measurements are recommended.
3. Equilibrate gas diode lasers and environmental controls (e.g., stage and objective heaters or incubation chambers) for at least 15 min prior to imaging.
4. Capture periodic motions such as a heartbeat or opening and closing of a heart valve at ten times per event (e.g., 30 fps for a 3 Hz heart beat). Increase acquisition rates for more complex or bimodal motions (see Note 23).
5. Position the mounted fish using brightfield illumination and bring the imaging target into view at the desired magnification.

A 63×/1.2 water-immersion objective is suitable for most heart imaging.

6. Configure the imaging channel(s) according to the selected fluorophore(s). Spinning disc confocals have internal software controlled excitation and emission filters.
7. The theoretical axial resolution limit is given by 0.61 λ/NA. For a 63×/N.A.1.2 water-immersion objective used to image EGFP samples with a 509 nm emission, this corresponds to 0.25 µm. This axial resolution is suitable to resolve the 0.2-µm diameter fluorospheres used in digital particle image velocimetry (DPIV) flow mapping with near-pixel resolution. The axial (z) resolution given by λ_n/NA^2 would be approximately 0.47 µm, but is somewhat less due to a slight mismatch between objective magnification and the fixed pinhole size. (The Yokogawa spinning disc systems have pinholes set to 1.0 Airy unit for a 100×/NA 1.4 objective). These resolution limits should be kept in mind when setting z-slice thickness and frame sizes to avoid under- or over-sampling which can cause image misrepresentation or unnecessarily reduced frame rates, respectively.
8. Open the live video preview. Set the exposure time and pixel area to achieve the desired frame rate (see Note 24). Binning may be required for high frame rate acquisitions.
9. Adjust the gain, binning, and offset levels to maximize usage of the camera's dynamic range while keeping sufficient resolution to see the imaging target. Open the image histogram for the live image stream and select an intensity-coded heat map preview. Adjust the offset to bring the minimum pixel intensity near the absolute black (0 pixel intensity) level. Adjust the gain upward until the peak intensity value is near to the absolute white or maximum intensity level (see Note 25). Repeat these adjustments until both intensity limits are achieved.
10. If the fluorescent signal is too weak even with moderate gain, set the binning to 2 × 2 or greater to increase signal intensity. This pixel averaging results in a corresponding loss of image resolution.
11. Alternatively, the frame rate may be reduced slightly in order to increase signal intensity without the need for binning-related loss of resolution. In these instances, a brief time-series acquisition should be captured to verify that the reduced temporal resolution has not caused too much blurring or streaking of heart wall borders.
12. Important: Acquire all images in a data set using the same acquisition parameters, especially if between group differences are being measured. Setting the acquisition parameters using the brightest sample is recommended to avoid pixel saturation.

13. Capture three or more motion periods (e.g., heartbeats) as a time-series of tiffs. Save data for later processing. Record all pertinent experimental parameters prior to saving so that this information is incorporated into the file metadata.
14. Export files as lossless tiffs if external data analysis is required.

3.5. Angiography

1. Inject fliGFP or flkGFP embryos with 0.02 μm carboxylate-modified red fluorescent (580 nm λ_{EX}, 605 nm λ_{EM}) from a diluted 0.2% working dilution of microspheres as described previously. Injected microspheres remain in circulation for several hours.
2. Performed whole body imaging (if needed) using an acquisition software tiling algorithm to together stitch multiple image z-stacks.
3. Two-channel (red/green) imaging highlights vessels that have no luminal blood flow (showing up as green only) and helps to better define the exact vessel wall location (defined as the red/green fluorescent border) (see Note 26).

3.6. 3D Imaging of Heart Wall Motions

1. Volumetric heart imaging may be accomplished by stitching together a series of planar or 2–3-slice time-series based on fiduciary landmark(s) or by straight volume capture (in a single x–y–t series) The former generally requires manual alignment and is tedious, time-consuming, and prone to user error (although efforts are being made to develop postacquisition synchronization algorithms for use with non-gated data (5, 6)). 3D time-series imaging utilizing spinning disc confocals is generally performed in this manner. The latter approach is more directly and readily performed using faster systems. For instance, the Zeiss 5Live is capable of 240 single image planes per second at corresponding to thirty 8-plane z-stacks per second at 256 × 512 pixel, suitable for 3D imaging of the 3 Hz heart beat in a 3–4-dpf zebrafish (see Note 27).

3.7. Negative-Contrast Particle Tracking Velocimetry

1. Particle tracking velocimetry (PTV) is an image analysis tool used to quantitatively map biofluid (e.g., blood) flow profiles by analyzing the motion of discrete particles as they move through a field of view.
2. Thaw the 0.001% Bodipy-FL C5-Ceramide stock solution and dilute 1:30 into egg water to achieve a final 0.001% Ceramide solution. Soak embryos 4 h to overnight the diluted Ceramide (see Note 28). The dye stains serum intensely leaving black RBC silhouettes that may be tracked manually or using PTV software (see Subheading 2.10, Fig. 2a).
3. Manual particle tracking can be performed in ImageJ by importing the video series and running the "Manual Tracker" add-on. Automated tracking can also be performed with the

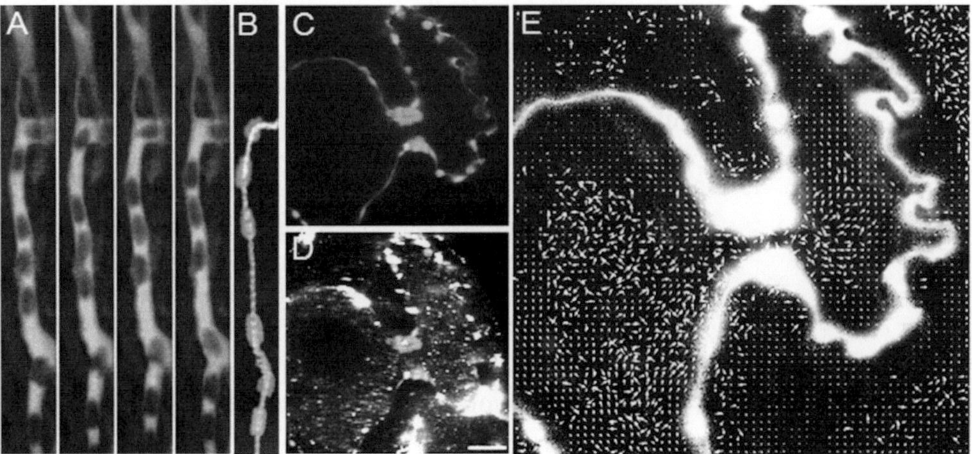

Fig. 2. High-speed confocal imaging of the zebrafish cardiovasculature. (**a**) Images of the dorsal longitudinal anastomotic vessel (DLAV) from a BODIPY-FL soaked fish video taken at 43 fps using a PerkinElmer CSU21 spinning disc confocal. RBC silhouettes used for velocity measurement are clearly evident. (**b**) Automated RBC tracking performed using intensity thresholding, shape recognition, and centroid determination performed in Improvision Volocity to obtain a 35 μm/s mean flow rate. (**c**, **d**) High-speed confocal image of a 3-dpf Fli:GFP zebrafish fluorescent heart wall acquired on a Zeiss 5Live confocal at 120 fps with a frame size of 512 × 512 (8-bit depth) acquired using a C-Apo 40×/1.20 W (**c**) and the corresponding red channel showing injected microspheres at a density of approximately 2,000 per field (**d**) (*Scale bar* indicates 15 μm). (**e**) DPIV analysis performed in Pixel Flow showing peak luminal blood flow with relatively little flow near heart walls.

"Spot Tracker" and "Particle Tracker" ImageJ algorithms. Improvision Volocity, Metamorph, and Imaris Bitplane have similar user-guided manual tracking capabilities as well as an automated tracking protocol that recognize RBC locations based on local pixel intensities derived using size and shape thresholding scripts (Fig. 2b) (7) (see Note 29).

3.8. Microsphere-Based PTV

1. Microsphere-based PTV is performed using a low to moderate seeding density of microspheres suitable for visual identification of particle locations in sequential images. To ensure accurate PTV measurements, the imaged particle diameters and corresponding seeding density should be such that the particles do not overlap. For particle diameters of 3 pixels, the optimal seeding density in a linear flow is roughly one particle per 33 pixels. This corresponds to 1,500 microspheres in the focal plane for a heart that takes up 1/5th of the image area in a 512 × 512 image series. Lower resolution PTV can, however, be performed at seeding densities down to 50 particles per image field. Inject fluorescent 0.5–1.0-μm diameter microspheres into the bloodstream as described previously.
2. With the appropriate seeding density achieved, remove the injection pipette and immediately transfer the fish to the high-speed confocal microscope for imaging. Microsphere deposition onto the vessel walls (most prominently observed in the

cardinal vein) diminishes the number of circulating particles making it necessary to move quickly from tracer injection to high-speed imaging.

3. Acquire images at a sufficient rate that each particle appears in at least three subsequent frames so that particle velocity and direction can be reliably measured. Maximizing the number of frames imaged per particle is nonetheless recommended, particularly in complex nonlinear flows (e.g., around the heart valve).
4. Utilize automated tracking algorithms per user preference.

3.9. Digital Particle Image Velocimetry

1. The DPIV approach is conceptually similar to PTV in that fluorescent markers suspended within the blood are assumed to move in a fashion representing plasma flow. However, the technique uses a higher density of smaller fluorescent microspheres (frequently referred to as "tracer particles") that are analyzed by matching up patterns in the distribution of particle clouds in one part of an image to nearby parts in the subsequent one. Unlike PTV, where individual particles are tracked, The DPIV uses interrogation windows to systematically isolate the same sub-image regions within sequential images, and performs a cross-correlation operation to obtain the average velocity vector of the groups of particles within the interrogation windows. The increased spatial resolution of DPIV makes it possible to more accurately measure relevant flow indices. Several thorough reviews of DPIV theory are available (8–11). Examples of the in vivo application of the DPIV methodology to microvessel flow mapping in the rat mesentery (12), ventricular blood flow in the embryonic chicken (13), and to the developing of zebrafish heart (14) provide a more detailed description of the approach.
2. Inject 0.1–0.5-μm fluorescent microspheres seeded at >2,000 tracers per image field. In vivo DPIV seeding densities are lower than those utilized for ex vivo applications by necessity because exceedingly high circulating tracer densities are both difficult to achieve and potentially detrimental to the animal.
3. Use specialized DPIV software to automate processing steps and assess the analysis quality. A typical analysis workflow is as follows:
   (a) *Cross-correlation*: Particle displacements between a pair of images are calculated.
   (b) *Outlier removal*: Particle displacements greater than an input threshold level (e.g., 3 pixels) are removed or corrected.
   (c) *Smoothing*: A median pixel filter is passed over the displacement data field. This removes high frequency jitter not attributed to the biofluid flow.

(d) *Window-shifting*: Initial cross-correlation particle displacements (step (a)) are used to locally displace interrogation windows, allowing for more accurate results on iterative cross-correlations passes. The displacement field is broken down into small blocks called "interrogation windows" which are compared in a manner similar to the initial cross-correlation. The comparisons are made by shifting the interrogation window across the larger image field at a rate of 1/3 its width with each move so that a high-accuracy displacement map.

(e) *Convert*: The particle displacement profiles are converted from the pixel domain to the real domain using predetermined calibration values (i.e., microns per pixel).

(f) *Vorticity calculation*: The vector data field is integrated to obtain the vorticity field associated with the vector field.

(g) *Strain rate calculation*: The vector data field is differentiated to obtain the strain rate field associated with the vector field.

4. An example of the results produced from DPIV analysis of zebrafish cardiac blood flow is shown in Fig. 2c–e.

4. Notes

1. Diurnal plant growth incubators provide reliable temperature control in near ambient conditions. The added diurnal lighting functionality makes it possible to more closely mirror natural cyclic lighting patterns. (This is particularly useful for behavioral studies such as the development of cardiovascular disease in response to alterations of circadian rhythms).
2. Alternatively, glass-bottom dishes may be prepared using: 12-mm circular number 1.5 (0.16–0.19 mm) cover glass (Fisher Scientific), clear marine silicone (Starbright, Fort Lauderdale, Florida), and standard 35 × 10 mm petri dishes (Fisher Scientific). Prepare dishes in an "assembly-line" fashion using a drill press and a backstop and a scrap wood blank (to minimize cracking of plastic during drill-through). Drill 11/32nd in. holes through the center of the petri dish bottoms using a high-speed steel drill bit (with dish upright). Smooth the rough edges lightly with emery cloth. Apply a small bead of silicone to the bottom side of the drilled holes using a large-gauge needle and a syringe filled with marine silicone. Do not get silicone on the center of the coverglass as this will interfere with imaging later. Firmly press the coverglass slides over the hole so that the edges seal completely and the coverglass is pressed firmly into the silicone and flat against the plastic dish. Allow dishes to dry overnight and rinse before use.

3. Small batches of approximately 20 mL are preferred to minimize the number of times the solid agarose is melted (by microwaving just to boiling in a 1,000 W microwave at full power for 10–15 s).
4. While commercial injection needles are available making access to a micropipette puller optional, the ability to tailor tip shapes and diameters to the age of the fish and the site of injection improves the quality and reproducibility of microinjection. Pipette tip "sagging" is not observed with horizontal pullers at the relatively large pipette tip diameters (2–4 μm internal diameter) used for tracer microinjections.
5. An injector capable of vacuum generation is useful for unclogging pipette tips during microinjection, but vacuum capability is not required. Positive pressure microinjector capable of delivering milliscecond long pulses at 2–10 psi will suffice.
6. Pipette beveling is generally not required for cardiovascular injections in embryonic or early larval zebrafish.
7. Injections may be performed on virtually any microscope irrespective of configuration, including upright or inverted styles and those with or without fluorescent capability. The optimal approach is to use an upright microscope which provides a direct view of the injection site combined with fluorescent illumination as a means of immediately verifying injection quality. Viewing pipette positioning *through* the fish body on an inverted microscope does work, particularly for tail vein injections into young embryos, but the utility of this approach diminishes quickly as the fish becomes more opaque and pigmented as it develops. A microscope with continuous zoom is beneficial when practicing tip placement so that the user can follow needle position without changing microscope objectives and risking tip breakage.
8. Larger-body micromanipulators with an extended range of motion are preferred to minimize tip vibration for stable remote access to the usually crowded sample viewing area. Small, postmounted manual manipulators flex more during tip placement and are recommended for use only with motorized control.
9. Carboxylated polystyrene fluorescent microspheres have a density of 1.05 g/mL, close to that of red blood cells (1.10 g/mL) and human serum (1.025 g/mL). These neutrally buoyant particles are of the proper size and density needed to accurately follow the microscale blood flow patterns through the zebrafish cardiovasculature. The carboxyl groups confer a net negative surface charge of 0.1 and 2.0 mEq/g and reduce binding to the negatively charged vessel wall proteins (15). The authors have observed no reduction in nonspecific binding to vessel walls with the addition of bovine serum albumin.

10. High contrast polystyrene microspheres may be used for crude bright-field flow mapping if a brightfield high-speed CMOS camera is available. This approach underestimates luminal fluid velocity somewhat because the slower near-wall tracer particles are included in the image field. A confocal approach is preferred because optical sectioning allows the user to more accurately measure how far particles are from the heart or vessel wall.
11. Imaging midline structures in the embryonic zebrafish (i.e., vasculature) at or near the working distance of the objective raises the risk that the objective will compress the fish body and disrupt normal physiology.
12. As ectotherms, many aspects of zebrafish physiology (such as core body temperature, heart rate, and blood velocity) are strongly influenced by the environment making stringent environmental control more important for these animals. A full environmental chamber that encloses the entire microscope stage and objective turret is preferred to minimize heat loss to the stage insert and objectives. If this is not available, then a stage and objective heater provide adequate temperature control.
13. Samples viewed under physiological medium or water (such as zebrafish embryos) are best viewed with objectives designed to accommodate refractive-index mismatches in the light path. Water-immersion objectives minimize the diffractive errors introduced at the refractive-index interfaces (e.g., air to glass, glass to water) that normally reduce the effective numerical aperture and introduce optical aberrations that reduce image quality, particularly as one moves deeper into the sample. The use of long working-distance water-immersion objectives, therefore, helps to maximize image quality in thick samples like the zebrafish heart and cardiovascular bed.
14. A variety of options are available for high-speed confocal imaging including Nipkow spinning disc scanners (e.g., Yokogawa CSU22), hybrid resonant point-scanner confocals (e.g., Nikon A1R or Leica TCS SP5), or fast line-scan systems (e.g., Zeiss 5Live). The spinning disc systems are ideal for single- or dual-channel imaging at 30 fps (512×512 pixels) up to a maximum 120 lines per second. The fixed-pinhole design results in a fixed "confocality" that works best when samples are brightly fluorescent. (Other systems allow the user to open the pinholes to increase the optical slice thickness to better handle dimly fluorescent samples). Resonant scanning systems offer additional laser line capability (up to five simultaneously imaged fluorophores for the Nikon A1R) at similar frame rates while allowing the user to adjust pinhole size in order to more effectively handle dim samples. The high-speed line-scanning Zeiss 5Live system has two single-line CCD sensors for dual-channel

acquisition at rates up to 120 fps (512 × 512 pixels) or 60,000 lines per second (1 × 512 pixels). All of these systems have sufficient temporal resolution to image heart wall motion in one optical plane or early blood flow (up to approximately 5 dpf depending on the vessel being imaged). Blood flow mapping, particularly in the heart and aortic outflow tract and/or at later developmental stages (>5 dpf), requires frame rates best accommodated by the most modern line-scanning systems.

15. Microspheres with different fluorescence spectra may be utilized as needed to match the available confocal laser lines.

16. There are two approaches to volumetric heart wall imaging, the application of which is based on the age of fish being imaged and on the maximal confocal acquisition rate. Most systems (including spinning disc systems) are capable of 2D, planar image capture at the needed frame rates. Volumetric imaging on these systems is accomplished by capturing a group of planar or 2–3-slice multiplane time-series. Individual time-series clips are then manually aligned using image landmarks as fiduciary references. This alignment is tedious, time-consuming, and prone to user error. A more direct approach is to utilize confocal capable of higher speed acquisition. The Zeiss 5Live confocal is capable of capturing 240 single image planes per second at 256 × 512 pixels, or thirty 8-plane z-stacks per second, suitable for 3D imaging of the 3 Hz heart beat in a 3–4-dpf zebrafish. The 3D reconstructions require a progressively larger time-shift as one moves down through the z-stack of images.

17. Open-source and freeware/shareware utilities provide virtually all of the functionality provided by the commercial software options, but require greater user input and (frequently) substantial programming knowledge.

18. Diffusive oxygen transport and the residual yolk material accommodate the metabolic needs of the embryos during the first 4 dpf, making it possible to perform time-lapse imaging experiments throughout this period without removing embryos from their mounts. It is good practice, however, to remove embryos from their mounts between imaging sessions whenever possible so that normal rearing and physiology predominate. Animals older than 6 dpf should not be held in a full agarose mount longer than necessary because diffusive oxygen transport alone is insufficient. Fish older than 6 dpf can be maintained in agarose by preparing the mounts as described below and cutting away the portion of the mount around the developing gills and mouth.

19. Aluminosilicate glass is generally too flexible for most embryo microinjections, but it may be useful for early stage (0–1 dpf) microinjections or injections directly into the pericardium. Borosilicate tubing is the most broadly applicable

because it is rigid enough to access almost all zebrafish injection targets. Quartz tubing is brittle resulting in a higher breakage rate than borosilicate. Filamented tubing may be useful for straight aqueous injections, but the authors have no empirical evidence to suggest that filamented glass reduces tip clogging for large particle suspensions such as fluorescent microspheres.

20. Centrifugation is beneficial for preparing microspheres suspensions with very small (<0.1-μm diameter) microspheres frequently used for angiography, and is not particularly useful for larger particles.

21. Vacuum filling is preferred if an injector system with a vacuum fill option is available since vacuum filling reduces clogging by dispersing debris in the tip. If a vacuum-enabled microinjector is not available, syringe MicroFil needles can be used to fill the pipette from inside near the tip. This approach requires care be taken to avoid air bubbles in the pipette tip. (A 25× jeweler's loop magnifier is particularly useful in verifying no air bubbles are present). Again, broken tips that eject fluid as they are inserted into the holder should be discarded.

22. An alternative approach is based on water droplet diameters in light mineral oil: Fill a small petri dish with a small amount of light mineral oil. Inject a single bolus from the injection pipette under the oil surface. Measure the droplet diameter with a 25–63× objective under transmitted light microscopy. Use stage and eyepiece micrometers work or software-based measurement tools to calculate the volume of the spherical droplet calculated using as $4/3\pi r^2$.

23. Most spinning disc systems can accommodate full-frame imaging at rates sufficient to record single-plane (2D) recordings of zebrafish heart wall motion through 5 dpf. Blood flow mapping requires much higher frame rates.

24. Frame rate and exposure time are not the mathematical inverse of one another due to equipment latencies. The frame rate of CCD cameras typically paired with spinning disc confocal scanners is line-limited. The desired camera frame rate is achieved by reducing the number of horizontal lines. Note: If multi-channel acquisition is being performed, the single image capture time will be the sum of the two exposure times plus the equipment latency time associated with filter changes.

25. The upper intensity limit for 8-bit images is 256 levels and 4,096 for 12-bit images.

26. Microsphere injection is preferred over fluorescent dye injection since dyes slowly migrate into the interstitial space and collect in the lymphatics making it difficult to identify structures as cardiovascular or lymphatic, particularly in fliGFP fish in which both beds fluoresce.

27. Each of the z-slices captured in this manner requires a time-shift correction for each z-plane to ensure accurate 3D reconstruction.
28. The dye crosses the chorion (if present).
29. PTV may also be performed with transgenic lines with fluorescent RBCs (such as *GATA1*:GFP). This approach, while it has the benefit of being noninvasive, requires lower frame rates to adequately capture the discrete RBC fluorescence. Fluorescent RBC walls are not easily recognized by automated tracking algorithms since the ring-shaped fluorescent cell wall is more difficult to identify using segmentation algorithms than a highly contrasted closed sphere.

Acknowledgments

The author would like to thank Steven Gilday and Jian Lu for their work in developing many of the protocols described herein. This work is supported by funding from the National Institutes of Health (R01 RR023190-01).

References

1. Forouhar, A. S., Liebling, M., Hickerson, A., Nasiraei-Moghaddam, A., Tsai, H. J., Hove, J. R., Fraser, S. E., Dickinson, M. E., and Gharib, M. (2006) The embryonic vertebrate heart tube is a dynamic suction pump, *Science 312*, 751–753.
2. Auman, H. J., Coleman, H., Riley, H. E., Olale, F., Tsai, H. J., and Yelon, D. (2007) Functional modulation of cardiac form through regionally confined cell shape changes, *Plos Biology 5*, 604–615.
3. Scherz, P. J., Huisken, J., Sahai-Hernandez, P., and Stainier, D. Y. (2008) High-speed imaging of developing heart valves reveals interplay of morphogenesis and function, *Development 135*, 1179–1187.
4. (2002) Zebrafish: A practical approach, in *Zebrafish: A practical approach* (Nuesslein-Volhard, C., and Dahm, R., Eds.), pp i–303, Oxford University Press.
5. Liebling, M., Forouhar, A. S., Gharib, M., Fraser, S. E., and Dickinson, M. E. (2005) Four-dimensional cardiac imaging in living embryos via postacquisition synchronization of nongated slice sequences, *J Biomed Opt 10*, 054001.
6. Liebling, M., Forouhar, A. S., Wolleschensky, R., Zimmermann, B., Ankerhold, R., Fraser, S. E., Gharib, M., and Dickinson, M. E. (2006) Rapid three-dimensional imaging and analysis of the beating embryonic heart reveals functional changes during development, *Dev Dyn 235*, 2940–2948.
7. Lima, R., Ishikawa, T., Imai, Y., Takeda, M., Wada, S., and Yamaguchi, T. (2009) Measurement of Individual Red Blood Cell Motions Under High Hematocrit Conditions Using a Confocal Micro-PTV System, *Annals of Biomedical Engineering 37*, 1546–1559.
8. Adrian, R. J. (1991) Particle-Imaging Techniques for Experimental Fluid-Mechanics, *Annual Review of Fluid Mechanics 23*, 261–304.
9. Dabiri, D. (2006) *Cross-Correlation Digital Particle Image Velocimetry - A Review*, ABCM.
10. Gharib, M., and Dabiri, D. (2000) *An Overview of Digital Particle Image Velocimetry in Flow Visualization: Techniques and Examples*, Imperial College Press, London.
11. Westerweel, J. (1993) *Digital particle image velocimetry: theory and application.*, Delft University Press.
12. Nakano, A., Sugii, Y., Minamiyama, M., and Niimi, H. (2003) Measurement of red cell velocity in microvessels using particle image velocimetry (PIV), *Clin Hemorheol Microcirc 29*, 445–455.

13. Vennemann, P., Kiger, K. T., Lindken, R., Groenendijk, B. C., Stekelenburg-de Vos, S., ten Hagen, T. L., Ursem, N. T., Poelmann, R. E., Westerweel, J., and Hierck, B. P. (2006) In vivo micro particle image velocimetry measurements of blood-plasma in the embryonic avian heart, *J Biomech 39*, 1191–1200.

14. Ohn, J., Tsai, H. J., and Liebling, M. (2009) Joint dynamic imaging of morphogenesis and function in the developing heart, *Organogenesis 5*, 166–173.

15. Product information: Working with Fluorspheres fluorescent microspheres: properties and modifications, revised June 02, 2004., Molecular Probes, Inc.

Chapter 27

Measurement of Electrical Conduction Properties of Intact Embryonic Murine Hearts by Extracellular Microelectrode Arrays

David G. Taylor and Anupama Natarajan

Abstract

The study of the embryonic development of the cardiac conduction system and its congenital and toxicological defects requires protocols to measure electrical conduction through the myocardium. However, available methods either lack spatial information, necessitate the hearts to be sliced and mounted, or require specialized equipment. Microelectrode arrays (MEAs) are plates with embedded surface electrodes to measure localized extracellular ionic currents (field potentials) created by the depolarization and repolarization of cultured cells and tissue slices. Here we describe a protocol using MEAs to examine electrical conduction through intact and beating cultured hearts isolated from mouse embryos at 10.5 days postcoitus. This method allows measurements of conduction time, estimates of conduction velocity, atrioventricular conduction delay and block, and heart rate and rhythmicity.

Key words: Mouse, Embryo, Cardiac conduction system, Microelectrode array, Field potentials, Conduction delay, Conduction velocity

1. Introduction

Defects in the development of the cardiac electrical conduction system are under increased scrutiny in order to explain prenatal and neonatal arrhythmias, heart failure, and lethality in genetic, pharmacological, and toxicity studies (1, 2). Unfortunately, many methods currently employed to examine electrical conduction through excitable tissues are impractical for very small organs, such as the embryonic hearts of common laboratory model rodents and birds. In the embryonic mouse, intracellular electrodes are limited to three simultaneously (3). Electrocardiograms are possible with only two external electrodes (atrium and ventricle) (4, 5), but they

Xu Peng and Marc Antonyak (eds.), *Cardiovascular Development: Methods and Protocols*,
Methods in Molecular Biology, vol. 843, DOI 10.1007/978-1-61779-523-7_27,

provide no spatial data. Optical mapping of the heart surface via voltage-sensitive intracellular dyes continues to be the most prominent method, providing good-to-excellent two-dimensional spatial resolution, although a photodiode array or sensitive high-speed CCD camera is necessary for good temporal resolution (3, 6). All these techniques require specialized equipment not available to many laboratories, and some must be performed within hours of dissection due to loss of cardiac viability (5).

In vitro microelectrode arrays (MEAs) are small plates, usually glass, containing a microscopic grid of surface microelectrodes capable of multichannel recording of extracellular field potentials (FPs) (7). FPs are the result of ionic currents in the medium during cell depolarization and repolarization. MEAs are commonly used to examine electrical activity and conduction in cultured cells (8–10) and flat neural tissue slices (11). Recent studies have shown their feasibility with slices of individual adult (12, 13) and embryonic (14) rodent heart chambers, although by necessity, tissue slicing of an embryonic heart requires dismembering the heart and embedding it in a solid medium, such as agarose (13).

Here, we describe a protocol to measure electrical conduction along the surface of an unpinned, intact, and beating embryonic mouse heart using basic MEA equipment increasingly found in electrophysiology laboratories. Although the spatial resolution of MEAs is lower than that of optical mapping, extracellular field potential signals can be sampled at high speed (<0.1 ms per sample, depending upon equipment). This method allows relatively rapid measurements of conduction time, estimates of conduction velocity, atrioventricular conduction delay and block, and heart rate and rhythmicity, although many finer electrical parameters, such as action potential duration, are not always quantifiable as they are in thin, flat samples (9, 15).

The following instructions assume the isolation of murine embryos at 10.5 days postcoitus (E10.5) (35–40 somite pairs (16)), although the basic principles are applicable to other species and stages, with appropriate alterations.

2. Materials

2.1. Preparation of Microelectrode Arrays

1. Commercial MEAs with central culture chamber (ring to contain medium) (such as #200/10iR-Ti-gr, Multichannel Systems; Reutlingen, Germany). If the available MEAs do not have an attached ring, it can be made by following steps 1–5 in Subheading 3.1. Once ringed MEAs are available, begin at step 6.
2. Sylgard 184 silicone encapsulant (Dow Corning, Midland, MI) (if needed).

3. 35-mm Cell culture dish (if needed).
4. 1,000-μL Micropipette tip and razor blade (if needed).
5. 0.1% Gelatin in water (Chemicon).

2.2. Preparation of Embryonic Hearts for Conduction Analysis

1. Clean and sterilized MEAs, treated with surface adhesion substrate (e.g., gelatin).
2. Dulbecco's Modified Eagle's Medium, high glucose with 1 mM sodium pyruvate (DMEM) (Invitrogen, Carlsbad, CA).
3. Heart medium for heart culture and experiments: DMEM supplemented with 10% fetal bovine serum (Hyclone, Logan, UT), 55 μM β-mercaptoethanol, 1% 100× α-minimum nonessential amino acids, penicillin G (100,000 U/L), streptomycin (100 mg/L), and 1.75 mM additional L-glutamine (Invitrogen).
4. Small dissection dishes or 100-mm Petri dishes filled with phosphate-buffered saline (PBS) (pH = 7.4).
5. Fine dissection tools: spring scissors and 1–2 #5 or #55 forceps.
6. 1,000-μL Micropipettor with tips, set at 100 μL.
7. 1.5-mL microcentrifuge tubes.
8. Gold electronmicroscopy index grids (Electron Microscopy Sciences, Hatfield, PA). These will serve as weights to hold the hearts to the MEA surface until they adhere to the gelatin substrate. The inert gold is nontoxic to the tissue, and the grid pores allow oxygenation and medium contact. Grids may be bent into an inverted-V shape to better lie on the hearts. Do not attempt to remove them from the hearts at any time as this will tear the hearts. Grids are reusable until they become too warped to lie atop the hearts and may be cleaned by soaking in acidic 70% ethanol, followed by washing with detergent and distilled water.

2.3. Recording of Electrical Activity from Beating Embryonic Hearts

1. Heart medium (see item 3 in Subheading 2.2).
2. 1,000-μL or greater micropipettor with tips.
3. 100% Ethanol and Kimwipes.

3. Methods

3.1. Preparation of Microelectrode Arrays

1. Cut the pipettor- (wide-) end of a 1,000-μL micropipette tip to ~1.5-cm in length. Place in the center of a 35-mm cell culture dish.
2. Prepare Sylgard 184 according to manufacturer's instructions and fill area surrounding micropipette tip. Wait 10 min.
3. Heat 20 min at 80°C. This can be performed in a hybridization oven. Sylgard ring will become a soft, sticky cushion-like solid.

4. Cut dish away from Sylgard ring and remove micropipette tip from center.
5. Place Sylgard ring around electrode center of MEA. The ring will adhere to MEA with gentle pressure.
6. Gently clean MEAs with glassware detergent and distilled water or according to manufacturer's instructions.
7. Sterilize MEAs by moving MEAs to a sterile biohood while totally immersed in 70% ethanol. Air dry under biohood.
8. Gelatin-coat MEAs by filling ring with gelatin solution for a minimum of 30 min (see Note 1). Place each MEA into a separate 100-mm Petri dish.
9. Fill MEA ring with heart medium in biohood, replace Petri dish lid, and place near dissecting microscope.

3.2. Preparation of Embryonic Hearts for Conduction Analysis

1. Beginning with the embryos in a dissection or Petri dish of PBS and using asceptic techniques as described in Note 2, cut and remove a forelimb bud to better access the heart.
2. Remove the bulbous heart from the body by cutting around the dorsal side.
3. While gently holding the superficial membrane with forceps, cut and remove the membrane with minimum contact with and manipulation of the heart.
4. Using the micropipettor, gently transfer each heart to a microcentrifuge tube filled with cold DMEM and store on ice or 4°C until placement on MEA. Do not pick up the heart with forceps.
5. Using the micropipettor, transfer each heart to an MEA filled with heart medium. Using forceps or small micropipette tips, gently push the heart to settle with the flat ventral surface in contact with electrodes (i.e., outflow tract projecting upward).
6. Immerse a gold grid in 70% ethanol and dry by air and touching a kimwipe until ethanol film is absent from all grid pores.
7. Gently place the grid over the heart. Applying excessive pressure is not required for contact and can damage the heart (see Fig. 1).
8. Replace the lid on the Petri dish and place into cell culture incubator. Walk very carefully and slowly as not to disturb the heart on the electrodes.
9. Culture 12–24 h (see Note 3).
10. Each heart will lie in a different location on the electrode grid. Prior to conduction experiments, carefully place each closed Petri dish on a microscope equipped with a camera and record a photomicrograph or movie in order to correlate each MEA electrode to heart location (see Fig. 1). This alone is often sufficient

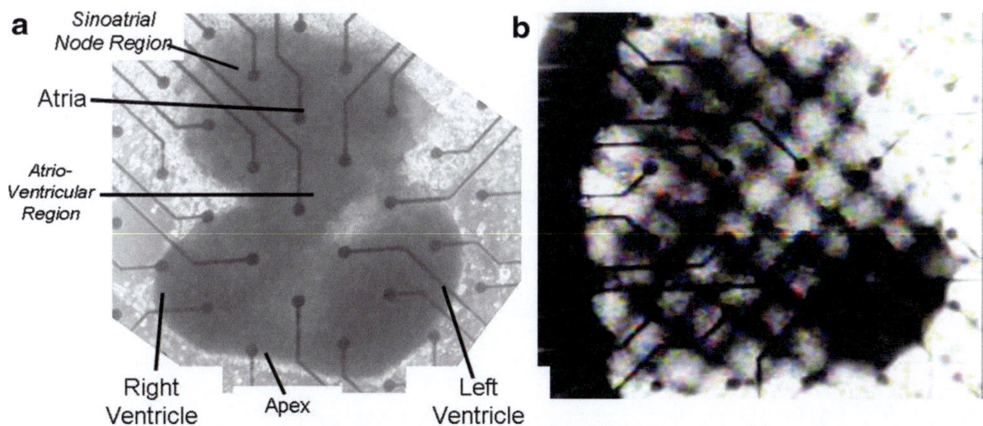

Fig. 1. Representative E10.5 mouse hearts on microelectrode arrays after overnight culture. Photomicrographs taken on an inverted light microscope with 4× objective in closed Petri dishes. Hearts exhibited regular spontaneous beating, indicating viability, although beating rate was dependent upon ambient temperature. (**a**) Heart without gold electronmicroscopy index grid for clarity and to identify major cardiac regions. Such images are rare, as moving the MEA from the workbench to the culture incubator typically shakes the heart away from the electrodes to settle elsewhere on the MEA. Hearts cannot be moved from their places of attachment after overnight culture without tearing. (**b**) Heart with recommended index grid to hold it in place. A series of images or film at multiple light intensities can reveal both the electrodes and shape of the heart.

to unambiguously identify major conduction areas, such as the sinoatrial nodal region and the apex, allowing measurement of conduction time and estimation of conduction velocity through the plane of the entire heart. Many commercial MEAs include a labeled coordinate system to identify individual electrodes directly on the MEA; otherwise, record any orienting marks on the MEA. A series of images or a film sequence from dark to overly bright allows visualization both of the electrodes and the outline of the heart. The temporal sequence of electrode signals obtained from the MEA data should reflect the known path of the cardiac conduction system, as revealed on these photomicrographs (see Fig. 2).

3.3. Recording of Electrical Activity from Beating Embryonic Hearts

1. Several hours prior to experiments, replace the heart medium on the MEA with fresh medium under a biohood. With a large micropipette set at maximum, gently remove the old medium in one motion at a location distant from the heart and microelectrodes. The heart should not move. Quickly and gently replace medium in one motion at same distant location. Return the MEAs to the incubator for tissue recovery from osmotic shock. This medium change will:
   (a) Replace used culture medium with fresh.
   (b) Replace medium of unknown volume (due to the addition of DMEM during the transfer of the heart from the

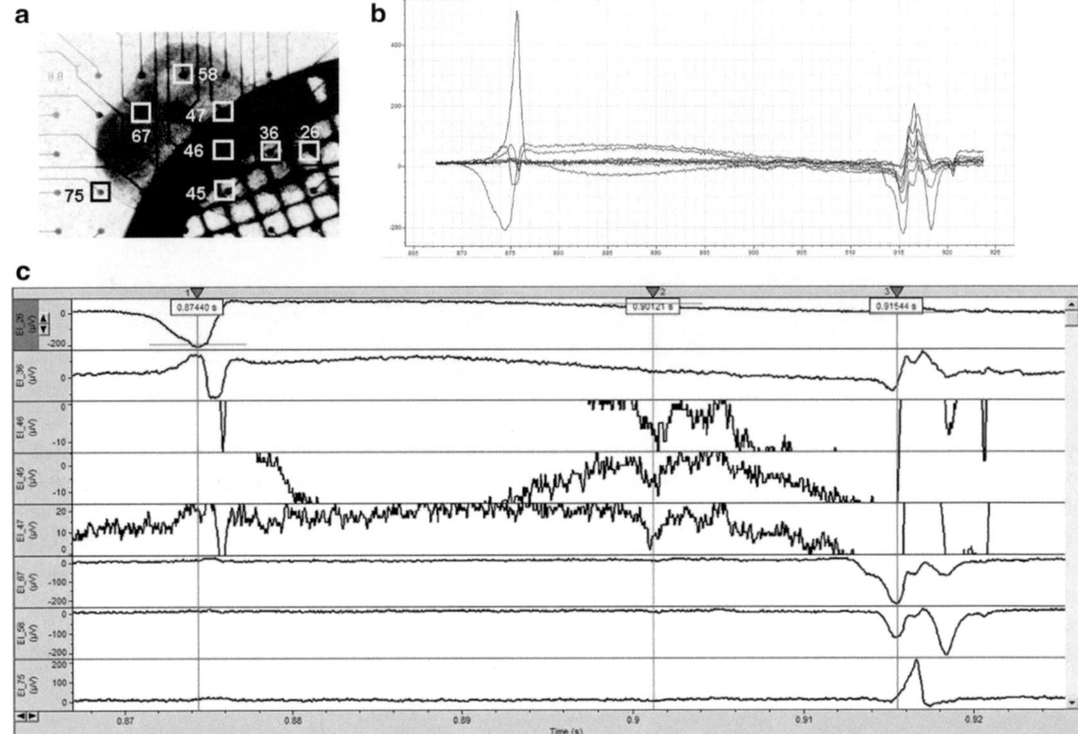

Fig. 2. Representative data from an E10.5 mouse heart obtained by extracellular MEA recording. Data collected by MC_Rack v3.5.10 (Multichannel Systems; Reutlingen, Germany) and analyzed by Clampfit v10 (Molecular Devices, Sunnyvale, CA). (**a**) Photomicrograph showing locations of representative electrodes: 26: First depolarizing electrode (Sinoatrial nodal region); 36: Downstream atria; 45–47: Atrioventricular region; 67: Epicardial breakthrough; 58: Downstream ventricle; 75: Noncontact electrode. (**b**) Overlapping signal traces of representative electrodes. Atrial depolarization is on the *left side*; ventricular depolarization is on the *right side*. Note the difference in signal magnitudes among the electrodes. (**c**) Individual electrode traces with Y-axis optimized for each trace. *Cursor lines* indicate time points for Electrode 26, atrioventricular region (FP_{min}s are within 0.5 ms of each other), and Electrode 67. Conduction time across the whole heart (sinoatrial nodal region to breakthrough) was 41 ms.

microcentrifuge tube to the MEA the day before) with medium of known volume to ensure proper concentration of drugs at the time of the experiment.

(c) Allow the replacement of CO_2-buffered medium with chemical-buffered medium, if desired (see Note 4).

2. Activate the temperature controller to preheat the heating plate on the amplifier to 37°C.
3. Gently and quickly wipe the contact pads along the outside edge of the MEA with 100% ethanol to remove any debris or medium. This will improve contact with the amplifier and the signal-to-noise ratio.
4. Carefully place the MEA on the headstage (amplifier), and place it such that the electrodes are always oriented the same way when recordings are taken (to ensure proper identification of electrodes).

5. In order to minimize electrical noise, use proper grounding and a Faraday cage.
6. Record data from all electrodes with proper software (such as MC_Rack, Multichannel Systems; Reutlingen, Germany) for 2 min at 10-min intervals (see Note 5).

3.4. Analysis of Field Potential Data

Due to the three-dimensional shape of the heart, the distance between the cells and surface electrodes, and the relatively large distance between the electrodes compared to the size of the embryonic heart, spatial resolution and the precision to relate signals to exact heart locations are limited. For the intact embryonic heart, MEAs are most precise when comparing conduction times over large distances, such as from the sinoatrial nodal region (first electrode to depolarize) to the epicardial breakthrough of the Purkinje fibers at the apex. However, the following principles can improve data analysis.

1. Measurement of conduction times for conduction velocity should be from FP_{min} (the time point of maximum negative deflection from baseline, corresponding to Phase 0 inward Na^{+} current of the action potential (9)) of one electrode to the FP_{min} of the next (FP delay) (15).
2. Magnitude of field potential deflection can vary due to electrode/heart contact, but should be consistent within each individual heart. A very weak signal compared to other electrodes can indicate a region of concave shape of the tissue surface (e.g., between atria and ventricles) or poor conduction to the surface. We make the choice of whether to accept this signal as being from the adjacent tissue or disregard as a conductive artifact (see step 3 below) largely on its relative magnitude compared to noise, whether its time of occurrence reflects known conduction pathways (e.g., if a signal from atrioventricular region occurs between sinoatrial nodal region and breakthrough, rather than near-simultaneously with either), if it occurs consistently and simultaneously through several nearby electrodes, and occurs at similar time points in multiple experimental preparations (see Fig. 2, Electrodes 45–47).
3. Because myocardium and cell medium are conductive, MEA electrodes will detect a field potential signal artifact even if not in contact with the depolarizing tissue (15, 17), although distance will weaken the artifact's magnitude compared to the original depolarization. These include both electrodes not in contact with the heart at all and those detecting signals from elsewhere in the heart. These signals can be identified and excluded in the following circumstances:
   (a) They are clearly outside the borders of the tissue as determined by the photomicrograph (see Fig. 2, Electrode 75).

These are frequently weak compared to signals from contact. However, hearts may move a small amount during transport and insertion into the amplifier headstage; if a noncontact electrode is very close to the heart border in the photomicrograph, it may be in contact during experimental readings.

(b) They are not shaped properly. Cell depolarizations typically appear as negative deflections (or traces with very strong negative components) in field potentials (9, 15, 18). Upward deflections are evidence of conductive artifact (see Fig. 2, Electrode 75).

(c) The signal trace includes two depolarizations—one strong and one weak, some duration apart. The stronger signal is the contact tissue. The weaker signal is from a strong signal elsewhere in the heart, usually the other cardiac chamber, and is easily identified as it occurs near-simultaneously with depolarization of the other chamber (see Fig. 2, Electrodes 26, 36, and 67) or other location (Electrode 58).

4. Because of fast conduction through gap junction-rich regions of the heart, it is often unnecessary to resolve the precise electrode for that region to acquire usable data. For example, the atrioventricular junction region is concave and often produces signals too imprecise to locate the atrioventricular node/bundle. However, the 2–4 electrodes within this region typically depolarize within <1 ms of each other, making their differences insignificant compared to conduction times within and between heart chambers (compare Electrodes 26 and 36, and the AVN electrodes in Fig. 2). This fact also allows the acquisition of data when an electrode may not be in direct contact with the precise region of interest (e.g., the sinoatrial node, breakthrough), because the delay to the electrode is usually insignificant provided that that electrode is in the direct path of the traveling action potential.

4. Notes

1. Gelatin has proven to be a successful and cost-effective substrate, providing adhesion sufficient for transporting murine embryonic hearts on MEAs around a laboratory with excellent electrode conduction and minimal cardiac cell proliferation and dispersion after 24–48 h. Other substrates, such as laminin and fibronectin, have not been tried.
2. All tissue preparation must be performed under aseptic techniques. Thoroughly clean workbench or lay surface protective covering. Tissue dishes, microcentrifuge tubes, and transfer

pipettes should be uncovered or exposed as little as possible. Media should be aliquoted under a sterile biosafety hood. Regularly mist area, dissection microscope and associated equipment, and closed dishes and tubes with 70% ethanol. Immerse tools and gold grids in 70% ethanol and remove ethanol by blotting on kimwipe prior to all tissue contact.

3. Hearts should regain spontaneous beating activity within hours in a cell culture incubator, with strong regular contractions within 12 h. A small percentage will not and should be excluded from experiments.
4. Although pH can be managed with chemical-buffered medium, the basic experiments are quick enough that we saw no difference in any examined electrical parameter in MEAs open to the air in bicarbonate-buffered or HEPES-buffered media.
5. Embryonic mouse hearts at E10.5 are very resistant to induced contraction by external field stimulation, so we performed the experiments with hearts at sinus rhythm. Stimulation may be attempted in other experiments, if appropriate.

Acknowledgments

The authors wish to thank Dr. Steven N. Ebert for the original idea and support to examine embryonic cardiac conduction by MEA and Drs. Peter Molnar and James J. Hickman for support and technical assistance.

References

1. Pennisi, D. J., Rentschler, S., Gourdie, R. G., Fishman, G. I., and Mikawa, T. (2002) Induction and patterning of the cardiac conduction system, *Int J Dev Biol 46*, 765–775.
2. Boukens, B. J., Christoffels, V. M., Coronel, R., and Moorman, A. F. (2009) Developmental basis for electrophysiological heterogeneity in the ventricular and outflow tract myocardium as a substrate for life-threatening ventricular arrhythmias, *Circ Res 104*, 19–31.
3. Rothenberg, F., Watanabe, M., Eloff, B., and Rosenbaum, D. (2005) Emerging patterns of cardiac conduction in the chick embryo: waveform analysis with photodiode array-based optical imaging, *Dev Dyn 233*, 456–465.
4. Rosa, A., Maury, J. P., Terrand, J., Lyon, X., Kucera, P., Kappenberger, L., and Raddatz, E. (2003) Ectopic pacing at physiological rate improves postanoxic recovery of the developing heart, *Am J Physiol Heart Circ Physiol 284*, H2384–2392.
5. Sarre, A., Maury, P., Kucera, P., Kappenberger, L., and Raddatz, E. (2006) Arrhythmogenesis in the developing heart during anoxia-reoxygenation and hypothermia-rewarming: an in vitro model, *J Cardiovasc Electrophysiol 17*, 1350–1359.
6. Chuck, E. T., Meyers, K., France, D., Creazzo, T. L., and Morley, G. E. (2004) Transitions in ventricular activation revealed by two-dimensional optical mapping, *Anat Rec A Discov Mol Cell Evol Biol 280*, 990–1000.
7. Fejtl, M., Stett, A., Nisch, W., Boven, K., and Moller, A. (2006) On Micro-Electrode Array Revival: Its Development, Sophistication of Recording, and Stimulation, in *Advances in Network Electrophysiology: Using Multi-Electrode Arrays* (Taketani, M., and Baudry, M., Eds.), pp 24–37, Springer, New York.
8. Chang, J. C., and Wheeler, B. C. (2006) Pattern Technologies for Structuring Neuronal Networks on MEAs, in *Advances in Network*

Electrophysiology: Using Multi-Electrode Arrays (Taketani, M., and Baudry, M., Eds.), pp 153–189, Springer, New York.

9. Halbach, M., Egert, U., Hescheler, J., and Banach, K. (2003) Estimation of action potential changes from field potential recordings in multicellular mouse cardiac myocyte cultures, *Cell Physiol Biochem 13*, 271–284.
10. Natarajan, A., Molnar, P., Sieverdes, K., Jamshidi, A., and Hickman, J. J. (2006) Microelectrode array recordings of cardiac action potentials as a high throughput method to evaluate pesticide toxicity, *Toxicol In Vitro 20*, 375–381.
11. Whitson, J., Kubota, D., Shimono, K., Jia, Y., and Taketani, M. (2006) Multi-Electrode Arrays: Enhancing Traditional Methods and Enabling Network Physiology, in *Advances in Network Electrophysiology: Using Multi-Electrode Arrays* (Taketani, M., and Baudry, M., Eds.), pp 38–68, Springer, New York.
12. Halbach, M., Pillekamp, F., Brockmeier, K., Hescheler, J., Muller-Ehmsen, J., and Reppel, M. (2006) Ventricular slices of adult mouse hearts–a new multicellular in vitro model for electrophysiological studies, *Cell Physiol Biochem 18*, 1–8.
13. Bussek, A., Wettwer, E., Christ, T., Lohmann, H., Camelliti, P., and Ravens, U. (2009) Tissue slices from adult mammalian hearts as a model for pharmacological drug testing, *Cell Physiol Biochem 24*, 527–536.
14. Pillekamp, F., Halbach, M., Reppel, M., Pfannkuche, K., Nazzal, R., Nguemo, F., Matzkies, M., Rubenchyk, O., Hannes, T., Khalil, M., Bloch, W., Sreeram, N., Brockmeier, K., and Hescheler, J. (2009) Physiological differences between transplanted and host tissue cause functional decoupling after in vitro transplantation of human embryonic stem cell-derived cardiomyocytes, *Cell Physiol Biochem 23*, 65–74.
15. Reppel, M., Pillekamp, F., Lu, Z. J., Halbach, M., Brockmeier, K., Fleischmann, B. K., and Hescheler, J. (2004) Microelectrode arrays: a new tool to measure embryonic heart activity, *J Electrocardiol 37 Suppl*, 104–109.
16. Kaufman, M. H. (1992) *The Atlas of Mouse Development*, Academic Press, Maryland Heights, MO.
17. Hescheler, J., Halbach, M., Egert, U., Lu, Z. J., Bohlen, H., Fleischmann, B. K., and Reppel, M. (2004) Determination of electrical properties of ES cell-derived cardiomyocytes using MEAs, *J Electrocardiol 37 Suppl*, 110–116.
18. Yeung, C. K., Sommerhage, F., Wrobel, G., Offenhausser, A., Chan, M., and Ingebrandt, S. (2007) Drug profiling using planar microelectrode arrays, *Anal Bioanal Chem 387*, 2673–2680.

INDEX

Xu Peng and Marc Antonyak (eds.), *Cardiovascular Development: Methods and Protocols*, Methods in Molecular Biology, vol. 843, DOI 10.1007/978-1-61779-523-7,

S

T

V

W

X

Z

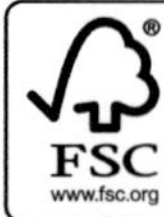

MIX
Papier aus verantwortungsvollen Quellen
Paper from responsible sources
FSC® C105338

If you have any concerns about our products,
you can contact us on
ProductSafety@springernature.com

In case Publisher is established outside the EU,
the EU authorized representative is:
Springer Nature Customer Service Center GmbH
Europaplatz 3, 69115 Heidelberg, Germany

Printed by Libri Plureos GmbH
in Hamburg, Germany